A Clinician's Guide to Childhood Obsessive-Compulsive and Related Disorders

This book provides mental health clinicians and trainees with an overview of the new category of obsessive-compulsive and related disorders as they apply to youth.

These disorders are highly impairing but can typically be overlooked in children and adolescents when they most often onset. This book draws attention to these disorders and provides an up-to-date review on the classification and development of these conditions in youth. Chapters explore the arguments for and against the new obsessive-compulsive related disorder DSM-5 category, provide reviews of transdiagnostic factors believed to underly these disorders, as well expert overviews of the clinical disorders that make up this category. An international team of contributors focuses on a range of topics such as: pediatric acute-onset neuropsychiatric syndrome, early-onset and tic-related OCD, common comorbid psychiatric conditions in youth, developmental neurobiology, and more.

This book is an essential read for clinicians who specialize in OCD and related disorders and treat children. It is also applicable to clinicians, trainees, and students across mental health disciplines such as: psychology, psychiatry, social work, mental health, and counselling.

Andrew G. Guzick is a clinical psychologist and assistant professor in the Center for the Treatment and Study of Anxiety at the University of Pennsylvania. His clinical and research focus is on children and adults with anxiety, obsessive-compulsive and related disorders, and misophonia. His work has also focused on anxiety among autistic individuals.

Eric A. Storch is professor and McIngvale presidential endowed chair in the Department of Psychiatry and Behavioral Sciences at Baylor College of Medicine. He serves as vice chair of psychology and specializes in the nature and treatment of childhood and adult obsessive-compulsive disorder, anxiety disorders, PTSD, and anxiety among youth with autism.

"An essential resource for clinicians, students and academics looking to understand OCRDs in childhood. Seamlessly blending easy to read and accessible information with depth of scientific knowledge, this book offers a comprehensive exploration of OCRDs, their common threads and distinctive nuances, developmental presentations, comorbidity, and treatment. Whether you're just stepping into the field or seeking fresh insights, this book has new knowledge for everyone."

Carly Johnco, *associate professor, PhD, School of Psychological Sciences, Macquarie University (Sydney, Australia)*

"Drs. Storch and Guzick are well established leaders in the field of childhood OCD and related disorders, and have gathered together an excellent set of equally well regarded chapter authors. The book's focus is much broader and more inclusive than other texts available, and should be an indispensable resource for students, clinicians, and researchers for years to come."

Caleb W. Lack, *PhD (he/him), professor of psychology, program coordinator, M.A. in Counseling Psychology and Practicum Coordinator, Counseling Psychology/MFT, University of Central Oklahoma*

"This fabulous book offers a cutting edge tour of OCRDs in children. Novice clinicians will gain a foundational overview of these challenging disorders, and seasoned clinicians will broaden their expertise and fine-tune their approach. This book will also help investigators advance much-needed research in pediatric OCRDs, several of which are woefully understudied. What a fantastic resource!"

Jedidiah Siev, *Swarthmore College*

"In this indispensable, comprehensive, and up-to-date book, Drs. Storch and Guzik assembled a cadre of international experts to provide a clear, balanced, and highly informative review of the Obsessive-Compulsive and Related Disorders (OCRDs) diagnostic category in youth. Uniquely, the book transcends existing OCRDs and critically examines additional conditions that may share features with OCD, including misophonia, hoarding and tic disorders, and even sensory dysregulation and health anxiety. This unique, authoritative book is an essential resource for pediatric mental health professionals."

Amitai Abramovitch, *PhD, associate professor, Texas State University*

"This book is a necessary addition for all those who work in mental health with children and adolescents, contributing to the understanding of areas that are still under study and development. The information provided, precise and clear, transforms this clinical guide into an undoubted theoretical and practical reference, which should be a basic reading recommended for therapists who want to nourish their knowledge and delve into topics of high interest today, both in research and in clinical practice."

"This splendid compilation is a resource that only comes around once a decade. Veterans of the field will delight in updates and guidance while serving as a starting point I could have only hoped for as a new clinician. While it is centered on children, much applies to adults. Its coverage of disgust, sensory dysregulation, tics, and significantly more provides insight for clinical practice so that already effective treatments can excel even further past current limitations. I joyfully welcome this book."

A Clinician's Guide to Childhood Obsessive-Compulsive and Related Disorders

Classification and Development

Edited by
Andrew G. Guzick and Eric A. Storch

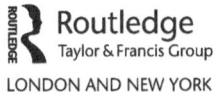
Routledge
Taylor & Francis Group

LONDON AND NEW YORK

Designed cover image: © Getty Images

First published 2025
by Routledge
4 Park Square, Milton Park, Abingdon, Oxon OX14 4RN

and by Routledge
605 Third Avenue, New York, NY 10158

Routledge is an imprint of the Taylor & Francis Group, an informa business

British Library Cataloguing-in-Publication Data
A catalogue record for this book is available from the British Library

Library of Congress Cataloging-in-Publication Data
Names: Guzick, Andrew G., editor. | Storch, Eric A., editor.
Title: A clinician's guide to childhood obsessive-compulsive and related disorders : classification and development / edited by Andrew G. Guzick, Eric A. Storch.
Identifiers: LCCN 2024032403 (print) | LCCN 2024032404 (ebook) |
Subjects: MESH: Obsessive-Compulsive Disorder | Compulsive Personality Disorder | Child | Adolescent
Classification: LCC RJ506.O25 (print) | LCC RJ506.O25 (ebook) | NLM WM 176 | DDC 618.92/85227–dc23/eng/20241112
LC record available at https://lccn.loc.gov/2024032403
LC ebook record available at https://lccn.loc.gov/2024032404

ISBN: 978-1-032-84919-5 (hbk)
ISBN: 978-1-032-84490-9 (pbk)
ISBN: 978-1-003-51742-9 (ebk)

DOI: 10.4324/9781003517429

Typeset in Times New Roman
by Taylor & Francis Books

Contents

Illustrations

Figures

Tables

Dedicated with love to Elle. Thank you for everything.

Andrew Guzick

Dedicated with love to my parents. Thank you all for your endless love and support.

Eric Storch

Contributors

Dr. Victoria Bacon, Ph.D., is currently a Postdoctoral Fellow at American Family Children's Hospital/University of Wisconsin Hospital and Clinics. She completed her Predoctoral Internship at Texas Children's Hospital/Baylor College of Medicine and her graduate training at the University of Nevada, Las Vegas. Her areas of specialty including working with children with medical complexities and their families. She is particularly interested in evidence-based interventions that address the intersection of physical and mental health.

Dr. Kelly Banneyer, Ph.D., is currently an Assistant Professor in the Psychology Division within the Department of Pediatrics at Baylor College of Medicine (BCM), as well as a licensed psychologist within the Obsessive-Compulsive and Anxiety Disorders Program at Texas Children's Hospital. Her areas of specialty including working with preschoolers, children, and adolescents with obsessive-compulsive disorder (OCD), panic disorder, social anxiety, selective mutism, separation anxiety, specific phobias, and generalized anxiety, including those with co-occurring symptoms of autism spectrum disorder. She uses evidence-based interventions, primarily exposure-based cognitive behavior therapy (ERP+CBT) and parent management training (PMT) to work with children and their families.

Dr. Steven T. Bellows, M.D., is a neurologist in Houston, Texas and is affiliated with Harris Health Ben Taub General and LBJ Hospitals. Dr. Bellows has expertise in treating Chronic Tic Disorders, Parkinson's disease, and non-Alzheimer's dementia.

Andreas Bezahler, B.S., is currently a doctoral student at Fordham University at the Compulsions, Obsessions, and Anxiety Program. Andreas' main research interest is improving treatment for OCD and related disorders, with a special focus on sexual and gender minority communities.

Dr. Liza Bonin, Ph.D., is a licensed psychologist in Texas, as well as an Associate Professor and Training Director in the Department of

Pediatrics, Division of Psychology at Baylor College of Medicine. Dr. Bonin provides assessment of and treatment for OCD/anxiety disorders via evidence-based practices. Her primary clinical focus is effective treatment of pediatric OCD and health anxiety via exposure-based cognitive behavioral therapy (ERP+CBT). Her academic interests include improving OCD treatment effectiveness, family resilience, quality improvement science, and excellence in clinical training.

Emily Braley, M.S., is a clinical doctoral student in the Clinical Child and Family Specialty Track at the University of Utah. Emily specializes in working with children and adolescences diagnosed with tic disorders, obsessive compulsive disorders, and other anxiety disorders using behavioral and cognitive-behavioral strategies.

Dr. Matti Cervin, Ph.D., is an Associate Professor at Lund University and Senior Clinical Psychologist in child and adolescent mental health services in Skåne. Dr. Cervin conducts clinical research in childhood OCD and related disorders, manages a training unit for psychology students, and supervises clinical psychologists.

Dr. Chacur Carina, MD, is a psychiatrist within the Obsessive, Compulsive, and Anxiety Spectrum Research Program at the Institute of Psychiatry of the Federal University of Rio de Janeiro (UFRJ).

Dr. Molly Church, Psy.D., is a Postdoctoral Fellow at Baylor College of Medicine on the OCD and Related Disorders Track. Her professional career interests include specializing in the treatment of OCD and related anxiety disorders, specifically the co-morbidity between OCD and eating disorders.

Augusto de las Casas is a fourth-year medical student at Baylor College of Medicine (class of 2024). After graduating from medical school, he will pursue a residency in psychiatry at Baylor College of Medicine.

Dr. Davide Fausto Borrelli is a resident doctor in psychiatry at the University Psychiatric Clinic of Parma. His fields of interest are OCD, Schizophrenia Spectrum disorders, and developmental psychopathology.

Dr. Brian Feinstein, Ph.D., is an Associate Professor in the Department of Psychology at Rosalind Franklin University of Medicine and Science who directs the Sexuality, Health, and Gender (SHAG) Lab. He obtained his Ph.D. in Clinical Psychology from Stony Brook University in 2015 after completing an APA-accredited internship at the University of Washington School of Medicine. He has also worked at the Feinberg School of Medicine and the Institute for Sexual and Gender Minority Health and Wellbeing at Northwestern University. Dr. Feinstein currently serves as an Associate Editor at Psychology of

Sexual Orientation and Gender Diversity, and he is a licensed psychologist in Illinois.

Madison Fitzpatrick, B.A., is the lead Research Assistant at the Yale OCD Research Clinic. Her research interests focus on the intersection of neuroscience and psychology, and she seeks to understand the underlying relationships between the brain and behavior that lead to OCRD symptomatology. In the future, she hopes to continue researching OCRDs and eventually become a doctor of Clinical Psychology, functioning as both a therapeutic provider and a researcher in the OCRD community.

Dr. Christoph Flessner, Ph.D., is a Professor in the Department of Psychological Sciences at Kent State University. He has been Director of the Pediatric Anxiety & Allergy Research Clinic (PAARC) at Kent State since 2011. Dr. Flessner's research focuses on biological and psychosocial risk factors that may be linked to the development of childhood anxiety and related problems—such as OCD, trichotillomania, and tic disorders—and how a better understanding of risk factors might be used to improve existing therapeutic interventions.

Dr. Leonardo F. Fontenelle has been a prolific clinical scientist in the obsessive-compulsive and related disorder field for decades. He is a Professor of Psychology at the Turner Institute for Brain and Mental Health, where he leads one of the most productive OCRD labs globally.

Dr. Frankovich, M.D., is a Clinical Professor in the Department of Pediatrics, Division of Allergy, Immunology Rheumatology (AIR) at Stanford University/Lucile Packard Children's Hospital (LPCH). Her clinical expertise is in systemic inflammatory and autoimmune diseases that co-occur with psychiatric symptoms. She completed her training in pediatrics, pediatric rheumatology, and clinical epidemiology at Stanford University/LPCH. She directs the Stanford PANS Program (since 2012) where she and her collaborators have created a longitudinal clinical database and large biorepository of patient and healthy control biospecimens. In addition to generating clinical data to better understand immune-behavioral health conditions, she is collaborating with ten basic science labs who aim to understand the immunological underpinnings of PANS and related conditions.

Chandni Fredrickson, MHA was a former clinical psychology graduate student at Kent State University. Her research interests include understanding the psychosocial impact of food allergy on affected children and their caregivers, along with examining the health disparities within pediatric food allergy outcomes.

Theresa (Tess) Gladstone, MA is a fifth-year clinical psychology graduate student at Kent State University. Tess's research focuses on risk factors, including anxiogenic parenting, for the development of child anxiety, as well as barriers to the implementation and dissemination of evidence-based care.

Andrew G. Guzick, Ph.D., is a clinical psychologist and Assistant Professor of Psychiatry at the University of Pennsylvania. His research and clinical specialization are in the assessment and treatment of children and adults with obsessive-compulsive, anxiety, and related disorders. He has published over 70 peer-reviewed publications in these areas and has received support from state, foundation, and federal grants for this work.

Dr. David Houghton, Ph.D., is Assistant Professor of Psychiatry and Behavioral Sciences and Center for Addiction Research at the University of Texas Medical Branch and Director of the HABITS Lab. He completed his Ph.D. in Clinical Psychology at Texas A&M University. After graduating, he conducted a post-doctoral fellowship at the Medical University of South Carolina. His areas of interest include OCD, addiction, anxiety disorders, and other neuropsychological conditions in children, adolescents, and adults. He has published over 20 peer-reviewed scientific articles as well as presented his works at various national and international scientific meetings.

Hannah Ishimuro, M.S., is a third year Clinical Psychology Ph.D. student at the University of Denver working in the Behavioral Research for Anxiety InterVention Efficiency (BRAVE) Lab. Before joining the BRAVE Lab, Hannah was a research volunteer at the Golden Bear Sleep and Mood Research Clinic at UC Berkeley and held a position as a research coordinator at the Youth Treatment and Evaluation of Anxiety and Mood Program at the New York State Psychiatric Institute. Hannah is interested in mechanism and treatment research targeting youth anxiety, OCD, and related disorders. More specifically, she is curious to explore cognitive and behavioral processes in response to distress, with the overall goal of improving treatment efficacy and equitable access to care for children and adolescents with anxiety disorders.

Lindsay Ives, Ph.D., is currently a postdoctoral fellow in the OCD and Anxiety Disorders Program in the Psychology Section at Texas Children's Hospital and Department of Pediatrics at Baylor College of Medicine. She specializes in the treatment of anxiety and related disorders in children and adolescents using exposure-based therapy, incorporating elements of mindfulness and acceptance.

Joseph Jankovic, M.D. is Professor of Neurology, Distinguished Chair in Movement Disorders, and Founder and Director of the Parkinson's Disease Center and Movement Disorders Clinic (PDCMDC) in the Department of Neurology at Baylor College of Medicine. Under the direction of Dr. Jankovic the PDCMDC has been recognized as "Center of Excellence" by the Tourette Association of America, Parkinson's Foundation, the Huntington Disease Society of America, and the Wilson Disease Association. Dr. Jankovic has published over 1,200 original articles and over 55 books.

Dr Amita Jassi is a Consultant Clinical Psychologist at the National and Specialist Obsessive-Compulsive Disorder, Body Dysmorphic Disorder (BDD), and Related Disorder Service for Children and Young People (South London and Maudsley National Health Service Trust). Amita is the lead for the BDD service as well as the Research Lead for the clinic. She is the Equality and Diversity Lead National Specialist CAMHS.

Dr. Yaman Kawamleh, D.O., is a licensed psychiatrist in Houston, Texas. He received his degree from New York Institute of Technology College of Osteopathic Medicine. He is currently affiliated with Baylor College of Medicine and Harris Health System.

Dr. Georgina Krebs, Ph.D., is an Associate Professor of Young People's Mental Health and Cognitive Behaviour Therapy (CBT) at University College London. Her expertise is in OCD, body dysmorphic disorder, and anxiety disorders, and she co-leads the Anxiety, self-Image and Mood (AIM) Lab and AIM Clinic.

Dr. Meiqian Ma, M.D., is a pediatric rheumatologist in Menlo Park, California and is affiliated with Lucile Packard Children's Hospital Stanford. She received her medical degree from Medical College of Wisconsin in 2013 and has been in practice for over ten years. Dr. Meiqian is also a Clinical Professor at Stanford Children's Health Specialty Services Sunnyvale. She is board certified in Pediatrics and Pediatric Rheumatology.

Katie Mangen, Ph.D., is a Postdoctoral Fellow at Baylor College of Medicine on the OCD and Related Disorders Track. Her clinical and research specialization is in obsessive-compulsive and related disorders.

Dr. Dean McKay, Ph.D., ABPP, is a Professor of Psychology at Fordham University, where he directs the Compulsive, Obsessive, and Anxiety Program. He has published over 200 peer reviewed articles and book chapters and is the editor or co-editor of over 19 books. He is board certified in Clinical and Cognitive-Behavioral Psychology from the American Board of Professional Psychology.

Emily graduated from Utah State University's Human Development and Family Studies department, Logan campus, in 2013 and currently works as an elementary school counselor. Part of her work includes teaching curriculum-based social and emotional topics relevant to the needs of the student body. She meets with students individually, as well as in small groups, and focuses on helping the students learn more about processing emotions.

Dr. Shankar Nandakumar, M.D., is a Psychiatry Resident at Baylor College of Medicine. He graduated from University of Texas Medical School at San Antonio in 2020.

Dr. Maria Morieria-de-Oliveira, PhD, is a psychology and neuroscience researcher within the Obsessive, Compulsive, and Anxiety Spectrum Research Program at the Institute of Psychiatry of the UFRJ.

Dr. Ogechi (Cynthia) Onyeka, Ph.D., is a Postdoctoral Fellow in the Obsessive Compulsive Disorders Program in the Menninger Department of Psychiatry & Behavioral Sciences at Baylor College of Medicine. She earned her Ph.D. in Clinical Psychology from Loyola University Chicago. Her research is focused on factors that promote resilience for youth of color, critical consciousness, and the relationship among socio-ecological stressors, internalizing symptoms, and psychosocial outcomes for minoritized populations. She is also interested in identifying biopsychosocial correlates of OCD from a community-based approach, primarily among individuals of Latine/x and African descent.

Dr. Grace Pham, Ph.D., is a Psychiatry Resident Physician at Baylor College of Medicine. She graduated with DO and PhD degrees from the University of North Texas Health Science Center.

Dr. Caitlin Pinciotti, Ph.D., is a licensed clinical psychologist in Texas and Wisconsin, and she currently serves as an assistant professor in the Department of Psychiatry & Behavioral Sciences at Baylor College of Medicine. Before arriving at BCM, she earned her doctorate in clinical psychology from Northern Illinois University with a specialization in trauma psychology, completed her internship and postdoc at Rogers Behavioral Health, and worked as a research psychologist at Rogers. Her research and clinical work focus on OCD, posttraumatic stress disorder (PTSD), and trauma. She has conducted research and provided evidence-based treatment with individuals with trauma and/or OCD at all levels of care ranging from Veterans' Administration and community outpatient centers to residential treatment facilities.

Dr. Ana Ribeiro, M.D., is a Chartered Clinical Psychologist and Mindfulness Teacher. She has many years of experience working across the life span in the National Health Service before moving to private practice. In her private practice, she has a wide range of international clients, and her main focus of work is with late adolescents and adults (age 16 years onwards). She offers therapy for a broad range of psychological difficulties including OCD, anxiety, panic attacks, depression, low self-esteem, work and school/UNI related stress (including management and prevention), sleeping problems, relationship difficulties, bereavement, and issues related to displacement and living away from home or in a foreign country.

Dr. Julia Ridgeway-Diaz is a staff psychiatrist in outpatient therapy at Menninger Clinic in Houston, TX. She is also a behavioral neurologist and neuropsychiatrist as well as an assistant professor in the Menninger Department of Psychiatry & Behavioral Sciences at Baylor College of Medicine. She has special expertise in neurocognitive disorders, movement disorders, autism spectrum disorder, sleep disorders, epilepsy, multiple sclerosis, and traumatic brain injury. She received her medical degree from University of California (San Francisco) School of Medicine and has been in practice for over eight years.

Dr. Michelle Rozenman, Ph.D., is an Assistant Professor at the University of Denver. She had previously been an Assisant Clinical Professor at the UCLA Semel Institute, and Associate Director of the UCLA Pediatric OCD Intensive Outpatient Program. Her research is focused on identifying and directly targeting basic cognitive biases in pediatric anxiety with novel experimental therapies, such as cognitive bias modification, as well as maximizing effectiveness of behavioral interventions for youth with anxiety and OCD.

Aditi Sabhlok, Ph.D., earned her doctoral degree in clinical psychology from the University of Texas at Austin in in 2023. She pursued her doctoral internship training at Texas Children's Hospital/Baylor College of Medicine.

Noelle Schlenk, M.A., is a Research Data Analyst I for Stanford Immune Behavioral Health Clinic / Research Team. She organizes, leads, and works as an analyst for projects aimed at understanding the genetic components of Pediatric Acute-Onset Neuropsychiatric Syndrome (PANS). She received her BS in Biology from the University of Kansas (2021) with University Honors, Departmental Honors, and a Certificate in Leadership Engagement. She then went on to receive her MA in Ecology & Evolutionary Biology from the University of Kansas (2023).

Karina Silva, M.A. is a doctoral student at the University of Houston and currently completing her externship at Texas Children's Hospital. She graduated from Florida International University in 2016, with a B.A. in Psychology and a minor in Education and received her M.A. at the

University of Houston in 2021. Her primary clinical and research interest is on the maintenance of childhood internalizing psychopathology among immigrant and undocumented populations, specifically focused on the risk and resilience factors that influence these relations.

Dr. Gudmundur Skarphedinsson, Ph.D., is a clinical child psychologist and professor at the Faculty of Psychology, University of Iceland, Reykjavik, Iceland. His research is dedicated to the evidence-based assessment and treatment of psychological disorders. Dr. Skarphedinsson's work notably focuses on evaluating and enhancing clinical assessments and treatments for OCD, anxiety disorders, and related conditions in children and adolescents.

Dr. Orri Smárason, Ph.D., is a clinical child and adolescent psychologist and researcher at the Department of Child and Adolescent Psychiatry, Landspitali National University Hospital, Iceland. His research interests include the assessment and treatments of obsessive-compulsive and related disorder, anxiety disorders, emotional dysregulation, and other psychiatric conditions in children and adolescents.

Dr. Samuel Spencer, Ph.D., is a Postdoctoral Fellow at Baylor College of Medicine on the OCD and Related Disorders Track. He received a Ph. D. in Clinical Psychology from the University of Hawaii at Manoa. His research interests broadly include acceptance and commitment therapy (ACT), psychotherapy process and outcome research, measurement of contextual behavioral science (CBS)-related constructs, and historical and philosophical traditions of CBT and CBS. He has co-authored over ten peer-review scientific papers since 2020.

Dr. Jordan Stiede, Ph.D., is a postdoctoral fellow in clinical psychology at Baylor College of Medicine. Dr. Stiede's research interests include understanding, improving, and disseminating behavioral interventions for children and adults with tic disorders. He has authored and co-authored numerous peer-reviewed scientific articles, as well as presented his findings at various regional, national and international scientific meetings.

Dr. Eric Storch, Ph.D. is Professor and McIngvale Presidential Endowed Chair in the Department of Psychiatry and Behavioral Sciences at Baylor College of Medicine (BCM). He serves as Vice Chair and Head of Psychology and co-directs the Obsessive-Compulsive and Related Disorders program at BCM. Dr. Storch specializes in the nature and treatment of childhood and adult OCD, anxiety disorders, PTSD, and anxiety among youth with autism. In addition to over 850 published articles and chapters and 22 books, he has received multiple federal grants to investigate treatment efficacy, mechanisms of action, genetics, bioethics, innovative approaches to phenotyping, and how to enhance outcomes for those struggling with OCD and related conditions.

Dr. Allison Vreeland, Ph.D., is licensed clinical psychologist who runs a private practice in California providing evidence-based care to youth, young adults, and families with PANS/PANDAS, OCD, and other behavioral challenges. After completing her clinical internship in Child Psychology at UCSF, she engaged in a two-year research fellowship in Clinical Psychology at Stanford University, receiving her Ph.D. in Clinical Psychological Science from Vanderbilt University in 2020. In addition to running a private practice, she also works as a clinical psychologist in the Immune Behavior Health Clinic at Stanford University School of Medicine, where her current research has focused on understanding the neural indices of Pediatric Acute Neuropsychiatric Syndrome (PANS).

Dr. Theresa Willett currently works at Stanford Medicine Children's Health as the Director of the Immune Behavioral Health Clinic. His research interests are focused on PANS/PANDAS. She received her PhD from Tufts University in 2002.

Dr. Brian Zaboski, Ph.D., is an Associate Research Scientist, licensed Connecticut psychologist, and a Nationally Certified School Psychologist at the Yale OCD Research Clinic. He currently serves the clinic as its Associate Director for Clinical Psychology. Dr. Zaboski's primary interests include the application of sophisticated quantitative methods to understanding the neurobiological networks in individuals afflicted by OCD, improving exposure therapy through translational neuroscience, and training clinicians in exposure-based techniques.

1 What is an OCRD? How These Disorders are and are Not Related, and Why We Should Care About Them in Children and Adolescents

Andrew G. Guzick and Eric A. Storch

What is an obsessive-compulsive related disorder (OCRD)?

The past several decades have seen an acceleration of clinical research in obsessive compulsive disorder (OCD), which has led to tremendous innovations in the scientific understanding of and treatment of this disorder. OCD can affect every aspect of a person's day-to-day life and cause tremendous psychological suffering. Although once thought to be relatively rare in youth, this misconception has been thoroughly and repeatedly debunked, with estimates now showing that about 2–3 percent of youth across the globe are affected by OCD (e.g., Barzilay et al., 2019; Canals et al., 2012).

As this literature developed, investigators and clinicians began to note how numerous other common clinical problems shared some intriguing features with OCD, as many other syndromes are characterized by repetitive thoughts or behaviors that are difficult to resist or control. A growing appreciation for commonalities across these disorders led to the introduction of formal categories in leading psychiatric diagnostic systems, including the Diagnostic and Statistical Manual for Mental Disorders-5th Edition (American Psychiatric Association, 2013) and the International Classification of Diseases-11th Edition (ICD-11; World Health Organization, 2019). These sections include body dysmorphic disorder (BDD), hoarding disorder (HD), excoriation or skin-picking disorder, trichotillomania or hair-pulling disorder. The ICD-11 also includes illness anxiety disorder and cross-lists Tourette syndrome in the OCRD chapter. Since the introduction of these chapters, awareness and clinical research in OCD and these possibly related disorders has continued to accelerate.

Unfortunately, while this body of work has taken off, research continues to lag behind significantly on OCRDs in childhood. This is particularly the case outside OCD and chronic tic disorders, despite the fact that these disorders most often onset in childhood or adolescence, and thus childhood is a prime opportunity for early intervention that has the potential to offset many of the significant negative downstream consequences of OCRDs (Fineberg et al., 2019). Despite this, we benefit from a very well-developed body of research in childhood OCD as well as

DOI: 10.4324/9781003517429-1

growing evidence on OCRDs. The goal of this book is to summarize the state of this research for mental health practitioners and trainees, provide an overview of the various OCRD presentations in childhood, describe trans-diagnostic psychological and neurobiological mechanisms, and highlight avenues for further research. The goal of this opening chapter is to set the stage for the rest of the book by defining the various OCRDs to be discussed and briefly reviewing evidence for and against their "relatedness."

The first section, "Obsessive-compulsive related disorders and psychological dimensions," provides an overview of the nature and theory of obsessive-compulsive related disorders as well as underlying, transdiagnostic psychological dimensions that may be implicated across these disorders, including compulsivity, impulsivity, response inhibition deficits (difficulties resisting behaviors associated with strong urges), habit formation, obsessiveness, disgust sensitivity; and sensory dysregulation. The second section focuses specifically on subtypes and developmental factors in childhood OCRDs, including pediatric acute-onset neuropsychiatric syndrome, early-onset/tic-related OCD, comorbidity in childhood OCRDs, neurobiology of childhood OCD and OCRDs, as well as issues related to sexual and gender minorities.

The book will conclude with considerations of future directions in OCRD research in childhood.

Proposed OCRD and presentation in childhood

A number of OCRDs have now been proposed, which are summarized in Table 1.1.

Table 1.1 Obsessive-compulsive and related disorders and considerations in childhood

Chapters 2–5: Obsessive-compulsive disorder (OCD)	OCD is characterized by obsessions (intrusive, distressing thoughts) and compulsions (repetitive, ritualistic, and/or excessive behaviors done to prevent a feared outcome or reduce distress associated with obsessions). OCD most often onsets during childhood or adolescence, with a subset experiencing a prepubescent onset that more strongly related to a family history and chronic tic disorders. Although the themes of symptoms vary widely, common themes in OCD include 1) contamination; 2) symmetry or incompleteness; 3) harm; 4) moral, sexual, or religious wrongdoing (Bloch et al., 2008).
Chapter 7: Health Anxiety/Illness Anxiety Disorder	Illness anxiety disorder is characterized by significant and excessive concerns with physical health. Compulsive behaviors such as checking and reassurance-seeking are extremely common in illness anxiety disorder. Although illness anxiety disorder is not very commonly studied in childhood *per se*, anxiety about health and illness is an extremely common theme in both OCD and generalized anxiety disorder, both of which are very common in childhood and adolescence.

Table 1.1 Obsessive-compulsive and related disorders and considerations in childhood

Chapter 8: Chronic tic disorders	Chronic tic disorders are characterized by persistent motor and/or vocal tics, which are defined as sudden, repetitive, non-rhythmic, semi-controllable movements of vocalizations, such as eye-blinking, shoulder shrugging, grimacing, grunting, snorting, or sniffing (Chang et al., 2009). These disorders most often onset during pre-adolescence, and sometimes reduce or remit by young adulthood. Tourette's disorder or Tourette's syndrome is specifically diagnosed when an individual experiences multiple motor tics and one or more vocal tics that have been present for a year or more.
Chapter 9: Skin-picking or excoriation disorder	Excoriation disorder is defined by repetitive skin-picking that results in skin lesions despite an individual's desire to reduce or stop. This disorder most often begins in adolescence.
Chapter 9: Hair-pulling disorder or trichotillomania	Trichotillomania is defined by repetitive hair-pulling despite an individuals' desire to reduce or stop. Trichotillomania also most often begins in adolescence.
Chapter 10: Body dysmorphic disorder (BDD)	BDD is characterized by an excessive preoccupation with perceived physical flaws and compensatory behaviors done to hide or correct these perceived defects, such as mirror-checking, camouflaging (e.g., wearing baggy clothing or excessive make-up), and reassurance-seeking. Body image concerns are very common in adolescence, and thus these concerns are overlooked and trivialized by parents and clinicians alike even when they reach a clinically significant threshold, which they often appear to during adolescence, with 2 percent reporting clinically elevated BDD-level symptoms (Schneider et al., 2017).
Chapter 11: Hoarding disorder	The core feature of hoarding disorder is difficulty discarding items of little intrinsic value. Although individuals with clinical hoarding most often present to clinical settings at older ages once the accumulation of possessions reaches a more severe threshold, sentimental attachment to objects is a common, normal part of childhood, and hoarding is a frequent associated feature of many common childhood disorders (e.g., autism spectrum disorder, attention-deficit/hyperactivity disorder). Adolescence is the most common age-of-onset when symptom begin, suggesting early intervention may be key (Guzick et al., 2020).

Table 1.1 Obsessive-compulsive and related disorders and considerations in childhood

Chapter 12: Misophonia	Misophonia is characterized by significant aversive emotional reactions to specific sounds, most often oral-motor sounds produced by others such as breathing, chewing, or humming, as well as their associated visual cues ("triggers") (Swedo et al., 2022). Children and adults with misophonia often use extensive measures to reduce contact with triggers, such as using noise-blocking headphones or covering their ears (Guzick et al., 2023). Misophonia has been found to most often begin in childhood (Swedo et al., 2022). Research is increasingly concluding that ***misophonia is not a subtype of OCD or appropriately classified as an OCRD***. Regardless, some have speculated misophonia may be usefully characterized as an OCRD, owing to the extensive protective behaviors (e.g., wearing headphones), hyper-fixation on emotional stimuli, and sensory distress that characterize misophonia. Given a rapidly growing body of research in misophonia and this current debate in academic and advocacy circles, we have also included a chapter on misophonia in this book, although its relatedness to the other OCRDs is least established.

Are these disorders related?

The introduction of this OCRD classification of disorders has not been without controversy. Proponents argue that high comorbidity among these disorders as well as similarities in clinical presentation/ phenomenology, genetics, neurocircuitry, and treatment response tie these disorders together (Bartz & Hollander, 2006; Fineberg et al., 2017; Fontenelle et al., 2022; Phillips et al., 2010). There has been comparatively less attention from a psychological perspective, which offers a particularly strong evidence base upon which to conceptualize these disorders through functional analysis, or analyzing *why* these repetitive behaviors continue by investigating what happens immediately before ("antecedents") or after ("consequences") them (Abramowitz, 2018; Storch et al., 2008). From this perspective, there is a strong case to continue to classify OCD with the anxiety disorders, a category to which OCD previously belonged, as avoidance and safety-seeking behaviors are negatively reinforced through relieving distress associated with upsetting or anxiety-provoking thoughts in OCD and all the anxiety disorders (Abramowitz, 2018; Storch et al., 2008). Further, much of the neurobiological, treatment response, and comorbidity data similarly suggest that OCD and anxiety disorders are at least as related to each other as OCD is to the putative OCRDs. Although not entirely conclusive, this debate has been a healthy one for science, as it has improved our understanding of compulsivity, impulsivity, obsessiveness and other transdiagnostic factors across these disorders.

The following sections will introduce each OCRD and briefly review evidence for how each proposed diagnostic category is or is not related to OCD or other OCRDs along several transdiagnostic levels of analysis, many of which are detailed in their own independent chapters in this book.

Illness Anxiety Disorder

Illness anxiety disorder, formerly known as hypochondriasis,[1] is characterized by recurrent distressing anxiety-provoking thoughts about having an illness, preoccupation with possible bodily signs of illness, and compensatory behaviors (reassurance-seeking, body-checking). There are clear overlaps in the phenomenology and clinical presentation with OCD, particularly contamination-related OCD, with both being characterized by recurrent, often anxiety-provoking thoughts about illness or contamination and repetitive behaviors done to relieve distress. Strong evidence for an overlap between illness anxiety and obsessive-compulsive disorders comes in a cognitive-behavioral conceptualization and treatment perspective, in which compulsions are conceptualized to maintain obsessions through negative reinforcement, and treatment is characterized by primarily exposure-based methods. Accordingly, illness anxiety disorder falls in the OCRD chapter in ICD-11, although it was retained in the Somatic Symptom and Related Disorders chapter in DSM-5, based on a lack of systematic research on the neurobiology and epidemiology of illness anxiety disorder and the extent to which it overlaps with OCD (Phillips et al., 2010). As little research as there continues to be on this disorder in general, there is minimal research on illness anxiety disorder in youth, despite health anxiety being a common concern among youth with OCD and anxiety disorders, and appears to share similar qualities as that in adults (e.g., anxiety sensitivity, intolerance of uncertainty). Chapter 7 reviews developmental considerations for the presentation and treatment of health anxiety in youth.

Chronic Tic Disorders

Chronic tic disorders are characterized by repeated and persistent tics, which are repetitive, semi-automatic, non-rhythmic movements (e.g., jerking, blinking, grimacing) or vocalizations (e.g., sniffing, grunting, throat-clearing). Tourette disorder or syndrome is a specific chronic tic disorder characterized by at least two motor and one vocal tic. Although chronic tic disorders are not categorized as an OCRD in the DSM-5, the biological relatedness of tic disorders and OCD is among the strongest of any of the possible ORCDs. Specifically, there has now been replicated, strong evidence for a genetic relatedness between these diagnoses among youth with early-onset/pre-pubescent OCD (see Chapters 8, 14, 15) as well as with body-focused repetitive behaviors (Lamothe et al., 2019; Monzani et al., 2014). When these diagnoses co-occur in the case of "Tourettic OCD," tics can often be conceptualized as serving a compulsive function in which they reduce distress caused by intrusive thoughts. Although there is strong evidence for a genetic overlap between these diagnoses among young children with OCD, tic disorders also share phenomenological and neurobiological similarities with body-focused repetitive behaviors, as both are characterized by an inability to inhibit an impulsive, self-oriented behavior, and more involvement of specific motor areas of the brain such as the supplementary motor area (Lamothe et al., 2019). Importantly, psychopharmacological and psychological treatment strategies tend to overlap more between tic disorders and body-focused repetitive behaviors, with the core behavioral technique in particular being habit reversal training in these diagnoses, compared to exposure in OCD and BDD.

Body-Focused Repetitive Behavior Disorders: Trichotillomania, Excoriation Disorder, and Others

Body-focused repetitive behavior (BFRB) disorders are characterized by excessive, repeated behaviors directed towards one's own body to the point that they cause distress, physical consequences (e.g., balding in the case of hair-pulling, lesions in the case of skin-picking), or other functional impairments. Although certain BFRBs are a normal part of childhood and are usually relatively harmless (e.g., thumb-sucking, nail-biting), skin-picking and hair-pulling are two BFRBs that more frequently lead to significant impairment and are termed "excoriation disorder" and "trichotillomania" when they pass this clinical threshold. Beyond their overlapping clinical presentation with OCD (i.e., sharing repetitive behaviors), large-scale factor analyses (a statistical technique to group a large number of variables into smaller number of parsimonious "latent constructs") have shed further light on appropriate categorization of BFRBs within the OCRD class. These studies tend to find strongest evidence for grouping OCD, BDD, and HD together, while BFRBs separate in an independent factor, suggesting that these two diagnoses may represent distinct underlying constructs (Fontenelle et al., 2022; Monzani et al., 2014; Snorrason et al., 2021). It is likely that these behaviors often exist on the impulsive end of a "compulsive-impulsive" spectrum (Hollander, 2005), with these behaviors frequently done to achieve a sense of a relief or pleasure, relative to OCD, BDD, or HD, in which behaviors are more often done to relieve distress or anxiety. Chapter 9 reviews BFRBs in childhood in more detail.

Body Dysmorphic Disorder

Body dysmorphic disorder (BDD) is characterized by persistent, distorted, distressing beliefs about one's appearance as well as repeated behaviors done in response to these beliefs (e.g., mirror-checking, mental comparisons with others, reassurance-seeking, or camouflaging concerning body parts with make-up, baggy clothing, or other measures). Body image concerns are extremely common among adolescents, although when these concerns begin to occupy a young person's mind excessively or interfere with their day-to-day functioning, they may become more appropriately considered clinical BDD. As noted, when factor analyzing all the proposed OCRDs together, BDD and OCD tend to be grouped together (Fontenelle et al., 2022; Monzani et al., 2014; Snorrason et al., 2021). Accordingly, there are clear overlaps in the phenomenology of these diagnoses, with the core characteristics of both being 1) intrusive, upsetting thoughts; and 2) repetitive behaviors done to relieve distress or prevent feared outcomes. OCD and BDD are highly comorbid and their pharmacological and psychological treatment strategies overlap considerably, with serotonin reuptake inhibitors and exposure therapy-focused CBT having the strongest evidence for both. Developmental considerations for BDD in youth are reviewed in Chapter 10.

Hoarding Disorder

Hoarding was formerly considered a subtype of OCD, although owing to its different clinical presentation, poorer response to treatment, and differences in proposed neurobiology, it separated as an independent "hoarding disorder" diagnosis. The core feature of hoarding disorder is difficulty throwing away objects that others would likely consider useless. One might believe hoarding disorder has limited relevance in childhood psychopathology, as individuals with the full diagnosis do not usually present for treatment until the accumulation of belongings becomes severe, and thus they have usually reached an older age. Adults with hoarding problems, however, consistently identify adolescence as the typical time-of-onset, and hoarding behaviors are often observed across forms of childhood psychopathology (and normal early child development, for that matter), and on rare occasions can independently reach a point of clinical significance. Thus, targeted early intervention should be considered within this diagnosis as well. Chapter 11 of this book reviews developmental considerations when assessing and treating potential hoarding problems in youth.

Misophonia

Misophonia is characterized by heightened emotional reactions to certain sounds (e.g., chewing, breathing noises, clicking) and associated visual stimuli. Although not recognized by any official psychiatric diagnostic system, misophonia can be highly impairing in youth, with age-of-onset estimates ranging from nine to 13 years old (Claiborn et al., 2020; Jager et al., 2020). Growing literature on misophonia has made it increasingly clear that it is independent of OCD or OCRDs, and that it is inappropriate to classify it under this category at this time. Historically, however, there has been a popular hypothesis that misophonia might be appropriately conceptualized as an OCRD, or perhaps even a subtype of OCD, with a fixation on trigger noises in misophonia as reflective of obsessions, and safety behaviors and active avoidance (e.g., covering ears, wearing headphones) as reflective of compulsions done to relieve distress. It also appears highly correlated with self-reported symptoms of OCD, obsessive-compulsive personality traits (in adults), and anxiety and depressive symptoms. While childhood misophonia research lags behind that of adults, there has been a rapid acceleration of research in this domain in recent years, and an updated review and consideration of its classification is included in Chapter 12. Although it seems clear that considering misophonia an OCRD is inappropriate at this time, given the popularity of this hypothesis in clinical and academic circles, we have chosen to include a chapter on this proposed diagnosis in our book.

Conclusion

Although there is a compelling case to be made both for an against the relatedness of the OCRDs, both as a general category as well as for specific diagnoses within it, it is without doubt that recognizing a class of "repetitive thought and behavior" disorders has brought them increased scientific and clinical attention. This debate has been healthy for spurring research in OCRDs including BDD, hoarding, body focused repetitive behavior disorders, tic disorders, and emerging areas as well, all of which are clinically meaningful areas for children and adolescents that often go overlooked in typical practice. Regardless of where one falls on this argument, it is undeniable that there have been important lessons learned related to theoretical models based on childhood OCD that could provide a useful framework as investigators pursue novel work in the related areas. Most of this research has focused on adults, leaving clinical practitioners and scientists without a firm understanding of developmental considerations for these disorders as they present in youth. This book aims to highlight this literature and consider where the field might go next.

Note

1 Slight modifications in diagnostic criteria for hypochondriasis to illness anxiety disorder were made in DSM-IV to DSM-5, although the core feature of a preoccupation on physical health despite no clear medical evidence to justify these concerns remains.

References

Abramowitz, J. S. (2018). Presidential Address: Are the Obsessive-Compulsive Related Disorders Related to Obsessive-Compulsive Disorder? A Critical Look at DSM-5's New Category. *Behavior Therapy*, 49(1), 1–11. doi:10.1016/j.beth.2017.06.002.

American Psychiatric Association. (2013). *Diagnostic and Statistical Manual of Mental Disorders, 5th Edition: DSM-5.*

Bartz, J. A. & Hollander, E. (2006). Is obsessive–compulsive disorder an anxiety disorder? *Progress in Neuro-Psychopharmacology and Biological Psychiatry*, 30 (3), 338–352. doi:10.1016/j.pnpbp.2005.11.003.

Barzilay, R., Patrick, A., Calkins, M. E., Moore, T. M., Wolf, D. H., Benton, T. D., Leckman, J. F., Gur, R. C., & Gur, R. E. (2019). Obsessive-Compulsive Symptomatology in Community Youth: Typical Development or a Red Flag for Psychopathology? *Journal of the American Academy of Child & Adolescent Psychiatry*, 58(2), 277–286.e4. doi:10.1016/j.jaac.2018.06.038.

Bloch, M. H., Landeros-Weisenberger, A., Rosario, M. C., Pittenger, C., & Leckman, J. F. (2008). Meta-Analysis of the Symptom Structure of Obsessive-Compulsive Disorder. *American Journal of Psychiatry*, 165(12), 1532–1542. doi:10.1176/appi.ajp.2008.08020320.

Canals, J., Hernández-Martínez, C., Cosi, S., & Voltas, N. (2012). The epidemiology of obsessive–compulsive disorder in Spanish school children. *Journal of Anxiety Disorders*, 26(7), 746–752. doi:10.1016/j.janxdis.2012.06.003.

Chang, S., Himle, M. B., Tucker, B. T. P., Woods, D. W., & Piacentini, J. (2009). Initial Psychometric Properties of a Brief Parent-Report Instrument for Assessing Tic Severity in Children with Chronic Tic Disorders. *Child & Family Behavior Therapy*, 31(3), 181–191. doi:10.1080/07317100903099100.

Claiborn, J. M., Dozier, T. H., Hart, S. L., & Lee, J. (2020). Self-identified misophonia phenomenology, impact, and clinical correlates. *Psychological Thought*, 13(2), Article 2. doi:10.37708/psyct.v13i2.454.

Fineberg, N. A., Apergis-Schoute, A. M., Vaghi, M. M., Banca, P., Gillan, C. M., Voon, V., Chamberlain, S. R., Cinosi, E., Reid, J., Shahper, S., Bullmore, E. T., Sahakian, B. J., & Robbins, T. W. (2017). Mapping Compulsivity in the DSM-5 Obsessive Compulsive and Related Disorders: Cognitive Domains, Neural Circuitry, and Treatment. *International Journal of Neuropsychopharmacology*, 21(1), 42–58. doi:10.1093/ijnp/pyx088.

Fineberg, N. A., Dell'Osso, B., Albert, U., Maina, G., Geller, D., Carmi, L., Sireau, N., Walitza, S., Grassi, G., Pallanti, S., Hollander, E., Brakoulias, V., Menchon, J. M., Marazziti, D., Ioannidis, K., Apergis-Schoute, A., Stein, D. J., Cath, D. C., Veltman, D. J., ... Zohar, J. (2019). Early intervention for obsessive compulsive disorder: An expert consensus statement. *European Neuropsychopharmacology*, 29(4), 549–565. doi:10.1016/j.euroneuro.2019.02.002.

Fontenelle, L. F., Destrée, L., Brierley, M.-E., Thompson, E. M., Yücel, M., Lee, R., Albertella, L., & Chamberlain, S. R. (2022). The place of obsessive–compulsive and related disorders in the compulsive–impulsive spectrum: A cluster-analytic study. *CNS Spectrums*, 27(4), 486–495. doi:10.1017/S109285292100033X.

Guzick, A. G., Cervin, M., Smith, E. E. A., Clinger, J., Draper, I., Goodman, W. K., Lijffijt, M., Murphy, N., Lewin, A. B., Schneider, S. C., & Storch, E. A.

(2023). Clinical characteristics, impairment, and psychiatric morbidity in 102 youth with misophonia. *Journal of Affective Disorders*, 324, 395–402. doi:10.1016/j.jad.2022.12.083.

Guzick, A. G., Schneider, S. C., & Storch, E. A. (2020). Future research directions in children and hoarding. *Children Australia*, 45(3), 175–181. doi:10.1017/cha.2020.13.

Hollander, E. (2005). Obsessive–compulsive disorder and spectrum across the life span. *International Journal of Psychiatry in Clinical Practice*, 9(2), 79–86. doi:10.1080/13651500510018347.

Jager, I., Koning, P. de, Bost, T., Denys, D., & Vulink, N. (2020). Misophonia: Phenomenology, comorbidity and demographics in a large sample. *PLOS ONE*, 15(4), e0231390. doi:10.1371/journal.pone.0231390.

Lamothe, H., Baleyte, J.-M., Mallet, L., & Pelissolo, A. (2019). Trichotillomania is more related to Tourette disorder than to obsessive-compulsive disorder. *Brazilian Journal of Psychiatry*, 42, 87–104. doi:10.1590/1516-4446-2019-0471.

Monzani, B., Rijsdijk, F., Harris, J., & Mataix-Cols, D. (2014). The Structure of Genetic and Environmental Risk Factors for Dimensional Representations of DSM-5 Obsessive-Compulsive Spectrum Disorders. *JAMA Psychiatry*, 71(2), 182–189. doi:10.1001/jamapsychiatry.2013.3524.

Phillips, K. A., Stein, D. J., Rauch, S. L., Hollander, E., Fallon, B. A., Barsky, A., Fineberg, N., Mataix-Cols, D., Ferrão, Y. A., Saxena, S., Wilhelm, S., Kelly, M. M., Clark, L. A., Pinto, A., Bienvenu, O. J., Farrow, J., & Leckman, J. (2010). Should an obsessive-compulsive spectrum grouping of disorders be included in DSM-V? *Depression and Anxiety*, 27(6), 528–555. doi:10.1002/da.20705.

Schneider, S. C., Turner, C. M., Mond, J., & Hudson, J. L. (2017). Prevalence and correlates of body dysmorphic disorder in a community sample of adolescents. *Australian & New Zealand Journal of Psychiatry*, 51(6), 595–603. doi:10.1177/0004867416665483.

Snorrason, I., Beard, C., Peckham, A. D., & Björgvinsson, T. (2021). Transdiagnostic dimensions in obsessive-compulsive and related disorders: Associations with internalizing and externalizing symptoms. *Psychological Medicine*, 51(10), 1657–1665. doi:10.1017/S0033291720000380.

Storch, E. A., Abramowitz, J., & Goodman, W. K. (2008). Where does obsessive–compulsive disorder belong in DSM-V? *Depression and Anxiety*, 25(4), 336–347. doi:10.1002/da.20488.

Swedo, S. E., Baguley, D. M., Denys, D., Dixon, L. J., Erfanian, M., Fioretti, A., Jastreboff, P. J., Kumar, S., Rosenthal, M. Z., Rouw, R., Schiller, D., Simner, J., Storch, E. A., Taylor, S., Werff, K. R. V., Altimus, C. M., & Raver, S. M. (2022). Consensus Definition of Misophonia: A Delphi Study. *Frontiers in Neuroscience*, 16. www.frontiersin.org/articles/10.3389/fnins.2022.841816.

World Health Organization. (2019). *International Classification of Diseases, Eleventh Revision (ICD-11)*. https://icd.who.int/browse11.

2 Compulsivity, Impulsivity, and Obsessiveness as Transdiagnostic Factors in Childhood Psychopathology

Maria E. Moreira-de-Oliveira, Ana P. Ribeiro, Carina Chacur and Leonardo F. Fontenelle

Introduction

Obsessive-compulsive and related disorders

Obsessive-compulsive disorder (OCD) is a disabling condition that may be found in up to 3% of the general population (Fontenelle et al., 2006). The hallmark of OCD is the existence of obsessions and/or compulsions. Obsessions are persistent and unwanted thoughts, images or urges that cause distress or anxiety. Compulsions are repetitive behaviors or mental acts that are performed in response to obsessions according to rigid rules, or to achieve a sense of completeness (Crego et al., 2015). One of the most notable aspects of OCD is that individuals affected by OCD more often than not recognize that their beliefs are exacerbated or probably not true (Robbins et al., 2019). In the general population, OCD is slightly more prevalent in females than males, however, in clinical settings, the ratio of females to males with OCD tends to be more balanced (Stein et al., 2019).

OCD typically starts early in life, having a bimodal incidence, with the first peak occurring in childhood (around 7–12 years old) and the second one in the early adult life (Geller et al., 1998). Phenotypically, OCD in children and adolescents is similar to OCD in adults (Alvarenga et al., 2019). Early onset symptoms' general themes tend to remain the same in chronic cases, but changes in symptom content have also been reported over the course of illness (Fernández de la Cruz et al., 2013; Mataix-Cols et al., 2005). A meta-analysis suggests that early onset OCD is more likely to occur in males, to have positive family history in first-degree relatives and to have higher comorbidity with tics, OC related disorders and personality disorders. In addition, early onset OCD is associated with greater OCD global severity and higher prevalence of sensory phenomena, just-right experiences and compulsive urges in the absence of obsessions (Taylor, 2011). Furthermore, compared to adults, it is more likely for children to lack insight regarding the irrationality of their obsessions and compulsions, presumably owing to underdeveloped meta-cognitive skills

DOI: 10.4324/9781003517429-2

(Krebs & Heyman, 2015). Insight in youth has been studied and correlation between poor insight and worse response to treatment was reported (Storch et al., 2014). Some studies also found that insight was inversely related to symptom severity, functional impairment, and family accommodation, as well as hoarding symptoms (Storch, et al., 2008). Please see Chapter 14: "Early-onset and tic-related OCD" for more details on unique developmental aspects of childhood OCD.

The long-term prognosis for OCD symptoms in children and adolescents is that, once treated, 40–60% will recover or no longer meet the criteria for OCD (Micali et al., 2010). However, certain factors such as the presence of comorbid disorders, earlier onset, longer duration of symptoms, poor response to medication, and parental psychopathology have been identified as predictors of a poorer outcome (Martin et al., 2017). The duration of untreated illness is a major factor that impairs clinical and health outcomes, highlighting the need for early identification (Dell'Osso et al., 2013). However, it is important to differentiate OCD from other obsessive-compulsive subclinical symptoms that are common during the development and that usually disappears with age. The urge to make things "just right" and symmetric, for instance, is a common behavior observed in children under the age of six. Other illustrative example is the fear of germs and contamination as well as checking behaviors observed in adolescents around 12 years old (Zohar & Bruno, 1997).

Given that many people have experienced intrusive thoughts or uncontrollable behavioral urges at some point in life, the diagnostic classification systems had to draw a line between OCD and subclinical OCD symptoms. For OCD to be diagnosed according to the Diagnostic and Statistical Manual of Mental Disorders, 5th Edition (DSM-5), obsessions or compulsions must be time-consuming (e.g., to take more than 1 hour per day) or cause clinically significant distress or impairment in social, occupational, or other important areas of functioning (American Psychiatric Association, 2013a). Among OCD symptom dimensions, most common ones are cleaning (contamination obsessions and cleaning compulsions); symmetry (symmetry obsessions and repeating, ordering, and counting compulsions); forbidden or taboo thoughts (e.g., aggressive, sexual, and religious obsessions and related compulsions); and harm (e.g., fears of harm to oneself or others and related checking compulsions).

The DSM-5 has also introduced a new category called Obsessive-Compulsive and Related Disorders (OCRDs) including obsessive-compulsive disorder (OCD), body dysmorphic disorder (BDD), hoarding disorder, trichotillomania (TTM; hair pulling disorder), and excoriation (skin-picking) disorder (American Psychiatric Association, 2013a). In these conditions, repetitive thoughts and behaviors focus on negative evaluation of one's own bodily appearance (BDD), the acquisition of or inability to discard personal items (hoarding disorder), and repetitive grooming behaviors (TTM and skin-picking disorder). The latest version of the International Classification of Diseases and Related Health Problems (ICD-11) also added olfactory reference disorder (ORD) and hypochondriasis to OCRDs (International Classification of Diseases, Eleventh Revision (ICD-11), n.d.). The establishment of the OCRDs chapter was supported by evidence showing that, although being a highly heterogeneous group, these disorders share similarities in terms of symptoms, neurobiological connections and patterns of comorbidity (Fineberg et al., 2011).

Transdiagnostic approaches in psychiatry

Historically, psychiatry nosology has defined mental disorders based largely on the description of signs and symptoms, their duration, and associated disabilities (Kendler, 2018). This approach was based on unitary diagnostic categories formally described in the DSM and the ICD. Since their creation, DSM and ICD refined psychiatric classification, reduced variations in prevalence estimates, and improved the diagnostic process and pragmatic decisions in the clinical setting, while providing a common language in the field (Kendell & Jablensky, 2003). More recently, DSM-5 and ICD-11 relaxed some of the diagnostic boundaries, increased acknowledgment of the variability within disorders, and encouraged incorporating validated and reliable biomarkers and neuroscience findings as they become available in the future. Recent work advocates that mental health symptoms are not all-or-none phenomena but are better conceptualized along continuous dimensions within the population as opposed to distinct categorical entities (Brown & Barlow, 2010). In fact, it has become clear that prototypical mental disorders seem to merge both into one another and into normality, with no demonstrable natural zones of rarity between them (Rounsaville et al., 2002).

However, these newer DSM and ICD classification systems still concur with some unsolved impasses that belong to their categorical nature. The high rates of comorbidity found in clinical and community samples (Kotov et al., 2017) and the heterogeneity of listed criteria and underlying pathological processes (Allsopp et al., 2019; Zimmerman et al., 2015) indicate that an approach to psychiatric nosology based on the description of signs and symptoms fails to represent psychopathology and its bases accurately (Goodwin, 2022). In the latter instance, the taxonomic approach instantiated in the DSM and ICD runs counter to the available clinical and research evidence and may hamper our understanding of mental illness and consequently how we manage and treat mental distress (Insel, 2014; Kotov et al., 2017). Therefore, psychiatry has been shifting its focus from classifying mental disorders as categorial diagnoses to utilizing empirical, dimensional models of mental illness.

Currently, there are no biological markers or cognitive processes that have been found to be uniquely linked to a specific disorder, yet they contribute to the signs and symptoms across a range of mental conditions. In this sense, such dimensions of disordered behavior, and their underlying biological factors, are considered "transdiagnostic" as it does not "respect" traditional diagnostic boundaries. Some have argued that deconstructing categorical diagnoses into dimensional constructs and identifying targetable transdiagnostic psychological and biological signatures of disorders could cut the way to new interventions and increase treatment effectiveness (Kelly et al., 2021; van Loo et al., 2019). With the aim to investigate such "transdiagnostic" constructs, the National Institute of Mental Health developed the Research Domain Criteria (RDoC).

The RDoC framework (Insel et al., 2010) intends to integrate knowledge from neuroscience with clinical practice, promoting research into valid neurocognitive phenotypes and dimensions. The main target of this initiative is to determine the mechanisms underlying normal-range functioning and then how disruptions correspond to psychopathology, irrespective of symptoms and diagnoses as currently conceptualized (Kraemer, 2015). Its infrastructure untangles mental health complexity into six domains: positive valence systems, negative valence systems, cognitive systems, systems for social process, arousal/modulatory systems, and sensorimotor systems, each divided into several constructs and subconstructs that can be interrogated at different units of analysis: genes, molecules, cells, circuits, physiology, behavior, self-reports, and paradigms.

And how does the "transdiagnostic" approach apply to OCRDs?

Obsessions and compulsions are present in a myriad of neuropsychiatric conditions and are considered the most important clinical constructs among OCRDs. Adopting the RDoC approach, they can be understood as final products of multiple disrupted cognitive processes and corresponding neurobiological systems (Fontenelle & Yücel, 2019). Indeed, consistently with the RDoC approach, the overlap within disorders in the OCRD group, in terms of genes and brain networks, has recently been demonstrated (Burton et al., 2021; Gillan & Seow, 2020; D. Liu et al., 2019; Parkes et al., 2020). Going one step above these constructs, we can find compulsivity, impulsivity, and obsessiveness as major endophenotypes of these thoughts and behaviors, represented in the RDoC matrix within positive, negative, and cognitive systems.

1 Compulsivity

Compulsivity refers to the extent to which a person feels driven to perform certain behaviors repetitively. It is a trait that is present in a wide spectrum of behaviors, ranging from ritualistic acts to substance abuse, gambling and eating disorders. Although the prototypical disorder associated with this construct is OCD, the idea that compulsivity is a crucial behavioral aspect that merits investigation across various disorders is becoming more widely accepted, and the number of studies on compulsivity has increased (Robbins et al., 2012). A team of renowned experts conducted a Delphi study to determine the RDoC constructs that were considered most crucial for understanding OCRDs (Fontenelle et al., 2020). Interestingly, compulsivity, although not originally listed in the matrix, was identified as essential when referring to OCRDs.

Most people have an intuitive understanding of what compulsive behavior entails. However, in science, defining compulsivity accurately is essential. The absence of an agreement on the definition of compulsivity leads to confusion in the field and hampers the comparison of compulsivity across psychiatric disorders (Luigjes & Denys, 2019). For instance, defining compulsivity as an inclination towards behavioral excesses lacks both clinical utility and treatment guidance, as it encompasses a significant number of symptoms in psychiatry, and there is no single approach that can efficiently treat all excessive behaviors (Fontenelle & Yücel, 2019). In fact, there may be multiple "compulsivities." While there are notable similarities among compulsive behaviors, their manifestation in different disorders may vary considerably (Luigjes et al., 2019). Hence, compulsivity has been theorized as a multidimensional construct, although the number and nature of these sub-constructs are not well established. In a study with more than 3000 subjects, Tiego et al. (2023) identified a two-factor structure of transdiagnostic compulsivity using the Cambridge–Chicago Compulsivity Trait Scale (CHI-T), namely "perfectionism" and "reward drive." This suggests that negative and positive reinforcement mechanisms may be crucial in various "compulsive" disorders.

Uncovering the underlying pathophysiological mechanisms of compulsivity as a transdiagnostic, neuropsychological domain would aid in the pursuit of new treatment targets and foster the creation of evidence-based treatments (Fineberg et al., 2013). So far, compulsive behaviors are thought to be rooted in disordered neural networks in the brain, specifically cortico-striato-thalamo-cortical circuits involved in reward processing, action selection, habit formation, and motor control. These circuits have both direct and indirect pathways and play a role in recognizing stimuli and regulating goal-directed responses, making them important for OCRDs (Fineberg et al., 2017). Therefore, the transdiagnostic view of compulsivity should stem from the overlap and interaction between these circuits. On the other hand, the possibility of differing mechanisms behind the development of compulsive behavior cannot be ruled out, owing to the absence of a widely accepted definition of compulsivity.

Recently, in an effort to attain a more cohesive definition, a study reviewed the different descriptions of "compulsive behavior" found in psychiatric literature (Luigjes et al., 2019). According to the authors, compulsive behavior is characterized by the feeling that one 'has to' perform a repetitive act that is not recognized to be in line with one's overall goal. This is an interesting definition, since it aligns with patients' reports of suffering resulting from the experience itself and feeling a loss of control. Although compulsive patients are fully aware that they are responsible for performing the compulsive act, they report as being 'coerced' to do so, as it doesn't "feel" like they have spontaneously chosen to perform the act (Luigjes & Denys, 2019).

Such controversial feeling suggests that free will may play an important role in compulsivity phenomenology. Although there are some conceptual discussions in literature (Denys, 2014; Karlsson, 2005; Meynen, 2012; Stein, 2012), only a few studies have investigated free will cognitions in patients with compulsive behaviors (Moreira-de-Oliveira et al., 2022; van der Salm et al., 2017; van Oudheusden et al., 2018; Vonasch et al., 2017). Regarding OCD, evidence suggests that a reduced sense of free will in adults with the disorder is linked to fundamental clinical features such as illness duration and severity, insight, and quality of life (van Oudheusden et al., 2018). In addition, some free will experiences seem to be associated with differential outcomes of symptoms in adults with OCD (Moreira-de-Oliveira et al., 2022). Yet, to our knowledge, no study has assessed perceptions of free will in children with compulsions.

However, compulsive disorders often start in childhood and the presentation of compulsive behavior in children is similar to that in adults (Mechler et al., 2018). Unsurprisingly, compulsivity in children and adolescents can lead to significant distress and interference in their daily lives, affecting their ability to participate in school and social activities (Lewin et al., 2006; McGuire et al., 2012). On the other hand, it is important to note that not all repetitive behaviors in childhood are indicative of compulsivity. Some degree of repetitive behavior is a normal part of child development and can serve important functions such as promoting learning and exploration. However, if repetitive behaviors become excessive, interfere with daily functioning and cause distress or impairment, they may be indicative of a compulsive disorder.

In the literature concerning children and adolescents, our review revealed a limited number of studies that specifically utilize the term "compulsivity" (Akkermans et al., 2019; Gooskens et al., 2019, 2021; Hollestein et al., 2020; Naaijen et al., 2017, 2018). In these studies, the authors utilized this terminology to denote a measure derived from the "compulsions" or "compulsive behavior" subscales of the Repetitive Behavior Scale/Repetitive Behavior Scale – Revised (RBS/RBS-R) questionnaires. These instruments were originally designed to capture the diverse range of restricted repetitive behaviors observed in individuals with autism spectrum disorder (ASD). Although these studies primarily investigated youths diagnosed with OCD and ASD, the precise definition of the term "compulsivity" was unclear. Their findings underline the importance of agreeing on what the term compulsivity actually means and what are the most appropriate instruments to assess its presence and/or severity.

2 Impulsivity

Impulsivity is a complex psychological construct involving a maladaptive tendency for fast, unplanned behavior with little foresight on the consequences of such behavior (Eysenck & Eysenck, 1977; Moeller et al., 2001). Clearly, impulsivity can sometimes be advantageous but is more likely to result in detrimental outcomes. Impulsivity is a central dimension of many behavioral disorders and a signature of developmental disorders, such as Attention Deficit Hyperactivity Disorder (ADHD) (Leffa et al., 2022). It has primarily been associated with disorders characterized by externalizing behaviors, including antisocial and aggressive behaviors (Beauchaine et al., 2017) and has also been consistently associated with addiction (Koob & Volkow, 2010; Potenza, 2014; Verdejo-Garcia et al., 2019).

More recently, impulsivity has been shown to play an important role in other disorders, including OCRDs (Brem et al., 2014; Grant & Chamberlain, 2021; Merz et al., 2018; Yang et al., 2021b). Subjects with OCD, especially the ones with aggressive and checking compulsions, have exhibited significantly elevated scores of cognitive impulsiveness using the Barratt Impulsiveness Scale (Ettelt et al., 2007). Similarly, disorders classically considered impulsive – such as Trichotillomania, Excoriation Disorder – have recently been regrouped with OCRDs, owing to neurobiological similarities with other compulsive disorders (Grant & Chamberlain, 2021).

Current framework considers impulsivity as a multidimensional construct. One possible way of classifying impulsivity includes at least four distinct factors, such as sense of urgency (urgency or negative urgency), lack of planning, lack of persistence (or perseverance), and sensation-seeking (Fischer & Smith, 2008; Whiteside & Lynam, 2001). These forms of impulsivity may be assessed with self-report questionnaires, such as the the Urgency, Premeditation, Perseverance, and Sensation-Seeking Scale (Whiteside et al., 2005) and other inventories (Claes et al., 2000; Vasconcelos et al., 2012). Although not in one-to-one correlation, these impulsivity factors seem to be expressions of problems with response inhibition (motor impulsivity), hyper-sensitivity to reward anticipation (reward impulsivity), and poor planning (reflection impulsivity) (Fineberg et al., 2009; Grant & Kim, 2014). Considering neuroimaging and functional study findings, these facets of impulsivity reflect altered connections between brain regions involved in impulse control, decision-making, and attention (Bari et al., 2013; Petitet et al., 2022).

Impulsivity can be understood as an imbalance between the top-down control, provided by the orbital frontal cortex and the anterior cingulated cortex (Clark et al., 2004) – which are involved in the adaptation of the behavior to social and future expectations and in predicting expectancies of reward and punishment –, and the bottom-up drives generated in limbic structures such as the amygdala, insula and the basal ganglia – which are involved in motivation and reward processing (Donnelly et al., 2014; Silva et al., 2020; Verdejo-Garcia & Albein-Urios, 2021).

Impulsivity can be a normal part of the development of children and adolescents and typically decreases as individuals mature (Churchwell & Yurgelun-Todd, 2013; Kray et al., 2021; Shaw et al., 2011).Clinically, it can be manifested in many ways, such as interrupting others while speaking, having difficulty waiting one's turn or delaying gratification, engaging in risky or dangerous behavior without considering the potential consequences, and making decisions without thinking through the available options (Moeller et al., 2001). Interestingly, there is evidence that pediatric patients with OCD display more persistent deficits in inhibitory control, suggesting that impulsivity can be bound to the chronicity and severity of the obsessive-compulsive symptoms in youth (Ettelt et al., 2007; Martinez-Loredo et al., 2018).

The phenotypic expression of impulsivity may derive from one or more of several sources and persist for different reasons later in life. ⊠Some studies have suggested that impulsivity may be related to differences in brain development, such as the timing of brain maturation or the rate of growth in specific brain regions (Arain et al., 2013; Ziegler et al., 2019). Also, interactive genetic factors (both heritable and nonheritable) (Bezdjian et al., 2011; Gustavson et al., 2020; Yang et al., 2021a) and environmental insults (Fenneman & Frankenhuis, 2020) seem to affect neural function and predispose it to greater impulsivity. Well-characterized influences on impulsive behavior include brain injuries, which may result from head trauma, hypoxia, or other central nervous system insults (Fullerton et al., 2019), and exposure to teratogenic agents such as alcohol and stimulant drugs of abuse (Bendix et al., 2019; J. Liu et al., 2013). Children and adolescents who grow up in stressful or chaotic environments, or who experience trauma or abuse, may be more likely to exhibit impulsive behavior as well (Mullet et al., 2022; Oshri et al., 2018).

3 Obsessiveness

'Obsession' is derived from the Latin word *"obsidere"*: being taken into possession, being occupied or preoccupied. In layman's language the term 'obsession' is polysemic and may refer to a variety of unpleasant, unwanted, or involuntary experiences such as anxious thoughts, ruminations, thought insertion, delusions, and obsession-like phenomena (Rasmussen & Parnas, 2022). For classic psychopathology, however, obsessions are described as ideas or representations which try to impose themselves on the conscience, in an unexpected, iterative, and persistent way, and which, owing to the peculiar nature of their contents are usually accompanied by a violent inner struggle and strong state of distress (Nobre de Melo, 1945; American Psychiatric Association, 2013a; Stein et al., 2019). Obsessions are not the same as worries or fears classically seen in anxiety disorders and should not be used as a synonym for delusional ideas present in psychotic disorders. Nevertheless, the clinical presentation of obsessiveness cannot always be clearly disentangled from those conditions.

Despite being one of the core features of OCRDs (especially OCD and BDD), obsessions may resemble common preoccupations and worries that are also seen in anxiety disorders (e.g., generalized anxiety disorder, hypochondria). Along with historical reasons, this clinical similarity probably justified the inclusion of OCD in the chapter of anxiety disorders until the past DSM-IV-TR. Also, some correspondence can be found between typical obsessions and the preoccupations with body form and appearance that are so characteristic of individuals with BDD and eating disorders. For all of these conditions, lack of insight and control into obsessive thoughts can blur the frontiers between these phenomena and delusions (Adelman & Lebowitz, 2012; Phillips et al., 1995; Starcevic, 2014; Vigne et al., 2014).

In DSM-5, the insight specifiers for OCRDs have been expanded to include a broader range of options, including delusional OCD beliefs, which could also be double coded as the psychotic disorders in the past (Eisen et al., 1999; Van Ameringen et al., 2014). Although significant in many psychiatric conditions, obsessive thoughts are common in the general population, and a large body of research indicates that the themes, content, and form of intrusive thoughts are the same among non-clinical and clinical samples, with differences remaining on the intensity and perceived distress related to the form of thoughts rather than just on their content (Abramowitz et al., 2014). Therefore, rather than a trait or a single symptom, obsessiveness should be better conceptualized as a dimensional phenotype.

Although we might consider obsessions as the most relevant phenomenon when dealing with obsessiveness, it is important to realize, however, that this dimension entails more than simply egodystonic obsessive thoughts. The preoccupation with details, perfectionism, rigidity, conscientiousness, and self-control seen in obsessive-compulsive personality disorder (OCPD) (American Psychiatric Association, 2013b) (Diedrich & Voderholzer, 2015; Grant & Chamberlain, 2019) may also be subsumed under the concept of "obsessiveness" and shared by other OCRDs, such as anorexia nervosa, in which obsessions about weight are coupled with strong rigidity need for control (Serpell, Livingstone, & Neiderman, 2002).

Similarly to the Delphi reviews described above that resulted in the proposal of compulsivity as one potential underlying construct shared by different OCRDs and disorders to addictive behaviors (Fontenelle et al., 2011; Luigjes et al., 2019), early attempts to identify constructs underlying obsessiveness were also performed (Obsessive Compulsive Cognitions

Working Group, 2005). These constructs, termed "obsessive beliefs," included three factors, namely: (a) overestimation of threat and responsibility (e.g., "I often think I am responsible for things that other people don't think are my fault"); (b) importance of and need to control thoughts (e.g., "If I don't control my unwanted thoughts, something bad is bound to happen"); and (c) perfectionism and need for certainty (e.g., "If I can't do something perfectly, I shouldn't do it at all") (Obsessive Compulsive Cognitions Working Group, 2005). These underlying constructs are typically assessed with self-report questionnaires such different versions of the Obsessive Beliefs Questionnaire, which was also developmentally adapted for youth in a child version and showed a similar underlying factor structure.

Neurobiological models of obsessions are lacking. One promising model implies that obsessions may be a consequence of dysfunction in fear conditioning processes, whereby patients cannot adequately extinguish fears that accompany normal intrusive thoughts and worries. In support of this hypothesis, impairments in extinction recall are evident in OCD, and the respective neural correlates also overlap on regions thought to be involved in the disorder (Milad et al., 2013). However, since patients with post-traumatic stress disorder (PTSD) have similar deficits in fear-extinction recall but do not typically present with obsessions, fear-conditioning abnormalities in OCD may reflect concomitant anxiety in OCD, rather than obsessions.

The identification of obsessive thoughts in children can be challenging, owing to their still-developing and variable abilities of self-observation (meta-cognition) or reduced insight. In terms of their typical themes/contents, one study comparing a sample of children and adolescents versus adults with OCD observed that youths had higher rates of aggressive/harm obsessions (including fears of catastrophic events, such as death or illness in self or loved ones) than adults (63 percent vs 69 percent vs 31 percent, p <.001). These fears were the most common obsessions in the pediatric age group. On the other hand, religious obsessions were over-represented in adolescents (36 percent) compared with children (15 percent) and adults (10 percent, p <.001), and sexual obsessions were under-represented in children (11 percent) compared with adolescents (36 percent) and adults (24 percent) (p =.011) (Geller et al., 2006).

General discussion

Compulsivity, impulsivity, and obsessiveness are important concepts in the field of psychiatry and psychology since they are often interrelated and frequently seen in clinical practice. The manifestations of these constructs in childhood can vary significantly, with some children exhibiting mainly compulsive or impulsive behaviors, while others may be obsessive. Some children may have symptoms that indicate perturbation in the three constructs. Although their definitions might be debatable (e.g., lack of consensus on what is compulsivity), these traits seem to be present as underlying mechanisms in OCRDs.

There is some evidence indicating that disorders involving compulsivity and impulsivity share a pattern of behavioral disinhibition, suggesting they may not be in opposition to each other. Instead, they may both be characterized by impaired prefrontal inhibitory control over subcortical structures, leading to exaggerated or uncontrollable behaviors. One way of differentiating these constructs is that compulsivity reflects persistent behavioral responses, whereas impulsivity refers to premature behavioral responses (Dalley et al., 2011). Some have postulated that with progression and chronicity, certain compulsive behaviors may become "impulsive compulsions" (Fontenelle et al., 2011) whereas impulsive actions may progressively turn into "compulsive impulsions" (Everitt & Robbins, 2005).

Another aspect to consider is the close relationship between obsessiveness and compulsivity. As pointed by Denys (2011), patients might not only be obsessed by a thought but also obsessed with an act that must be performed (compulsion). Early behavioral theories of OCD proposed that obsessions were the primary trigger for compulsive rituals, with compulsions serving as a means of reducing anxiety caused by the obsession (Rachman & Hodgson, 1980). However, this anxiety reduction hypothesis had difficulty explaining why some compulsions actually increased anxiety, such as checking rituals that paradoxically reduce memory confidence and induce further checking (Radomsky et al., 2014). In this sense, some researchers have suggested that compulsions may actually be the core feature of OCD, with obsessions arising as a result of compulsive behaviors (Gillan et al., 2014; Gillan & Sahakian, 2015).

However, it's important to note that, particularly in children, compulsions, obsessions and impulsive acts can manifest along a continuum that may not necessarily be pathological. Therefore, distinguishing between normal developmental repetitive behavior, like bedtime rituals, and persistent distressing thoughts and compulsions is crucial (Boileau, 2011). It is likely that some early subclinical compulsivity, impulsivity or obsessiveness increase the risk for future OCRDs or disorders to addictive behaviors. However, it is unclear whether these traits are cross diagnostic and represent common prodromes for these disorders. It can also be difficult to determine where to draw the line between what should or not be treated (Fontenelle & Yücel, 2019). Whether subclinical traits require early intervention to decrease conversion to clinical disorders is still debatable.

Given the potential challenges associated with early use of medications or behavioral interventions (e.g., costs and/or potential side effects) for mild symptoms, lifestyle interventions may represent a promising approach for addressing subclinical OCRD. However, there is currently insufficient evidence regarding which lifestyle factors should be targeted to prevent the development of mental illness (Firth et al., 2020). Despite the limited number of well-designed randomized controlled trials targeting unhealthy lifestyles in OCRDs, a recent review found that meditation-based therapies and interventions focusing on eliminating sedentarism show promise as potential treatments. The authors suggest that these strategies may represent valid alternatives for individuals with subthreshold symptoms of OCRDs (Brierley et al., 2021; Fontenelle et al., 2018). In addition, when considering children with compulsions, obsessions and impulsive acts, it is crucial to take into account the impact of family factors on symptom expression, as families can inadvertently maintain and exacerbate symptoms through their involvement and accommodation; thus, it is imperative that parents are equipped with supportive and effective strategies to manage their child's behaviors.

Summary

Psychiatry has traditionally defined mental disorders based on signs and symptoms, resulting in discrete diagnostic categories. Although this DSM- and ICD-approaches have been useful, recent research suggests that mental health symptoms should be conceptualized as continuous dimensions within the population rather than distinct categorical entities. The high rates of comorbidity found in clinical and community samples indicate that an approach to psychiatric nosology based on the description of signs and symptoms fails to represent psychopathology and its bases accurately. Therefore, mental health is shifting its focus to utilizing empirical, dimensional models of mental illness, such as the RDoC, which aims to integrate knowledge from neuroscience with clinical practice to identify transdiagnostic biosignatures of disorders.

Compulsivity, impulsivity and obsessiveness are important constructs in a variety of neuropsychiatric conditions and can be understood as products of disrupted cognitive processes and neurobiological systems according to the RDoC approach. These constructs overlap within disorders in the OCRD group, as demonstrated by recent research. In general, compulsivity reflects persistent behavioral responses and impulsivity refers to premature behavioral responses. In contrast, while obsessions and compulsions are closely related, identifying obsessive thoughts in children can be challenging, owing to their limited ability of self-observation or reduced insight. In children, it is important to distinguish between normal repetitive behaviors and persistent distressing thoughts and OC symptoms, and it is unclear whether subclinical traits require early intervention to decrease conversion to clinical disorders.

References

Abramowitz, J. S., Fabricant, L. E., Taylor, S., Deacon, B. J., McKay, D., & Storch, E. A. (2014). The relevance of analogue studies for understanding obsessions and compulsions. *Clinical Psychology Review*, 34(3), 206–217. doi:10.1016/j.cpr.2014.01.004.

Adelman, C. B. & Lebowitz, E. R. (2012). Poor insight in pediatric obsessive compulsive disorder: Developmental considerations, treatment implications, and potential strategies for improving insight. *Journal of Obsessive-Compulsive and Related Disorders*, 1(2), 119–124. doi:10.1016/j.jocrd.2012.02.003.

Akkermans, S. E. A., Rheinheimer, N., Bruchhage, M. M. K., Durston, S., Brandeis, D., Banaschewski, T., Buitelaar, J. K., van Rooij, D., Oldehinkel, M., de Ruiter, S. W., Naaijen, J., Mennes, M., Zwiers, M. P., Ilbegi, S., Glennon, J. C., van de Vondervoort, I. I. G. M., Havenith, M. N., Franke, B., Poelmans, G. J. V., Bralten, J. B., Heskes, T., Groot, P., Schwalber, A., & Auby, P. (2019). Frontostriatal functional connectivity correlates with repetitive behaviour across autism spectrum disorder and obsessive-compulsive disorder. *Psychological Medicine, 49(13)*, 2247–2255.

Allsopp, K., Read, J., Corcoran, R., & Kinderman, P. (2019). Heterogeneity in psychiatric diagnostic classification. *Psychiatry Research*, 279(April), 15–22. doi:10.1016/j.psychres.2019.07.005.

Alvarenga, P., Mastroros, R., & Rosário, M. (2019). Obsessive compulsive disorder in children and adolescents. In J. M. Rey & A. Martin (Eds), *JM REY'S IACAPAP e-Textbook of Child and Adolescent Mental Health*. International Association for Child and Adolescent Psychiatry and Allied Professions.

American Psychiatric Association. (2013a). *Diagnostic and Statistical Manual of Mental Disorders: DSM 5* (5th Ed.). American Psychiatric Association.

American Psychiatric Association. (2013b). DSM-5 Diagnostic Classification. In *Diagnostic and Statistical Manual of Mental Disorders*. doi:10.1176/appi.books.9780890425596.x00diagnosticclassification.

Arain, M., Haque, M., Johal, L., Mathur, P., Nel, W., Rais, A., Sandhu, R., & Sharma, S. (2013). Maturation of the adolescent brain. *Neuropsychiatric Disease and Treatment*, 9, 449–461. doi:10.2147/NDT.S39776.

Bari, A., Robbins, T. W., Andrea, Q., & Robbins, T. W. (2013). Inhibition and impulsivity: Behavioral and neural basis of response control. *Progress in Neurobiology*, 108, 44–79. https://doi.org/10.1016/j.pneurobio.2013.06.005.

Beauchaine, T. P., Zisner, A. R., & Sauder, C. L. (2017). Trait impulsivity and the externalizing spectrum. *Annual Review of Clinical Psychology*, 13, 343–368.

Bendix, I., Hadamitzky, M., Herz, J., & Felderhoff-Müser, U. (2019). Adverse neuropsychiatric development following perinatal brain injury: from a preclinical perspective. *Pediatric Research*, 85(2), 198–215. https://doi.org/10.1038/s41390-018-0222-6.

Bezdjian, S., Baker, L. A., & Tuvblad, C. (2011). Genetic and environmental influences on impulsivity: A meta-analysis of twin, family and adoption studies. *Clinical Psychology Review*, 31(7), 1209–1223. doi:10.1016/j.cpr.2011.07.005.

Boileau, B. (2011). A review of obsessive-compulsive disorder in children and adolescents. *Dialogues in Clinical Neuroscience*, 13(4), 401–411. doi:10.31887/DCNS.2011.13.4/bboileau.

Brem, S., Grünblatt, E., Drechsler, R., Riederer, P., & Walitza, S. (2014). The neurobiological link between OCD and ADHD. *ADHD Attention Deficit and Hyperactivity Disorders*, 6(3), 175–202. doi:10.1007/s12402-014-0146-x.

Brierley, M. E. E., Thompson, E. M., Albertella, L., & Fontenelle, L. F. (2021). Lifestyle Interventions in the Treatment of Obsessive-Compulsive and Related

Disorders: A Systematic Review. *Psychosomatic Medicine*, 83(8), 817–833. doi:10.1097/PSY.0000000000000988.

Brown, T. A. & Barlow, D. H. (2010). *A Proposal for a Dimensional Classification System Based on the Shared Features of the DSM-IV Anxiety and Mood Disorders: Implications for Assessment and Treatment.* 21(3), 256–271. doi:10.1037/a0016608.A.

Burton, C. L., Lemire, M., Xiao, B., Cor, E. C., Erdman, L., Bralten, J., Poelmans, G., Yu, D., Shaheen, S., Goodale, T., Sinopoli, V. M., Working, O. C. D., Consortium, P. G., Soreni, N., Hanna, G. L., Fitzgerald, K. D., Rosenberg, D., Nestadt, G., Paterson, A. D., ... Crosbie, J. (2021). *Genome-wide association study of pediatric obsessive-compulsive traits: shared genetic risk between traits and disorder.* doi:10.1038/s41398-020-01121-9.

Churchwell, J. C. & Yurgelun-Todd, D. A. (2013). Age-related changes in insula cortical thickness and impulsivity: Significance for emotional development and decision-making. *Developmental Cognitive Neuroscience*, 6, 80–86. doi:10.1016/j.dcn.2013.07.001.

Claes, L., Vertommen, H., & Braspenning, N. (2000). Psychometric properties of the Dickman Impulsivity Inventory. *Personality and Individual Differences*, 29 (1), 27–35. doi:10.1016/S0191-8869(99)00172-00175.

Clark, L., Cools, R., & Robbins, T. W. (2004). The neuropsychology of ventral prefrontal cortex: Decision-making and reversal learning. *Brain and Cognition*, 55(1), 41–53. doi:10.1016/S0278-2626(03)00284-00287.

Crego, C., Samuel, D. B., & Widiger, T. A. (2015). The FFOCI and Other Measures and Models of OCPD. *Assessment*, 22(2), 135–151. doi:10.1177/1073191114539382.

Dalley, J. W., Everitt, B. J., & Robbins, T. W. (2011). Impulsivity, Compulsivity, and Top-Down Cognitive Control. *Neuron*, 69(4), 680–694. doi:10.1016/j.neuron.2011.01.020.

Dell'Osso, B., Benatti, B., Buoli, M., Altamura, A. C., Marazziti, D., Hollander, E., Fineberg, N., Stein, D. J., Pallanti, S., Nicolini, H., Ameringen, M. Van, Lochner, C., Hranov, G., Karamustafalioglu, O., Hranov, L., Menchon, J. M., & Zohar, J. (2013). The influence of age at onset and duration of illness on long-term outcome in patients with obsessive-compulsive disorder: A report from the International College of Obsessive Compulsive Spectrum Disorders (ICOCS). *European Neuropsychopharmacology*, 23(8), 865–871. doi:10.1016/j.euroneuro.2013.05.004.

Denys, D. (2011). Obsessionality & compulsivity: A phenomenology of obsessive-compulsive disorder. *Philosophy, Ethics, and Humanities in Medicine*, 6(1), 3. doi:10.1186/1747-5341-6-3.

Denys, D. (2014). Compulsivity and free will. *CNS Spectrums*, 19(1), 8–9. doi:10.1017/S1092852913000412.

Diedrich, A. & Voderholzer, U. (2015). Obsessive–Compulsive Personality Disorder: a Current Review. *Current Psychiatry Reports*, 17(2). doi:10.1007/s11920-014-0547-8.

Donnelly, N. A., Holtzman, T., Rich, P. D., Nevado-Holgado, A. J., Fernando, A. B. P., Van Dijck, G., Holzhammer, T., Paul, O., Ruther, P., Paulsen, O., Robbins, T. W., & Dalley, J. W. (2014). Oscillatory activity in the medial prefrontal cortex and nucleus accumbens correlates with impulsivity and reward outcome. *PLoS ONE*, 9(10), 14–17. doi:10.1371/journal.pone.0111300.

Eisen, J. L., Phillips, K. A., & Rasmussen, S. A. (1999). Obsessions and delusions: The relationship between obsessive-compulsive disorder and the psychotic disorders. *Psychiatric Annals*, 29(9), 515–522).

Ettelt, S., Ruhrmann, S., Barnow, S., Buthz, F., Hochrein, A., Meyer, K., Kraft, S., Reck, C., Pukrop, R., Klosterkötter, J., Falkai, P., Maier, W., Wagner, M., Freyberger, H. J., & Grabe, H. J. (2007). Impulsiveness in obsessive-compulsive disorder: results from a family study. *Acta Psychiatrica Scandinavica*, 115(1), 41–47. doi:10.1111/j.1600-0447.2006.00835.x.

Everitt, B. J. & Robbins, T. W. (2005). Neural systems of reinforcement for drug addiction: From actions to habits to compulsion. *Nature Neuroscience*, 8(11), 1481–1489. doi:10.1038/nn1579.

Eysenck, S. B. G. & Eysenck, H. J. (1977). The place of impulsiveness in a dimensional system of personality description. *British Journal of Social and Clinical Psychology*, 16(1), 57–68.

Fenneman, J. & Frankenhuis, W. E. (2020). Is impulsive behavior adaptive in harsh and unpredictable environments? A formal model. *Evolution and Human Behavior*, 41(4), 261–273. doi:10.1016/j.evolhumbehav.2020.02.005.

Fernández de la Cruz, L., Micali, N., Roberts, S., Turner, C., Nakatani, E., Heyman, I., & Mataix-Cols, D. (2013). Are the symptoms of obsessive-compulsive disorder temporally stable in children/adolescents? A prospective naturalistic study. *Psychiatry Research*, 209(2), 196–201. doi:10.1016/j.psychres.2012.11.033.

Fineberg, N. A., Apergis-Schoute, A. M., Vaghi, M. M., Banca, P., Gillan, C. M., Voon, V., Chamberlain, S. R., Cinosi, E., Reid, J., Shahper, S., Bullmore, E. T., Sahakian, B. J., & Robbins, T. W. (2017). Mapping Compulsivity in the DSM-5 Obsessive Compulsive and Related Disorders: Cognitive Domains, Neural Circuitry, and Treatment. *International Journal of Neuropsychopharmacology*, 21(1), 42–58. doi:10.1093/ijnp/pyx088.

Fineberg, N. A., Baldwin, D. S., Menchon, J. M., Denys, D., Grünblatt, E., Pallanti, S., Stein, D. J., & Zohar, J. (2013). Manifesto for a European research network into obsessive-compulsive and related disorders. *European Neuropsychopharmacology*, 23(7), 561–568. doi:10.1016/j.euroneuro.2012.06.006.

Fineberg, N. A., Potenza, M. N., Chamberlain, S. R., Berlin, H. A., Menzies, L., Bechara, A., Sahakian, B. J., Robbins, T. W., Bullmore, E. T., & Hollander, E. (2009). Probing Compulsive and Impulsive Behaviors, from Animal Models to Endophenotypes: A Narrative Review. *Neuropsychopharmacology*, 35(3), 591–604. doi:10.1038/npp.2009.185.

Fineberg, N. A., Saxena, S., Zohar, J., & Craig, K. J. (2011). Obsessive-Compulsive Disorder: Boundary Issues. In E. Hollander, J. Zohar, P. J. Sirovatka, & D. A. Regier (Eds), *Obsessive-Compulsive Spectrum Disorders: Refining the Research Agenda for DSM-V*. American Psychiatric Publishing.

Firth, J., Solmi, M., Wootton, R. E., Vancampfort, D., Schuch, F. B., Hoare, E., Gilbody, S., Torous, J., Teasdale, S. B., Jackson, S. E., Smith, L., Eaton, M., Jacka, F. N., Veronese, N., Marx, W., Ashdown-Franks, G., Siskind, D., Sarris, J., Rosenbaum, S., … Stubbs, B. (2020). A meta-review of "lifestyle psychiatry": the role of exercise, smoking, diet and sleep in the prevention and treatment of mental disorders. *World Psychiatry*, 19(3), 360–380. doi:10.1002/wps.20773.

Fischer, S. & Smith, G. T. (2008). Binge eating, problem drinking, and pathological gambling: Linking behavior to shared traits and social learning. *Personality and Individual Differences*, 44(4), 789–800. doi:10.1016/j.paid.2007.10.008.

Fontenelle, L. F., Mendlowicz, M. V., & Versiani, M. (2006). The descriptive epidemiology of obsessive-compulsive disorder. *Progress in Neuro-Psychopharmacology and Biological Psychiatry*, 30(3), 327–337. doi:10.1016/j. pnpbp.2005.11.001.

Fontenelle, L. F., Oldenhof, E., Eduarda Moreira-de-Oliveira, M., Abramowitz, J. S., Antony, M. M., Cath, D., Carter, A., Dougherty, D., Ferrão, Y. A., Figee, M., Harrison, B. J., Hoexter, M., Soo Kwon, J., Küelz, A., Lazaro, L., Lochner, C., Marazziti, D., Mataix-Cols, D., McKay, D., ... Yücel, M. (2020). A transdiagnostic perspective of constructs underlying obsessive-compulsive and related disorders: An international Delphi consensus study. *Australian & New Zealand Journal of Psychiatry*, 54(7). doi:10.1177/0004867420912327.

Fontenelle, L. F., Oostermeijer, S., Harrison, B. J., & Pantelis, C. (2011). Obsessive-Compulsive Disorder, Impulse Control Disorders and Drug Addiction Common Features and Potential Treatments. *Drugs*, 71(7), 827–840.

Fontenelle, L. & Yücel, M. (2019). A Transdiagnostic Approach to Obsessions, Compulsions and Related Phenomena. In *A Transdiagnostic Approach to Obsessions, Compulsions and Related Phenomena* (pp. 1–13). Cambridge University Press.

Fontenelle, L. F., Zeni-Graiff, M., Quintas, J. N., & Yücel, M. (2018). Is There A Role For Lifestyle Interventions In Obsessive-Compulsive And Related Disorders? *Current Medicinal Chemistry*, 25(41), 5698–5711. doi:10.2174/0929867325666180104150854.

Fullerton, A. F., Jackson, N. J., Tuvblad, C., Raine, A., & Baker, L. A. (2019). Early childhood head injury attenuates declines in impulsivity and aggression across adolescent development in twins. *Neuropsychology*, 33(8), 1035–1044. doi:10.1037/neu0000570.

Geller, D. A., Biederman, J., Jones, J., Shapiro, S., Schwartz, S., & Park, K. S. (1998). Obsessive-Compulsive Disorder in Children and Adolescents: A Review. *Harvard Review of Psychiatry*, 5(5), 260–273. doi:10.3109/10673229809000309.

Geller, D. A., Doyle, R., Shaw, D., Mullin, B., Coffey, B., Petty, C., Vivas, F., & Biederman, J. (2006). A quick and reliable screening measure for OCD in youth: reliability and validity of the obsessive compulsive scale of the Child Behavior Checklist. *Comprehensive Psychiatry*, 47(3), 234–240. https://doi.org/10.1016/j. comppsych.2005.08.005.

Gillan, C. M., Morein-Zamir, S., Urcelay, G. P., Sule, A., Voon, V., Apergis-Schoute, A. M., Fineberg, N. A., Sahakian, B. J., & Robbins, T. W. (2014). Enhanced avoidance habits in obsessive-compulsive disorder. *Biological Psychiatry*, 75(8), 631–638. doi:10.1016/j.biopsych.2013.02.002.

Gillan, C. M. & Sahakian, B. J. (2015). Which is the driver, the obsessions or the compulsions, in OCD? *Neuropsychopharmacology*, 40(1), 247–248. doi:10.1038/npp.2014.201.

Gillan, C. M. & Seow, T. X. F. (2020). Carving Out New Transdiagnostic Dimensions for Research in Mental Health. *Biological Psychiatry: Cognitive Neuroscience and Neuroimaging*, 5(10), 932–934. doi:10.1016/j. bpsc.2020.04.013.

Goodwin, G. M. (2022). The overlap between anxiety, depression, and obsessive-compulsive disorder. doi:10.31887/DCNS.2015.17.3/ggoodwin.

Gooskens, B., Bos, D. J., Mensen, V. T., Shook, D. A., Bruchhage, M. M., Naaijen, J., ... & Durston, S. (2019). No evidence of differences in cognitive control in children with autism spectrum disorder or obsessive-compulsive disorder: An fMRI study. *Developmental cognitive neuroscience, 36*, 100602.

Gooskens, B., Bos, D. J., Naaijen, J., Akkermans, S. E., Kaiser, A., Hohmann, S., ... & Durston, S. (2021). The development of cognitive control in children with autism spectrum disorder or obsessive-compulsive disorder: A longitudinal fMRI study. *Neuroimage: Reports, 1*(2), 100015.

Grant, J. E. & Chamberlain, S. R. (2019). Obsessive compulsive personality traits: Understanding the chain of pathogenesis from health to disease. *Journal of Psychiatric Research*, 116(May), 69–73. doi:10.1016/j.jpsychires.2019.06.003.

Grant, J. E. & Chamberlain, S. R. (2021). Trichotillomania and Skin-Picking Disorder: An Update. *Focus (American Psychiatric Publishing)*, 19(4), 405–412. https://doi.org/10.1176/appi.focus.20210013.

Grant, J. E. & Kim, S. W. (2014). Brain circuitry of compulsivity and impulsivity. *CNS Spectrums*, 19(1), 21–27. doi:10.1017/S109285291300028X.

Gustavson, D. E., Friedman, N. P., Fontanillas, P., Elson, S. L., Palmer, A. A., & Sanchez-Roige, S. (2020). The Latent Genetic Structure of Impulsivity and Its Relation to Internalizing Psychopathology. *Psychological Science*, 31(8), 1025–1035. https://doi.org/10.1177/0956797620938160.

Hollestein, V., Buitelaar, J. K., Brandeis, D., Banaschewski, T., Kaiser, A., Hohmann, S., ... & Naaijen, J. (2021). Developmental changes in fronto-striatal glutamate and their association with functioning during inhibitory control in autism spectrum disorder and obsessive compulsive disorder. *NeuroImage: Clinical, 30*, 102622.

Insel, T. R. (2014). The NIMH Research Domain Criteria (RDoC) Project: precision medicine for psychiatry. *The American Journal of Psychiatry*, 171(4), 395–397. doi:10.1176/appi.ajp.2014.14020138.

Insel, T. R., Cuthbert, B., Garvey, M., Heinssen, R., Pine, D., Quinn, K., Sanislow, C., & Wang, P. (2010). Research Domain Criteria (RDoC): Toward a New Classification Framework for Research on Mental Disorders. *American Journal of Psychiatry Online*, July, 748–751. doi:10.1176/appi.ajp.2010.09091379.

International Classification of Diseases, Eleventh Revision*(ICD-11)*. (n.d.). World Health Organization.

Karlsson, H. (2005). Psychiatry, neuroscience and free will. *Nordic Journal of Psychiatry*, 59(1), 5. doi:10.1080/08039480510018869.

Kelly, J. R., Gillan, C. M., Prenderville, J., Kelly, C., Harkin, A., Clarke, G., & O'Keane, V. (2021). Psychedelic Therapy's Transdiagnostic Effects: A Research Domain Criteria (RDoC) Perspective. *Frontiers in Psychiatry*, 12(December). https://doi.org/10.3389/fpsyt.2021.800072.

Kendell, R. &Jablensky, A. (2003). Distinguishing Between the Validity and Utility of Psychiatric Diagnoses. *Am J Psychiatry*, 160, 4–12. doi:10.1007/11946465_44.

Kendler, K. S. (2018). Classification of psychopathology: conceptual and historical background. *World Psychiatry*, 17(3), 241–242. doi:10.1002/wps.20549.

Koob, G. F. & Volkow, N. D. (2010). Neurocircuitry of addiction. *Neuropsychopharmacology*, 35(1), 217–238. doi:10.1038/npp.2009.110.

Kotov, R., Waszczuk, M. A., Krueger, R. F., Forbes, M. K., Watson, D., Clark, L. A., Achenbach, T. M., Althoff, R. R., Ivanova, M. Y., Michael Bagby, R., Brown, T. A., Carpenter, W. T., Caspi, A., Moffitt, T. E., Eaton, N. R., Forbush, K. T., Goldberg, D., Hasin, D., Hyman, S. E., ... Zimmerman, M. (2017). The hierarchical taxonomy of psychopathology (HiTOP): A dimensional alternative to traditional nosologies. *Journal of Abnormal Psychology*, 126(4), 454–477. doi:10.1037/abn0000258.

Kraemer, H. C. (2015). Research Domain Criteria (RDoC) and the DSM—Two Methodological Approaches to Mental Health Diagnosis. *JAMA Psychiatry*, 72 (12), 1163–1164. doi:10.1001/jamapsychiatry.2015.2134.

Kray, J., Kreis, B. K., & Lorenz, C. (2021). Age differences in decision making under known risk: The role of working memory and impulsivity. *Developmental Psychology*, 57(2), 241–252. doi:10.1037/dev0001132.

Krebs, G. & Heyman, I. (2015). Obsessive-compulsive disorder in children and adolescents. *Archives of Disease in Childhood*, 100(5), 495–499. doi:10.1136/archdischild-2014-306934.

Leffa, D. T., Caye, A., & Rohde, L. A. (2022). ADHD in Children and Adults: Diagnosis and Prognosis. *Current Topics in Behavioral Neurosciences*, 57, 1–18. doi:10.1007/7854_2022_329.

Lewin, A. B., Storch, E. A., Geffken, G. R., Goodman, W. K., & Murphy, T. K. (2006). A neuropsychiatric review of pediatric obsessive-compulsive disorder: Etiology and efficacious treatments. *Neuropsychiatric Disease and Treatment*, 2 (1), 21–31.

Liu, D., Cao, H., & Kural, K. C. (2019). Integrative analysis of shared genetic pathogenesis by autism spectrum disorder and obsessive-compulsive disorder. *BioSci Rep*, 39(12), 1–9.

Liu, J., Lester, B. M., Neyzi, N., Sheinkopf, S. J., Gracia, L., Kekatpure, M., & Kosofsky, B. E. (2013). Regional brain morphometry and impulsivity in adolescents following prenatal exposure to cocaine and tobacco. *JAMA Pediatrics*, 167(4), 348–354. doi:10.1001/jamapediatrics.2013.550.

Luigjes, J. & Denys, D. (2019). The Philosophy of Compulsive Disorders: Compulsivity and Free Will. In L. F. Fontenelle & M. Yücel (Eds), *A Transdiagnostic Approach to Obsessions, Compulsions and Related Phenomena* (pp. 14–18). Cambridge University Press. doi:10.1017/9781108164313.003.

Luigjes, J., Lorenzetti, V., de Haan, S., Youssef, G. J., Murawski, C., Sjoerds, Z., van den Brink, W., Denys, D., Fontenelle, L. F., & Yücel, M. (2019). Defining Compulsive Behavior. *Neuropsychology Review*, 29(1), 4–13. https://doi.org/10.1007/s11065-019-09404-9.

Martin, A., Bloch, M. H., & Volkmar, F. R. (Eds). (2017). *Lewis's Child and Adolescent Psychiatry: A Comprehensive Textbook* (5th Ed.). LWW.

Martinez-Loredo, V., Fernandez-Hermida, J. R., De La Torre-Luque, A., & Fernandez-Artamendi, S. (2018). Trajectories of impulsivity by sex predict substance use and heavy drinking. *Addictive Behaviors*, 85(May), 164–172. doi:10.1016/j.addbeh.2018.06.011.

Mataix-Cols, D., Do Rosario-Campos, M. C., & Leckman, J. F. (2005). A multi-dimensional model of obsessive-compulsive disorder. *American Journal of Psychiatry*, 162(2), 228–238. doi:10.1176/appi.ajp.162.2.228.

McGuire, J. F., Kugler, B. B., Park, J. M., Horng, B., Lewin, A. B., Murphy, T. K., & Storch, E. A. (2012). Evidence-based assessment of compulsive skin picking, chronic tic disorders and trichotillomania in children. *Child Psychiatry and Human Development*, 43(6), 855–883. doi:10.1007/s10578-012-0300-7.

Mechler, K., Häge, A., Schweinfurth, N., Glennon, J. C., Dijkhuizen, R. M., Murphy, D., Durston, S., Williams, S., Buitelaar, J. K., Banaschewski, T., Dittmann, R. W., De Ruiter, S., Akkermans, S., Mennes, M., Zwiers, M., Ilbegi, S., Hennissen, L., Naaijen, J., Van De Vondervoort, I., ... Auby, P. (2018). Glutamatergic agents in the treatment of compulsivity and impulsivity in child and adolescent psychiatry: A systematic review of the literature. *Zeitschrift Fur Kinder- Und Jugendpsychiatrie Und Psychotherapie*, 46(3), 246–263. doi:10.1024/1422-4917/a000546.

Merz, E. C., He, X., & Noble, K. G. (2018). Anxiety, depression, impulsivity, and brain structure in children and adolescents. *NeuroImage: Clinical*, 20(July), 243–251. doi:10.1016/j.nicl.2018.07.020.

Meynen, G. (2012). Obsessive-Compulsive Disorder, Free Will, and Control. *Philosophy, Psychiatry, & Psychology*, 19(4), 323–332. doi:10.1353/ppp.2012.0053.

Micali, N., Heyman, I., Perez, M., Hilton, K., Nakatani, E., Turner, C., & Mataix-Cols, D. (2010). Long-term outcomes of obsessive-compulsive disorder: Follow-up of 142 children and adolescents. *British Journal of Psychiatry*, 197(2), 128–134. doi:10.1192/bjp.bp.109.075317.

Milad, M. R., Furtak, S. C., Greenberg, J. L., Keshaviah, A., Im, J. J., Falkenstein, M. J., Jenike, M., Rauch, S. L., & Wilhelm, S. (2013). Deficits in conditioned fear extinction in obsessive-compulsive disorder and neurobiological changes in the fear circuit. *JAMA Psychiatry*, 70(6), 608–618. doi:10.1001/jamapsychiatry.2013.914.

Moeller, F. G., Barratt, E. S., Dougherty, D. M., Schmitz, J. M., & Swann, A. C. (2001). Psychiatric aspects of impulsivity. *American Journal of Psychiatry*, 158 (11), 1783–1793. doi:10.1176/appi.ajp.158.11.1783.

Moreira-de-Oliveira, M. E., de Menezes, G. B., Laurito, L. D., Loureiro, C. P., dos Santos-Ribeiro, S., & Fontenelle, L. F. (2022). A longitudinal evaluation of free will related cognitions in obsessive–compulsive disorder. *BMC Psychiatry*, 22(1), 463. doi:10.1186/s12888-022-04108-6.

Mullet, N., Hawkins, L. G., Tuliao, A. P., Snyder, H., Holyoak, D., McGuire, K. C., Earl, A. K., & McChargue, D. (2022). Early Trauma and Later Sexual Victimization in College Women: A Multiple Mediation Examination of Alexithymia, Impulsivity, and Alcohol Use. *Journal of Interpersonal Violence*, 37(19–20), NP18194–NP18214. doi:10.1177/08862605211035876.

Naaijen, J., de Ruiter, S., Zwiers, M. P., Glennon, J. C., Durston, S., Lythgoe, D. J., ... & Buitelaar, J. K. (2016). COMPULS: design of a multicenter phenotypic, cognitive, genetic, and magnetic resonance imaging study in children with compulsive syndromes. *BMC psychiatry*, 16, 1–10.

Naaijen, J., Lythgoe, D. J., Amiri, H., Buitelaar, J. K., & Glennon, J. C. (2015). Fronto-striatal glutamatergic compounds in compulsive and impulsive syndromes: a review of magnetic resonance spectroscopy studies. *Neuroscience & Biobehavioral Reviews*, 52, 74–88.

Nobre de Melo, A. L. (1945). Introdução à Psiquiatria. *Liv. Odeon, Rio.*

Obsessive Compulsive Cognitions Working Group. (2005). Psychometric validation of the obsessive belief questionnaire and interpretation of intrusions inventory—Part 2: Factor analyses and testing of a brief version. *Behaviour Research and Therapy*, 43(11), 1527–1542. doi:10.1016/j.brat.2004.07.010.

Oshri, A., Kogan, S. M., Kwon, J. A., Wickrama, K. A. S., Vanderbroek, L., Palmer, A. A., & MacKillop, J. (2018). Impulsivity as a mechanism linking child abuse and neglect with substance use in adolescence and adulthood. *Development and Psychopathology*, 30(2), 417–435. doi:10.1017/S0954579417000943.

Parkes, L., Satterthwaite, T. D., & Bassett, D. S. (2020). Towards precise resting-state fMRI biomarkers in psychiatry: synthesizing developments in transdiagnostic research, dimensional models of psychopathology, and normative neurodevelopment. *Current Opinion in Neurobiology*, 65, 120–128. doi:10.1016/j.conb.2020.10.016.

Petitet, P., Zhao, S., Drew, D., Manohar, S. G., & Husain, M. (2022). Dissociable behavioural signatures of co-existing impulsivity and apathy in decision-making. *Scientific Reports*, 12(1),21476. doi:10.1038/s41598-022-25882-z.

Phillips, K. A., Kim, J. M., & Hudson, J. I. (1995). Body image disturbance in body dysmorphic disorder and eating disorders: Obsessions or delusions? *Psychiatric Clinics of North America*, 18(2), 317–334. doi:10.1016/s0193-953x(18)30057-30051.

Potenza, M. R. M. & Potenza, M. N. (2014). Addictions and Personality Traits: Impulsivity and Related Constructs. *Curr Behav Neurosci Rep.*, 1(1), 1–12. doi:10.1007/s40473-013-0001-y.

Rachman, S. & Hodgson, R. J. (1980). *Obsessions and compulsions.* Prentice Hall.

Radomsky, A. S., Dugas, M. J., Alcolado, G. M., & Lavoie, S. L. (2014). When more is less: Doubt, repetition, memory, metamemory, and compulsive checking in OCD. *Behaviour Research and Therapy*, 59, 30–39. doi:10.1016/j.brat.2014.05.008.

Rasmussen, A. R. & Parnas, J. (2022). What is obsession? Differentiating obsessive-compulsive disorder and the schizophrenia spectrum: Obsession and differential diagnosis. *Schizophrenia Research*, 243(July 2021), 1–8. doi:10.1016/j.schres.2022.02.014.

Robbins, T. W., Gillan, C. M., Smith, D. G., de Wit, S., & Ersche, K. D. (2012). Neurocognitive endophenotypes of impulsivity and compulsivity: Towards dimensional psychiatry. *Trends in Cognitive Sciences*, 16(1), 81–91. doi:10.1016/j.tics.2011.11.009.

Robbins, T. W., Vaghi, M. M., & Banca, P. (2019). Obsessive-Compulsive Disorder: Puzzles and Prospects. *Neuron*, 102(1), 27–47. doi:10.1016/j.neuron.2019.01.046.

Rounsaville, B., Alarcón, R., Andrews, G., Jackson, J., Kendell, R., & Kendler, K. (2002). Basic Nomenclature Issues for DSM-V. In D. J. Kupfer, M. B. First, & D. A. Regier (Eds), *A Reserach Agenda for DSM-V.* American Psychiatric Association.

Serpell, L., Livingstone, A., Neiderman, M., & Lask, B. (2002). Anorexia nervosa: Obsessive–compulsive disorder, obsessive–compulsive personality disorder, or neither? *Clinical Psychology Review*, 22, 647–669. doi:10.1016/S0272-7358(01)00112-X.

Shaw, P., Gilliam, M., Liverpool, M., Weddle, C., Malek, M., Sharp, W., Greenstein, D., Evans, A., Rapoport, J., & Giedd, J. (2011). Cortical development in typically developing children with symptoms of hyperactivity and impulsivity:

Support for a dimensional view of attention deficit hyperactivity disorder. *American Journal of Psychiatry*, 168(2), 143–151. doi:10.1176/appi. ajp.2010.10030385.

Silva, B., Canas-Simião, H., & Cavanna, A. E. (2020). Neuropsychiatric Aspects of Impulse Control Disorders. *Psychiatric Clinics of North America*, 43(2), 249–262. doi:10.1016/j.psc.2020.02.001.

Starcevic, V. (2014). 4 Relationships with Other Psychopathology and Differential Diagnosis of Hypochondriasis. In *Hypochondriasis and health anxiety: A guide for clinicians*. Oxford University Press.

Stein, D. J. (2012). Philosophy and Obsessive–Compulsive Disorder. *Philosophy, Psychiatry, & Psychology*, 19(4), 339–342.

Stein, D. J., Costa, D. L. C., Lochner, C., Miguel, E. C., Reddy, Y. C. J., Shavitt, R. G., van den Heuvel, O. A., & Simpson, H. B. (2019). Obsessive–compulsive disorder. *Nature Reviews Disease Primers*, 5(1), 52. doi:10.1038/s41572-019-0102-3.

Storch, E. A., Milsom, V. A., Merlo, L. J., Larson, M., Geffken, G. R., Jacob, M. L., Murphy, T. K., & Goodman, W. K. (2008). Insight in pediatric obsessive-compulsive disorder: Associations with clinical presentation. *Psychiatry Research*, 160(2), 212–220. doi:10.1016/j.psychres.2007.07.005.

Storch, E. A., De Nadai, A. S., Jacob, M. L., Lewin, A. B., Muroff, J., Eisen, J., Abramowitz, J. S., Geller, D. A., & Murphy, T. K. (2014). Phenomenology and correlates of insight in pediatric obsessive–compulsive disorder. *Comprehensive Psychiatry*, 55(3), 613–620. doi:10.1016/j.comppsych.2013.09.014.

Taylor, S. (2011). Early versus late onset obsessive-compulsive disorder: Evidence for distinct subtypes. *Clinical Psychology Review*, 31(7), 1083–1100. doi:10.1016/j.cpr.2011.06.007.

Tiego, J., Trender, W., Hellyer, P. J., Grant, J. E., Hampshire, A., & Chamberlain, S. R. (2023). Measuring Compulsivity as a Self-Reported Multidimensional Transdiagnostic Construct: Large-Scale (N = 182,000) Validation of the Cambridge–Chicago Compulsivity Trait Scale. *Assessment*. doi:10.1177/10731911221149083.

Van Ameringen, M., Patterson, B., & Simpson, W. (2014). DSM-5 obsessive-compulsive and related disorders: Clinical implications of new criteria. *Depression and Anxiety*, 31(6), 487–493. doi:10.1002/da.22259.

van der Salm, S. M., Cath, D. C., Rootselaar, A.-F. van, Koelman, J. H., de Haan, R. J., Tijssen, M. A., & Meynen, G. (2017). Clinician and patient perceptions of free will in movement disorders: mind the gap. *Journal of Neurology, Neurosurgery & Psychiatry*. doi:10.1136/jnnp-2016-315152.

van Loo, H. M., Romeijn, J. W., & Kendler, K. S. (2019). Changing the definition of the kilogram: Insights for psychiatric disease classification. *Philosophy, Psychiatry and Psychology*, 26(4), E97–E108. doi:10.1353/ppp.2019.0046.

van Oudheusden, L. J. B., Draisma, S., van Der Salm, S., Cath, D., van Oppen, P., van Balkom, A. J. L. M., & Meynen, G. (2018). Perceptions of free will in obsessive-compulsive disorder: A quantitative analysis. *BMC Psychiatry*, 18(1), 1–9. doi:10.1186/s12888-018-1985-3.

Vasconcelos, A. G., Malloy-Diniz, L., & Correa, H. (2012). Systematic review of psychometric proprieties of barratimpulsiveness scale version 11 (BIS-11). *Clinical Neuropsychiatry*, 9(2), 61–74.

Verdejo-Garcia, A. & Albein-Urios, N. (2021). Impulsivity traits and neurocognitive mechanisms conferring vulnerability to substance use disorders.

Neuropharmacology, 183(October 2020), 108402. doi:10.1016/j. neuropharm.2020.108402.

Verdejo-Garcia, A., Garcia-Fernandez, G., & Dom, G. (2019). Cognition and addiction. *Dialogues in Clinical Neuroscience*, 21(3), 281–290. doi:10.31887/ DCNS.2019.21.3/gdom.

Vigne, P., de Menezes, G. B., Harrison, B. J., & Fontenelle, L. F. (2014). A study of poor insight in social anxiety disorder. *Psychiatry Research*, 219(3), 556–561. doi:10.1016/j.psychres.2014.05.033.

Vonasch, A. J., Clark, C. J., Lau, S., Vohs, K. D., & Baumeister, R. F. (2017). Ordinary people associate addiction with loss of free will. *Addictive Behaviors Reports*, 5, 56–66. doi:10.1016/j.abrep.2017.01.002.

Whiteside, S. P. & Lynam, D. R. (2001). The five factor model and impulsivity: Using a structural model of personality to understand impulsivity. *Personality and Individual Differences*, 30(4), 669–689. doi:10.1016/S0191-8869(00)00064-00067.

Whiteside, S. P., Lynam, D. R., Miller, J. D., & Reynolds, S. K. (2005). Validation of the UPPS impulsive behaviour scale: A four-factor model of impulsivity. *European Journal of Personality*, 19(7), 559–574. doi:10.1002/per.556.

Yang, Z., Wu, H., Lee, P. H., Tsetsos, F., Davis, L. K., Yu, D., Lee, S. H., Dalsgaard, S., Haavik, J., Barta, C., Zayats, T., Eapen, V., Wray, N. R., Devlin, B., Daly, M., Neale, B., Børglum, A. D., Crowley, J. J., Scharf, J., ... Paschou, P. (2021a). Investigating Shared Genetic Basis Across Tourette Syndrome and Comorbid Neurodevelopmental Disorders Along the Impulsivity-Compulsivity Spectrum. *Biological Psychiatry*, 90(5), 317–327. doi:10.1016/j.biopsych.2020.12.028.

Ziegler, G., Hauser, T. U., Moutoussis, M., Bullmore, E. T., Goodyer, I. M., Fonagy, P., Jones, P. B., Lindenberger, U., & Dolan, R. J. (2019). Compulsivity and impulsivity traits linked to attenuated developmental frontostriatal myelination trajectories. *Nature Neuroscience*, 22(6), 992–999. doi:10.1038/s41593-019-0394-3.

Zimmerman, M., Ellison, W., Young, D., Chelminski, I., & Dalrymple, K. (2015). How many different ways do patients meet the diagnostic criteria for major depressive disorder? *Comprehensive Psychiatry*, 56, 29–34. doi:10.1016/j. comppsych.2014.09.007.

Zohar, A. H. & Bruno, R. (1997). Normative and Pathological Obsessive-compulsive Behavior and Ideation in Childhood: A Question of Timing. *Journal of Child Psychology and Psychiatry*, 38(8), 993–999. doi:10.1111/j.1469-7610.1997. tb01616.x.

3 Disgust, Disgust Sensitivity, and Contamination-Related Obsessive-Compulsive Disorder

Dean McKay

Contamination obsessions are commonly reported among children and adolescents with obsessive-compulsive disorder (OCD) (Selles, Storch, & Lewin, 2014). The base rate of contamination symptoms in youth with OCD closely resembles that in adult samples, which is roughly half of all individuals with the disorder (Demet, et al., 2005; Sasson, et al., 1997). Most major models depicting the emotional components that drive avoidance in OCD emphasize anxiety (Taylor, Abramowitz, & McKay, 2007), research over the past two decades have suggested a significant role for disgust in contamination obsessions and washing compulsions (McKay & Moretz, 2009). In light of the growing evidence that disgust plays a prominent role in contamination obsessions, recent research has further shown facets of disgust are implicated in contamination obsessions in youth (Knowles, Jessup, & Olatunji, 2018; Olatunji, et al., 2017).

Considering the prevalence of contamination obsessions among individuals with OCD, and the growing evidence that disgust contributes significantly to the manifestation of this specific symptom, this chapter has the following aims: first, to describe the ways in which disgust is meaningfully related to contamination obsession; second, to present a framework that accounts for the manifestation of contamination obsessions; and third, describe treatment directions for disgust in youth contamination obsessions. Given that the research on disgust in youth contamination obsessions is still in the nascent stages of development, much of the empirical evidence relied on in this chapter comes from adult samples.

Overview of disgust

Disgust has gained increased recognition in the past three decades as a critical emotion in a wide range of psychopathology, particularly conditions marked by avoidance (Olatunji & McKay, 2009). At its core, disgust serves the function of preventing the oral ingestion of potential toxins, but in typical human development, this emotional reaction generalizes to several classes of stimuli. These classes of stimuli, called disgust elicitors, are: food, which encompasses rotting food as well as food that is

DOI: 10.4324/9781003517429-3

culturally unfamiliar; insects and animals, particularly ones associated with decomposition or decaying food; body products, such as feces, urine, mucous, and blood; death; sex, particularly culturally non-normative acts; and body envelope violations, which relates to any imagery of piercing of skin or other physical covering that conceals organs or other internal functioning body parts. Further, disgust is a 'communicable emotion,' in that the elicitors follow the 'laws of sympathetic magic.' Specifically, objects associated with disgust can transmit disgust through either the "Law of Contagion," where incidental contact with an otherwise neutral object is rendered disgusting; or the "Law of Similarity," where an object that is 'clean' evokes disgust by resembling a disgust elicitor (summarized in McKay, 2017; Rozin & Fallon, 1987).

In addition to disgust elicitors, it has been shown that there are individual differences in disgust reactions. One of these factors is disgust propensity, which connotes the degree one is disgusted by any stimuli from the aforementioned elicitors. The other, disgust sensitivity, reflects the extent that one attributes specific physical sensations to disgust (van Overveld, et al., 2006).

Disgust propensity and sensitivity as contamination indicators

The aversion to putative pathogens was originally ascribed to general neuroticism (summarized in Oosterhoff, Shook, & Iyer, 2018). This association led to research to elucidate the distinction between general negative affectivity and disgust in the prediction of behavioral avoidance in general, and contamination concerns in particular. On the former, it has been shown that disgust can be uniquely attributed to avoidance, particularly in anxiety disorders (Olatunji, Armstrong, & Elwood, 2017). As to contamination obsessions, disgust propensity appears to play a significant maintenance role (Melli, et al., 2019), while disgust sensitivity plays a prominent role in promoting contamination obsessions (Deacon & Olatunji, 2007; Olatunji, 2010).

In youth OCD, research has begun to accumulate to show that disgust in general is the best predictor of contamination fear, and that it is specific when compared to other anxiety disorders (Cervin et al., 2021). Further, recent findings show that disgust propensity is predictive of contamination obsessions, while disgust sensitivity is associated with moral-based obsessions (i.e., intrusive thoughts of harm or blasphemy) (Georgiadis, et al., 2020). These findings are among the earliest in the child OCD literature that carefully examine the relationship between disgust propensity and sensitivity in relation to contamination obsessions, and while in contrast to the aforementioned associated in adult samples, further research will likely clarify these associations.

Pathogen disgust

Experts in OCD recognize that contamination obsessions can take a wide range of forms, from concerns with personal infections, to risk of infecting others, to contamination by 'concepts' such as moral degradation or loss of identity (Rachman, 2004). Recent findings suggest that individuals make appraisals of potential social contacts based on a range of perceived 'pathogens,' including the social costs from affiliation as well as more fundamental concerns with physical infection (Kupfer & Tybur, 2017). Modern conceptualizations of disgust encompass interpersonal reactions, including moral dimensions. As a result, disgust in evoking contamination obsessions is highly complex, extending beyond everyday contaminants.

As a result of this broader definition of contamination, assessment of situations that might evoke behavioral avoidance, as a result of pathogens, should encompass the broadest range of potential stimuli and situations. One compelling model that addresses the broad range of potential contaminants and how avoidance may develop is the behavioral immune system (BIS) (Schaller & Park, 2011). The BIS describes a process whereby protective mechanisms develop when there is an anticipated unseen pathogen present. This process has implications for how individuals may avoid others, out of perceived concerns different groups may pose pathogen risk. While the BIS is useful in explaining facets of xenophobia, it also has proximal consequences around anticipated risks of infection. For example, during the COVID-19 pandemic, disgust sensitivity and anxiety sensitivity were found to activate the BIS and explain extent of avoidance of public places, checking behaviors related to infection risk, and level of anticipated danger of contracting the illness (Paluszek, et al., 2021).

Contamination obsessions: not just disgust

The behavioral manifestation of contamination fear involves a range of complex avoidance strategies and compensatory acts that collectively minimize the perceived risk of contact with perceived harmful stimuli. While the BIS is a useful conceptual framework to understand how contamination obsessions emerge, along with specific client characteristics that may predict severity, it lacks one core element. Relying on disgust alone implies that the pathogen may enter through the mouth. This is largely because the majority of disgust conceptualizations emphasize oral incorporation (see McKay, 2017). Even in the moral dimension, disgust is viewed as primarily preventing entry through the mouth, even if primarily metaphorical (Rozin, Haidt, & Fincher, 2009).

Youth with contamination obsessions typically avoid perceived contaminated objects by avoiding touch, or really any skin contact. This is in reference to an understood method of pathogen transmission, namely transdermally. This connotes that disgust may be expressed at the prospect of entry through the skin, and not just orally. There are two closely related recent constructs that describe the unique blend of disgust and fear. One, the chills, captures this phenomena and has been shown to be associated with neuroticism (Maruskin, Thrash, & Elliot, 2012). While this construct has not yet been carefully examined in contamination obsession adults or youth, it has recently demonstrated a predictor of clinician hesitation in providing exposure therapy during the COVID pandemic (McKay, Minaya, & Storch, 2020).

Another conceptualization that describes the conjoint role of disgust and fear, the heebie-jeebies (Blake et al., 2017), sounds like it is an emotional blend ready made for children. However, the available research is still with adults. Whereas the chills has been assessed as a phenomena that overcomes and individual from time to time, and that might be associated with a perceived risk of skin penetration, the heebie jeebies is more proximal and experienced at the sight of implied presence of a known pathogen. Recent findings suggest that the heebie jeebies can be provoked in the lab using stimuli such as bloodworms, and that these reactions are distinct from disgust (handwashing with soap the color and shape of feces) and fear (placing one's hand in a dark box without knowing the contents), and further, that avoidance for heebie jeebies stimuli was significantly associated with contamination obsessions (Mancusi & McKay, 2021).

Disgust in youth contamination obsessions

The aforementioned research collectively points to a strong need for additional investigation into how disgust functions in contamination obsessions in youth. Disgust begins with bitter taste in infants and develops through social learning to encompass increasingly complex objects and interpersonal situations. The emotion develops over the early years and is fully realized in experience and facial recognition by approximately eight years of age (Widen & Russell, 2013). Interestingly, longitudinal findings suggest that intensity of infant disgust reactions to bitter taste predict disgust propensity in adolescence (Christensen & Lewis, 2021). In light of research demonstrating that disgust propensity may be a predictor of contamination obsessions, bitter taste reactions could serve as a putative risk factor. Interestingly, children with earlier onset of OCD have a higher rate of contamination obsessions (or cleaning compulsions) compared with individuals whose symptom onset was in adolescence or adulthood (Butwicka & Gmitrowicz, 2009). However, there are inconsistencies in this body of research, as other findings suggest a preponderance of contamination obsessions in later onset OCD (Grover, et al., 2018), and other findings suggest that early onset is associated with greater severity across all symptom dimensions (Anholt et al., 2014). Assuming disgust, and emotional processes associated with disgust, play a role in the development and maintenance of contamination obsessions, additional research is warranted that clarifies the developmental trajectories for each and their influences on one another.

In addition to the developmental trajectory connecting bitter taste recognition in infants to disgust propensity in adolescence, moral disgust develops through a range of social learning forces in connection with basic disgust reactions (Kurth, 2021). Experimental research has demonstrated that physical transgressions lead to specific moral judgements and disgust reactions (reviewed in Chapman & Anderson, 2013). The available research suggests that provoked disgust (such as through olfactory offenses) produce small but detectable effects on moral disgust (Landy et al., 2015). When connected to moral development, the role of disgust as a socially influenced emotional reaction can extend from contamination concerns (and obsessions) up to broad existential concerns that govern avoidance. In this way, disgust can be employed as an overarching consideration for the full range of contamination obsessions, whether regarding personal infection or the transmission of disease, through to the loss of social integrity by affiliation with socially defined morally debased others.

There is one more dimension to consider when evaluating the role of disgust in contamination obsessions, namely scrupulosity. In everyday discourse, scrupulosity is often associated with high degrees of religious or spiritual standards. As a psychological process, it has been characterized as pathological, encompassing distressing levels of guilt at perceived transgressions from one's own religious or spiritual values, and potentially compulsions aimed at correcting these perceived errors (Hedges & Hedges, 2008). As a morally dictated cognitive-emotional phenomena, scrupulosity may involve cleanliness compulsions, as is commonly prescribed in numerous religious traditions. Indeed, recently this connection has been made explicit. In an analysis comparing high and low scrupulous participants of the Muslim faith, those with high scrupulosity rated perceived contaminated stimuli more disgusting and had a higher urge to neutralize this experience (such as through washing) than the low scrupulosity participants (Inozu et al., 2017).

Treatment implications

Disgust has been shown resistant to interventions. This has been largely attributed to the persistence of associations through evaluative conditioning, a process where conditioned emotional reactions can be strengthened through specific labeling processes (Hofmann, et al., 2010). Considering the discussion in this chapter that connects disgust to socially prescribed stimuli, situations, and behaviors, the role of evaluative conditioning has been a pronounced facet of conceptualization. This specific form of conditioning has been described as particularly resistant to habituation or extinction efforts such as those involved in exposure therapy (i.e., Olatunji, Forsyth, & Cherian, 2007). As a result, efforts to reduce disgust reactions has been considered challenging.

Over ten years ago, there was a detailed summary of the available evidence for treatments to alleviate disgust (Mason & Richardson, 2012). That review suggested that exposure methods, which are widely understood as evidence-based for alleviating anxiety for all ages (see meta-analysis of exposure for childhood anxiety; Whiteside et al., 2020), it is not necessarily the case for reducing disgust. At the time of that review, exposure models of treatment emphasized habituation (Foa & Kozak, 1986). Further, in a recent meta-analysis, exposure interventions result in small positive effects for disgust (Pascal, Podina, & Nedelcea, 2020). Shortly after the Mason and Richardson review of disgust interventions, the inhibitory learning model (ILM) to exposure emerged as a dominant alternative model (Craske et al., 2014). This model stresses the development of new learning that competes with the former avoidance responses as a central mechanism of change, and thus numerous methods of exposure have been described. Among the methods of exposure that form the basis of the ILM include: changes in expectancies through connecting the avoided situation with a different emotional reaction; removal of safety signals, which are discrete stimuli that indicate the circumstances surrounding the avoided stimuli lack the perceived dangerousness; 'deepened extinction,' a process of systematically combining situational cues associated with the avoided stimuli to procure more adaptive reactions; exposure in multiple contexts, employed to ensure greater generalization of treatment; and variability, which involves randomly presenting exposure stimuli from different points on the hierarchy, and to mimic the everyday experience of encounters with the avoided stimuli. The full range of ILM approaches have been more recently described as parts of a treatment sequence (Craske et al., 2022). As of this writing, there have been no systematic applications of the ILM in the reduction of disgust reactions for any psychological condition. However, it does serve as a promising option to consider when addressing disgust in contamination obsessions in youth.

Aside from exposure, the other major approach to alleviating disgust that has accumulated support is counterconditioning. The approach underlying counterconditioning involves connecting aversive stimuli is paired with an incompatible emotional response or behavior. Until recently, the application of counterconditioning was considered either inefficient or ineffective in producing change (Kerkhof, et al., 2010). As evidence has accumulated to show that exposure alone produced modest changes in disgust reactions, however, counterconditioning has enjoyed renewed attention. This emergent line of work remains limited by (a) reliance on self-report rather than behavioral indices; (b) non-clinical or subclinical samples; and (c) heterogeneous incompatible paired stimuli, it appears at this point counterconditioning can reduce disgust reactions specifically in contamination obsessions (Ludvik, Boschen, & Neumann, 2015). To date, no systematic or case based illustrations of counterconditioning in youth contamination obsessions have appeared in the research literature.

Summary

The role of touch is central in the contraction of disgust and serves as a mechanism for provoking contamination obsessions. The nature of disgust, a response that begins at birth with reactions to bitter taste, grows in complexity over the lifespan to encompass not only concerns over contraction of illness but also morally prohibited behaviors and individual qualities. The full range of disgust reactions have important implications for the treatment of contamination obsessions. The scope of how to conceptualize and treat disgust in youth with contamination obsessions has not been systematically investigated. It is hoped that this chapter will serve as a means for stimulating research on this underexamined emotional state (McKay, 2017), and provide a refined means for providing treatment.

References

Anholt, G. E., Aderka, I. M., van Balkom, A. J. L. M., Smit, J. H., Schruers, K., van der Wee, N. J. A., Eikelenboom, M., De Luca, V., & van Oppen, P. (2014). Age of onset in obsessive-compulsive disorder: Admixture analysis a youth sample. *Psychological Medicine*, 44, 185–194.

Blake, K. R., Yih, J., Zhao, K., Sung, B., & Harmon-Jones, C. (2017). Skin-transmitted pathogens and the heebie jeebies: Evidence for a subclass of disgust stimuli that evoke a qualitatively unique emotional response. *Cognition & Emotion*, 31, 1153–1168.

Butwicka, A. & Gmitrowicz, A. (2009). Symptom clusters in obsessive-compulsive disorder (OCD): Influence of age and age of onset. *European Child & Adolescent Psychiatry*, 19, 365–370.

Cervin, M., Perrin, S., Olsson, E., Claesdotter-Knutsson, E., & Lindvall, M. (2021). Involvement of fear, incompleteness, and disgust during symptoms of pediatric-obsessive-compulsive disorder. *European Child & Adolescent Psychiatry*, 30, 271–281.

Chapman, H. A. & Anderson, A. K. (2013). Things rank and gross in nature: A review and synthesis of moral disgust. *Psychological Bulletin*, 139, 300–327.

Christenen, R. E. & Lewis, M. (2021). The development of disgust and its relationship to adolescent psychosocial functioning. *Child Psychiatry and Human Development*, 53, 1309–1318.

Craske, M. G., Treanor, M., Conway, C. C., Zbozinek, T., & Vervliet, B. (2014). Maximizing exposure therapy: An inhibitory learning approach. *Behaviour Research and Therapy*, 58, 10–23.

Deacon, B. & Olatunji, B. O. (2007). Specificity of disgust sensitivity in the prediction of behavioral avoidance in contamination fear. *Behaviour Research and Therapy*, 45, 2110–2120.

Craske, M.G., Treanor, M., Zbozinek, T.D., & Vervliet, B. (2022). Optimizing exposure therapy with an inhibitory retrieval approach and the OptEx Nexus. *Behaviour Research and Therapy*, 152, 104069.

Demet, M. M., Deveci, A., Taskin, E. O., Ermertcan, A. T., Yurtsever, F., Deniz, F., Bayraktar, D., & Ozturkcan, S. (2005). Obsessive-compulsive disorder in a dermatology outpatient clinic. *General Hospital Psychiatry*, 27, 426–430.

Foa, E. B. & Kozak, M. J. (1986). Emotional processing of fear: Exposure to corrective information. *Psychological Bulletin*, 99, 20–35.

Georgiadis, C., Schreck, M., Gervasio, M., Kemp, J., Freeman, J., Garcia, A., & Case, B. (2020). Disgust propensity and sensitivity in childhood anxiety and obsessive-compulsive disorder: Two construct differentially related to obsessional content. *Journal of Anxiety Disorders*, 76, 102294.

Grover, S., Sarkar, S., Gupta, G., Kate, N., Ghosh, A., Chakrabarti, S., & Avasthi, A. (2018). Factor analysis of symptom profile in early onset and late onset OCD. *Psychiatry Research*, 262, 631–635.

Hedges, C. H. & Hedges, D. W. (2008). Scrupulosity disorder: An overview and introductory analysis. *Journal of Anxiety Disorders*, 22, 1042–1058.

Hofmann, W., de Houwer, J., Perugini, M., Baeyens, F., & Crombez, G. (2010). Evaluative conditioning in humans: A meta-analysis. *Psychological Bulletin*, 136, 390–421.

Inozu, M., Eremsoy, E., Cicek, N. M., & Ozcanli, F. (2017). The association of scrupulosity with disgust propensity and contamination based obsessive-compulsive symptoms: An experimental investigation using highly scrupulous Muslims. *Journal of Obsessive-Compulsive and Related Disorders*, 15, 43–51.

Kerkhof, I., Vansteenwegen, D., Baeyens, F., & Hermans, D. (2010). An effective technique for changing conditioned preferences. *Experimental Psychology*, 58, 31–38.

Knowles, K. A., Jessup, S. C., & Olatunji, B. O. (2018). Disgust in anxiety and obsessive-compulsive disorders: Recent findings and future directions. *Current Psychiatry Reports*, 20, 68.

Kupfer, T. R. & Tybur, J. M. (2017). Pathogen disgust and interpersonal personality. *Personality and Individual Differences*, 116, 379–384.

Kurth, C. (2021). Cultivating disgust: Prospects and moral implications. *Emotion Review*, 13, 101–112.

Landy, J. F. & Goodwin, G. P. (2015). Does incidental disgust amplify moral judgment? A meta-analytic review of experimental evidence. *Perspectives on Psychological Science*, 10, 518–536.

Ludvik, D., Boschen, M. J., & Neumann, D. L. (2015). Effective behavioural strategies for reducing disgust in contamination-related OCD: A review. *Clinical Psychology Review*, 42, 116–129.

Mancusi, L. & McKay, D. (2021). Behavioral avoidance tasks for eliciting disgust and anxiety in contamination fear: An examination of a test for a combined disgust fear reaction. *Journal of Anxiety Disorders*, 78, 102366.

Maruskin, L. A., Thrash, T. M., & Elliot, A. J. (2012). The chills as a psychological construct: Content universe, factor structure, affective composition, elicitors, trait antecedents, and consequences. *Journal of Personality and Social Psychology*, 103, 135–157.

Mason, E. C. & Richardson, R. (2012). Treating disgust in anxiety disorders. *Clinical Psychology: Science & Practice*, 19, 180–194.

McKay, D. (2017). Presidential address: Embracing the repulsive: The case for disgust as a functionally central emotional state in the theory, practice, and dissemination of cognitive-behavior therapy. *Behavior Therapy*, 48, 731–738.

McKay, D., Minaya, C. & Storch, E. A. (2020). Conducting exposure and response prevention treatment for contamination fears during COVID-19: The behavioral immune system impact on clinician approaches to treatment. *Journal of Anxiety Disorders*, 74, 102270.

McKay, D. & Moretz, M. W. (2009). The intersection of disgust and contamination fear. In B. O. Olatunji & D. McKay (Eds), *Disgust and Its Disorders (pp. 211–227)*. Washington, DC: American Psychological Association Press.

Melli, G., Poli, A., Chiorri, C., & Olatunji, B. O. (2019). Is heightened disgust propensity truly a risk factor for contamination-related obsessive-compulsive disorder? *Behavior Therapy*, 50, 621–629.

Olatunji, B. O. (2010). Changes in disgust correspond with changes in symptoms of contamination-based OCD: A prospective examination of specificity. *Journal of Anxiety Disorders*, 24, 313–317.

Olatunji, B. O., Armstrong, T., & Elwood, L. (2017). Is disgust proneness associated with anxiety and related disorders? A qualitative review and meta-analysis of group comparisons and correlational studies. *Perspectives on Psychological Science*, 12, 613–648.

Olatunji, B. O., Ebesutani, C., Kim, J., Riemann, B. C., & Jacobi, D. M. (2017). Disgust proneness predicts obsessive-compulsive disorder symptom severity in a clinical sample of youth: Distinctions from negative affect. *Journal of Affective Disorders*, 213, 118–125.

Olatunji, B. O., Forsyth, J. P., & Cherian, A. (2007). Evaluative differential conditioning of disgust: A sticky form of relational learning that is resistant to extinction. *Journal of Anxiety Disorders*, 21, 820–834.

Olatunji, B. O. & McKay, D. (2009). *Disgust and its disorders*. Washington, DC: American Psychological Association Press.

Oosterhoff, B., Shook, N. J., Iyer, R. (2018). Disease avoidance and personality: A meta-analysis. *Journal of Research in Personality*, 77, 47–56.

van Overveld, W. J. M., de Jong, P. J., Peters, M. L., Cavanagh, K., & Davey, G. C. L. (2006). Disgust propentisve and disgust sensitivity: Separate constructs that are differentially related to specific fears. *Personality and Individual Differences*, 41, 1241–1252.

Paluszek, M. M., Asmundson, A. J. N., Landry, C. A., McKay, D., Taylor, S., & Asmundson, G. J. G. (2021). Effects of anxiety sensitivity, disgust, and intolerance of uncertainty on the COVID stress syndrome: A longitudinal assessment of transdiagnostic constructs and behavioral immune system. *Cognitive Behaviour Therapy*, 50, 191–203.

Pascal, S. A., Podina, I. R., & Nedelcea, C. (2020). A meta-analysis on the efficacy of exposure-based treatment in anxiety disorders: Implications for disgust. *Journal of Evidence-based Psychotherapies*, 20, 31–49.

Rachman, S. (2004). Fear of contamination. *Behaviour Research and Therapy*, 42, 1227–1255.

Rozin, P. & Fallon, A. E. (1987). A perspective on disgust. *Psychological Review*, 94, 23–41.

Rozin, P., Haidt, J., & Fincher, K. (2009). From oral to moral. *Science*, 323, 1179–1180.

Sasson, Y., Zohar, J., Chopra, M., Lustig, M., Iancu, I., & Hendler, T. (1997). Epidemiology of obsessive-compulsive disorder: A world view. *Journal of Clinical Psychiatry, 58 (Suppl 12)*, 7–10.

Schaller, M. & Park, J. H. (2011). The behavioral immune system (and why it matters). *Current Directions in Psychological Science*, 20, 99–103.

Selles, R. R., Storch, E. A., & Lewin, A. B. (2014). Variations in symptom prevalence and clinical correlates in younger versus older youth with obsessive-compulsive disorder. *Child Psychiatry and Human Development*, 45, 666–674.

Taylor, S., Abramowitz, J. S., & McKay, D. (2007). Cognitive-behavioral models of OCD. In M. M. Antony, C. Purdon, & L. Summerfeldt (Eds), *Psychological treatment of OCD: Fundamentals and beyond (pp. 9–29)*. Washington, DC: American Psychological Association Press.

Whiteside, S. P. H., Sim, L. A., Morrow, A. S., Farah, W. H., Hilliker, D. R., Murad, M. H., & Wang, Z. (2020). A meta-analysis to guide the enhancement of CBT for childhood anxiety: Exposure over anxiety management. *Clinical Child and Family Review*, 23, 102–121.

Widen, S. C. & Russell, J. A. (2013). Children's recognition of disgust in others. *Psychological Bulletin*, 139. 271–299.

4 Incompleteness and Not Just Right Experiences in Children and Adolescents with Obsessive-Compulsive Disorder

Matti Cervin and Davide Fausto Borrelli

Emotion as a driver of compulsions

What drives the compulsive behaviors characteristic of OCD? The emotion researcher Peter J. Lang famously stated that emotions are action dispositions (Lang, 1995). Thus, in Lang's view, the core function of emotions is to initiate and guide behavior and to direct attention to the most salient aspects of the internal and external environment. This is in line with recent models of human behavior where emotions are considered superordinate mechanisms that coordinates a range of other mechanisms such as attention, perception, physiology, energy allocation, and behavior (Al-Shawaf et al., 2016). Emotion is also intricately interwoven within the diagnostic criteria of OCD, as both the 5th version of the Diagnostic and Statistical Manual of Mental Disorders (DSM-5) (American Psychiatric Association, 2013, 2022) and the 11th revision of the International Classification of Diseases (ICD-11) (World Health Organization, 2019) stress that obsessions are characterized by distress or anxiety and that compulsions often serve the function of reducing distress.

But which emotions drive compulsive behavior in OCD? Contemporary cognitive-behavioral models emphasize the central role of fear and anxiety (Abramowitz et al., 2009; Rachman, 1997). That is, intrusive thoughts (e. g., what if I push this person in front of the train) generate anxiety which triggers compulsions or avoidance, when performed lead to short-term anxiety relief. Anxiety is also central to exposure-based cognitive behavioral therapy (CBT) of OCD, where core fears should be identified and then actuated using exposures, leading to behavioral pressure to perform compulsions or engage in avoidance (Foa & McLean, 2016). When compulsions and avoidance are repeatedly resisted, improvement is typically observed (Reid et al., 2021; Öst et al., 2022; Öst et al., 2016), allegedly through fear extinction learning (Foa et al., 2006).

Fear and anxiety are interconnected yet distinct concepts. While fear is a response to immediate threat, anxiety arises in anticipation of potential threat, often in the form of future possibilities, and may persist even in

DOI: 10.4324/9781003517429-4

the absence of acute threat (American Psychiatric Association, 2013). It is easy to understand why OCD can be considered an anxiety disorder, as obsessions often revolve around potential harm (e.g., what if I hurt someone), responsibility (e.g., what if forgot to turn off the stove), or moral or personal failure (e.g., what if I am sexually attracted to young children) (Cervin et al., 2021). But do all OCD patients experience fear or anxiety? In the seminal DSM-IV Field Trial study by Foa and Kozak (1995), 41 percent of adults with OCD reported that their primary obsessions did not involve fear of a harmful consequence. Accordingly, in a sample of 124 children and adolescents interviewed about their emotions during OCD symptoms, 16 percent reported that they experienced no or just a little fear or anxiety and an additional 22 percent reported only moderate fear or anxiety (Cervin et al., 2020b). Similarly, in a sample of 170 children and adolescents with OCD, Schreck et al. (2021) found that 18 percent experienced no fear or anxiety as part of their symptoms. Thus, anxiety seems to be common but not necessary in OCD, which was one of the reasons that OCD was removed from the anxiety disorders chapter in DSM-5 and placed at the center of a new chapter termed Obsessive-Compulsive and Related Disorders (Stein et al., 2010).

Incompleteness and not just right experiences in OCD

If emotion drives compulsions and anxiety is common but not necessary in OCD, what other emotional mechanisms are involved? A feature distinguishing OCD from the anxiety disorders is compulsions, which are repetitive behaviors or mental acts (American Psychiatric Association, 2013, 2022). An emotion-related construct that may help explain the repetitive nature of compulsions is OCD is the feeling of incompleteness, which refers to a sensation of dissatisfaction and things being "not just right" as well as emotional urges to adjust the internal or external environment to reach a sense of completeness (Pallanti et al., 2017).

The link between feelings of incompleteness and OCD is not new. As early as the 1900s, the French neurologist Pierre Janet documented cases of patients exhibiting OCD-like symptoms and noted that compulsive behaviors were often motivated by a sense of imperfection or incompleteness and often repeated until the patient felt the behaviors had been completed in a satisfactory way (Pitman, 1984). Even though feelings of incompleteness and not just right experiences may distinguish OCD from other mental disorders – including anxiety disorders – the emotional construct of incompleteness has received relatively little attention in contemporary OCD research.

Incompleteness has been defined as an "internal state of imperfection" (Cougle & Lee, 2014) and a "sense or feeling that one's actions, intentions, or experiences have not been properly achieved" (Taylor et al., 2014b). A closely related construct is that of not just right experiences, which have been defined as a "subjective sense that something isn't just as it should be" (Coles et al., 2003) and a "mismatch between perceptions of a desired state and a current state" (Fergus, 2014). Another related construct is sensory phenomena, which refers to a broad range of mental or sensory experiences preceding or accompanying repetitive behaviors, including just-right perceptions, feelings of incompleteness, and not just-right phenomena (Ferrao et al., 2012). In a sample of 1,001 adults with OCD, over 60 percent reported that they experienced sensory phenomena during their OCD symptoms (Ferrao et al., 2012). Furthermore, in a large cross-national study on the heterogeneity of OCD, 89.5 percent of individuals with OCD reported at least one symptom under the broad incompleteness dimension that comprised not just right behaviors, preoccupations with accuracy, and perceptual phenomena (Cervin et al., 2021). Of note, in the latter study, incompleteness was the dimension with most unique associations with other symptom dimensions, indicating that incompleteness may play a central role in OCD.

Feelings of incompleteness and not just right experiences are common in the general population, with one study reporting that 83 percent of undergraduate students had experienced at least on such experience during the last month (Ghisi et al., 2010). In relation to psychiatric symptoms, studies indicate that feelings of incompleteness and not just right experiences are particularly strongly linked to OCD. Most research on the diagnostic specificity of incompleteness has compared adults with OCD to adults with anxiety disorders and results have showed that incompleteness is more elevated in individuals with OCD (Chik et al., 2010; Ecker et al., 2014; Ghisi et al., 2010). Incompleteness also distinguishes adults with OCD from those with depression (Ecker et al., 2014) and gambling and eating disorders but not hair-pulling disorder (Sica et al., 2015). Furthermore, incompleteness and not just right experiences show unique associations with self-reported OCD symptoms in both clinical and non-clinical samples, even after accounting for general distress and other psychiatric symptoms (Belloch et al., 2016; Ecker & Gonner, 2008; Sica et al., 2012; Taylor et al., 2014b). In contrast, no unique associations between incompleteness and not just right experiences and worry, depressive symptoms, or anxiety symptoms have emerged (Apa et al., 2022; Coles et al., 2005), albeit with some exceptions (Fergus, 2014). Not just right experiences are also common in individuals with OCD and co-occurring Tourette's syndrome, with 81 percent of individuals struggling with both conditions reporting such experiences, with the corresponding frequency in those with Tourette's syndrome alone being 56 percent (Leckman et al., 1994). Interestingly, not just right experiences have also been linked to body dysmorphic disorder, skin picking disorder, and trichotillomania (Cerea et al., 2022; Ricketts et al., 2021; Wetterneck et al., 2020), providing support for the inclusion of these disorders in the new Obsessive-Compulsive and Related Disorders chapter in DSM, although more research is needed in this field, particularly with pediatric samples.

The core dimensions model of OCD: harm avoidance and incompleteness

Based on the existing empirical evidence in support of the role of incompleteness and not just right experiences in OCD and building on the work by Rasmussen and Eisen (1992), Summerfeldt et al. (2014) developed a model of OCD known as the core dimensions model. In the model, Summerfeldt and colleagues emphasized the heterogeneity of OCD and that OCD symptoms appear to cluster around several major symptom dimensions. However, they also pointed out that there is considerable overlap between different symptom dimensions and that many symptoms are related to several dimensions. They concluded that a major limitation of the current symptom dimension models of OCD is that the dimensions are based solely on topographic information, that is, what a person does. Instead, they argued that a model based on why a person does a certain behavior (functional information) would be of more relevance to the onset, maintenance, and treatment of OCD. Accordingly, the core dimensions model is an attempt to provide such a model, in part to help explain the vast heterogeneity of OCD. According to the core dimensions model, much of the topographic heterogeneity of OCD can be explained by variation alongside two basic affective-motivational dimensions: harm avoidance and incompleteness (Summerfeldt et al., 2014).

In the core dimensions model, harm avoidance refers to a trait-like tendency to perceive threats, experience fear and anxiety, and engage in avoidance of potential harm (Schreck et al., 2021). In contrast, incompleteness refers to the sensations described above, that is, distressing feelings of imperfection, that things are not just right, or that intentions or actions have not been fully completed (Summerfeldt et al., 2014). The two dimensions are not mutually exclusive. Rather, most individuals with OCD experience both, but to different degrees, and according to Summerfeldt et al. (2014), individual variation across these two dimensions gives rise to the heterogeneity of OCD.

A major advantage of combining harm avoidance and incompleteness in the understanding of OCD is that the same topographic symptom can be motivated by different underlying processes. Consider the example of a person repetitively washing his or her hands. What drives the behavior? The person can engage in the repetitive hand washing, owing to a strong fear of catching a serious illness. However, the exact same behavior can also be driven by an urge to reach a sense of completeness. It is also possible that both harm avoidance and incompleteness are involved. For example, the hand washing can be initiated by a fear of catching a serious illness but then repeated because of feelings of incompleteness.

Empirical studies have mainly supported the postulates of the core dimensions model. First, harm avoidance and incompleteness have been found to be psychometrically separate constructs (Pietrefesa & Coles, 2008; Summerfeldt et al., 2014; Taylor et al., 2014a). Second, the two constructs appear to be distributed differently in different individuals. For example, in a sample of 85 individuals with OCD, Bragdon and Coles (2017) found evidence for four broad groups of individuals: those with higher incompleteness than harm avoidance (35 percent of the sample), those with high scores on both motivational dimensions (26 percent), those who were low on both motivational dimensions (22 percent), and those with higher harm avoidance than incompleteness (16 percent). Furthermore, it has been shown that self-reported trait levels of harm avoidance and incompleteness in individuals with OCD adequately capture the emotions they experience during symptoms (Cervin & Perrin, 2019; Summerfeldt et al., 2014), suggesting that self-report questionnaires of more trait-like tendencies for harm avoidance and incompleteness can be used to study the role of these dimensions in OCD.

Incompleteness, not just right experiences, and harm avoidance in pediatric OCD

Very few studies have examined feelings of incompleteness and not just right experiences in children and adolescents with OCD. The first study was conducted by Cervin and colleagues. They recruited clinical samples of treatment-seeking youth with either principal OCD or a principal anxiety disorder as well as a sample of youth without psychiatric disorders. All participants completed a self-report scale of trait-like tendencies for harm avoidance and incompleteness, the Obsessive-Compulsive Trait Core Dimensions Questionnaire (OCTCDQ), developed by Summerfeldt et al. (2014). In addition, all clinical participants were interviewed about the degree to which they experienced harm avoidance/anxiety, incompleteness, or disgust during their symptoms. This interview also followed the procedures developed by Summerfeldt et al. (2014).

In a first report, Cervin and colleagues examined the psychometric properties of the OCTCDQ, as this was the first time the measure was used in children and adolescents. Findings showed that the scale worked well and that harm avoidance and incompleteness were separate constructs (Cervin & Perrin, 2019). These findings are promising as they suggest that young people can identify and discriminate between the emotional/affective experiences of incompleteness and harm avoidance.

In a second report, Cervin and colleagues examined whether self-reported levels of incompleteness distinguished youth with OCD from those with anxiety disorders. In line with the core dimensions model, they expected trait incompleteness to be elevated in youth with OCD compared to youth with anxiety disorders as well as compared with non-clinical youth. Further, it was expected trait harm avoidance would be elevated in both OCD and anxiety disorders compared to non-clinical youth. Both hypotheses were confirmed. Youth with OCD reported much higher levels of incompleteness than the other two groups (Cervin et al., 2020a). Furthermore, compared to non-clinical youth, harm avoidance was elevated in youth with OCD as well as in youth with anxiety disorders, with no significant difference between the two clinical groups. The authors also analyzed the degree to which incompleteness and harm avoidance were associated with self-reported severity of OCD, using the Obsessive Compulsive Inventory-Child Version (OCI-CV) (Aspvall et al., 2020; Foa et al., 2010). Importantly, they accounted for anxiety and depression in these analyses. Structural equation modeling showed that trait harm avoidance was uniquely associated with OCD, anxiety, and depression while incompleteness was uniquely associated only with OCD. With respect to the symptom dimensions of OCD, incompleteness was most strongly associated with the OCI-CV dimensions of doubting/checking, ordering, and neutralizing while harm avoidance was most strongly associated with doubting/checking, obsessing, and washing.

In a third report, Cervin and colleagues analyzed the degree to which youth with OCD and anxiety disorders experienced harm avoidance, incompleteness, and disgust during their symptoms. Each participant was asked to recall a symptom episode during the last week and was then introduced to the three emotional concepts and asked to report how much they experienced each of the emotions during their symptoms (Cervin & Perrin, 2019; Cervin et al., 2020b). Importantly, all participants with OCD were classified according to their major symptom dimension (aggressive/disturbing thoughts, symmetry, contamination) and all participants with an anxiety disorder had either social anxiety disorder or generalized anxiety disorder. Among youth with OCD, 85 percent report moderate to severe feelings of incompleteness during symptoms (Cervin et al., 2020b). For comparison, 75 percent reported moderate to severe levels of harm avoidance. Further, all three subtypes of OCD were associated with elevated levels of incompleteness compared to social and generalized anxiety disorder, with the most elevated levels being observed in the symmetry group. In contrast, only youth with OCD with the aggressive/disturbing thoughts subtype reported similar high levels of harm avoidance as youth with social or generalized anxiety disorder (Cervin et al., 2020b).

Schreck and colleagues have also studied incompleteness in children and adolescents with OCD. In their study, the core obsessional theme of 170 youth with OCD was analyzed by clinicians who then rated whether the compulsions were primarily driven by harm avoidance or incompleteness (Schreck et al., 2021). They found that a majority of patients (56 percent) were motivated by a combination of harm avoidance and incompleteness, while 25 percent were primarily motivated by harm avoidance, and 18 percent primarily motivated by incompleteness. In line with Cervin et al. (2020a), Schreck et al. (2021) found that incompleteness was uniquely associated with the OCI-CV dimensions of doubting/ checking, ordering, and neutralizing and harm avoidance with doubting/ checking, obsessing, and neutralizing.

Taken together, the current findings on incompleteness and not just right experiences in children and adolescents with OCD clearly indicate that these experiences are common and distinguishes pediatric OCD from pediatric anxiety disorders. Further, while incompleteness appears to be elevated across all major symptom dimensions of pediatric OCD, it seems to be specifically linked to symmetry/ordering and doubting and checking, which is consistent with research in adults (Coles & Ravid, 2016; Ferrão et al., 2012; Nissen & Parner, 2018; Sibrava et al., 2016).

Treatment outcomes

Few studies have examined whether incompleteness and not just right experiences affect treatment outcome in individuals with OCD. As exposure-based CBT for OCD is based on a fear-centric model and because most treatment protocols lack modules designed to address incompleteness-related symptoms (Schwartz, 2018), it is reasonable to assume that individuals with OCD whose symptoms are primarily driven by incompleteness may fare poorer in CBT. In adults, some evidence supports poorer outcomes for those with symmetry symptoms (Abramowitz et al., 2003; Schwartz, 2018) and both Foa et al. (1999) and Eisen et al. (2013) have reported that OCD patients whose obsessions do not include a feared outcome have poorer treatment outcomes than those with a feared outcome. Importantly, incompleteness and not just right experiences were not specifically assessed in these studies.

Regarding children and adolescents, three relevant studies have been published. Nissen and Parner (2018) analyzed naturalistic treatment outcomes in 317 children and adolescents with OCD and observed that baseline severity of not just right experiences increased the risk of relapse. In Cervin et al. (2020b), small to moderate reductions in self-reported levels of incompleteness were observed following naturalistic treatment, and change in incompleteness was strongly associated with change in overall OCD severity. Furthermore, Cervin and Perrin (2020) found that youth who reported high levels of incompleteness as part of their baseline symptoms had poorer naturalistic treatment outcomes while levels of harm avoidance at baseline did not predict outcome.

The third study did not examine treatment outcomes, but rather asked the question why feelings of incompleteness may be associated with poorer outcomes. Building on the work by Foa et al. (1999) and Cervin and Perrin (2020), Milgram et al. (2022) examined whether incompleteness-related distress differed from fear-related distress in youth with OCD who received exposure and response prevention (ERP). ERP is the key ingredient in exposure-based CBT for OCD and is typically used to elicit obsession-related fear while helping the patient to refrain from compulsions and avoidance. Milgram and colleagues suggested that there may be several reasons that individuals with incompleteness-driven OCD may experience poorer outcomes of ERP. First, because incompleteness is not linked to a feared outcome, distress levels may not be elevated enough for effective ERP to occur. Second, incompleteness-related distress may not vary or habituate in the same way as fear-related distress, which could affect outcomes (Craske et al., 2014). To examine these possibilities, Milgram et al. (2022) recorded 831 ERP sessions in 280 youth with severe OCD and noted whether each exposure targeted harm avoidance or incompleteness. By analyzing subjective distress during ERP, they found that exposure tasks aimed to elicit incompleteness generated less severe distress than exposure task aimed to elicit harm avoidance. Further, incompleteness-generated distress was more stable over time (i.e., showing a flatter distress/habituation curve), although decreases in distress were the norm during both incompleteness and harm avoidance exposure tasks. In sum, the findings by Milgram and colleagues suggest that incompleteness and harm avoidance are distinct emotional processes, and that exposure-based CBT for OCD could be strengthened by including more direct guidance on how to work with patients primarily driven by incompleteness.

The brain and incompleteness, not just right experiences, and sensory phenomena

To our knowledge, only two studies have attempted to investigate specific neuroanatomical substrates of incompleteness, not just right experiences, and sensory phenomena in OCD. In the first study, Subirà et al. (2015) compared individuals with OCD with and without sensory phenomena and found that those with sensory phenomena evidenced a grey matter volume increase in the medial aspect of the sensorimotor cortex. These results were confirmed also after excluding patients with a history of tic disorders, supporting the interpretation that sensory phenomena in OCD are independent of the presence of tics. However, the authors found no significant correlation between regional grey matter volumes and the severity of sensory phenomena.

Brown et al. (2019) used a "body-focused" video task designed to elicit activation in interoception and sensorimotor brain regions (e.g., a video of a person's throat while swallowing) in individuals with OCD. Results indicated that the severity of sensory phenomena was positively associated with activation in left mid-posterior insula as well as right mid-anterior insula, bilateral somatosensory cortex (postcentral gyri), left posterior temporal cortex, bilateral middle orbitofrontal cortex, and left dorsal prefrontal regions. These associations were independent of OCD severity and other disorder-relevant clinical characteristics (e.g, general anxiety, depression, harm avoidance).

In a broader sense, evidence suggests that OCD symptoms arise from structural and functional brain abnormalities in the cortico-striato-thalamo-cortical circuit, which is involved in the control of motor behaviors and integration of sensory information (Shephard et al., 2021; van den Heuvel et al., 2016). Importantly, sensory phenomena and not just right experiences are very common in Tourette's syndrome as "sensory tics" (Reese et al., 2014) and have been linked to "urges-for-action" experiences (e.g., the urge to blink) (Jackson et al., 2011). In line with these observations, a recent neuroimaging study demonstrated that OCD patients exhibited increased activity in mid and anterior insula and cingulate motor area during eyeblink suppression (Stern et al., 2020).

The underlying neurophysiological mechanisms involved in incompleteness, not just right experiences, and sensory phenomena are largely unknown. Feelings of incompleteness have been associated with maladaptive action repetition and impaired inhibitory control (Coles & Ravid, 2016; Fergus, 2014). Accordingly, Dominke et al. (2021) found that high trait-like feelings of incompleteness in healthy individuals were associated with a reduced N200 amplitude, an electrophysiological marker of response inhibition.

Taken together, current findings suggest that incompleteness, not just right experiences, and sensory phenomena are both functionally and structurally related to somatosensory areas. Furthermore, as argued by Brown et al. (2019), because these experiences encompass multiple sensory domains (e.g., somatosensory, interoceptive, auditory and visual), it cannot be ruled out that different manifestations may be underpinned by different neural mechanisms. However, the current research base is small, and more studies are needed to reach a more precise understanding of the neural substrates associated with the different phenotypic expressions of incompleteness, not just right experiences, and sensory phenomena in OCD.

Sensory processing as a potential overarching framework

An overarching framework that can help explain incompleteness, not just right experiences, and sensory phenomena and how and why they are linked to OCD is provided by the investigation of sensory processing difficulties. Growing evidence shows that people with OCD have difficulties in the integration of interoceptive/proprioceptive signals (Ezrati et al., 2019; Lazarov et al., 2012; Stern, 2014) and sensory-motor cues (Rossi et al., 2005; Russo et al., 2014) and some authors have underscored the role of sensory processing abnormalities in youth with OCD (Cervin, 2022; Van Hulle et al., 2019), as well as in youth with compulsive behaviors

(Bart et al., 2017; Dar et al., 2012). In this regard, it has been speculated that incompleteness and not just right experience may represent an impaired ability to use sensory feedback to guide behavior (Summerfeldt et al., 2015). This suggestion is coherent with increasing evidence showing that a sense of agency may constitute an integrative building block for understanding OCD features, including the emergence of sensory phenomena (Szalai, 2019). The sense of agency construct refers to the feeling of control over voluntary actions and their outcomes (Moore, 2016) and is the product of computational procedures that combine bottom-up sensory data with top-down contextual knowledge, searching for a match between expected and actual outcomes in the subjective experience of performing an action (Moore & Fletcher, 2012; Salomon, 2017). This integration process is due mainly to a comparator model of motor control (Frith et al., 2000), which compares the prediction of the outcome of an action with sensory feedback signals that provide information about the action being performed and its effects (Sarah-Jayne et al., 2000). Considering this comparator model, if there is no mismatch between the predicted and observed effect, the predicted effect is "removed" from the experience. Examining EEG responses to self-generated versus externally generated visual stimuli, Gentsch et al. (2012) found that the suppression of the N1 component (a hallmark of this sensory attenuation) was reduced in OCD participants compared to healthy controls. Thus, individuals with OCD failed to predict and suppress the sensory consequences of their own actions, which persist as "noisy" signals. The authors speculated that this discrepancy may lead to persistent "feelings of incompleteness." Coherently, Szalai (2019) argued that this mechanism may induce repetitive behaviors to achieve an outcome congruent with what was predicted.

In a similar vein, Poletti and colleagues (Poletti et al., 2022; Poletti, Gebhardt, & Raballo, 2022) suggested a possible pathophysiological role for altered corollary discharges (i.e., copies of motor commands used to form a prediction of sensations from self-generated actions) in the emergence of sensory phenomena in OCD. However, the literature on this topic is still scarce and no research has attempted to investigate sensory processing mechanisms in pediatric OCD, nor to directly analyze the association with incompleteness and not just right experiences. This is unfortunate, because a better understanding of these mechanisms may help young OCD patients with sensory phenomena in achieving correct levels of self-efficacy and reducing the urge to compulsive behaviors.

Implications and limitations of the current research

OCD is a heterogenous disorder implying a heterogenous emotional architecture. Growing evidence suggests that feelings of incompleteness, not just right experiences, and sensory phenomena may be important or even crucial building blocks of this architecture. Several studies indicate that incompleteness, not just right experiences, and sensory phenomena are clearly elevated in individuals with OCD, also in children and adolescents, and that such experiences may be specific to OCD and potentially to other disorders included in the Obsessive-Compulsive and Related Disorders chapter in DSM. There is also evidence that individuals with OCD whose symptoms are driven by incompleteness may have poorer outcomes than those whose obsessions revolve around specific fears, and the largest study to date observed this in youth receiving CBT for OCD (Cervin & Perrin, 2020). A limitation of the treatment outcome literature is that it has been conducted in naturalistic clinical settings with limited control over interventions. Further, the overall literature about incompleteness, not just right experiences, and sensory phenomena is limited by three broad concepts that refer to largely overlapping phenomena, and the lack of clear guidelines about how to assess these phenomena in OCD is hindering progress. Moving forward, it would be beneficial to agree upon common definitions and which measures should be used to assess the constructs. Such advances would also benefit research into the neural underpinnings of incompleteness, not just right experiences, and sensory phenomena in OCD.

While advances in definitions and assessment tools could benefit future research, the current evidence has concluded that incompleteness, not just right experiences, and sensory phenomena are common in OCD, including in children and adolescents, and that they are of clear clinical relevance. Clinicians should therefore be aware of these concepts and assess to which degree they are relevant for the person in front of them.

References

Abramowitz, J. S., Franklin, M. E., Schwartz, S. A., & Furr, J. M. (2003). Symptom presentation and outcome of cognitive-behavioral therapy for obsessive-compulsive disorder. *J Consult Clin Psychol*, 71(6), 1049–1057. doi:10.1037/0022-006x.71.6.1049.

Abramowitz, J. S., Taylor, S., & McKay, D. (2009). Obsessive-compulsive disorder. *Lancet*, 374(9688), 491–499. doi:10.1016/s0140-6736(09)60240–60243.

Al-Shawaf, L., Conroy-Beam, D., Asao, K., & Buss, D. M. (2016). Human emotions: An evolutionary psychological perspective. *Emotion Review*, 8(2), 173–186.

American Psychiatric Association. (2013). *Diagnostic and Statistical Manual of Mental Disorders* (5th Ed.).

American Psychiatric Association. (2022). *Diagnostic and statistical manual of mental disorders, fifth edition, text revision*. American Psychiatric Association.

Apa, F., Tumkaya, S., Yucens, B., & Kashyap, H. (2022). Are "not just-right experiences" trait and/or state marker for obsessive-compulsive disorder? *The European Journal of Psychiatry*, 36(1), 51–59. doi:10.1016/j.ejpsy.2021.09.003.

Aspvall, K., Cervin, M., Andrén, P., Perrin, S., Mataix-Cols, D., & Andersson, E. (2020). Validity and clinical utility of the Obsessive Compulsive Inventory-Child Version: Further evaluation in clinical samples. *BMC psychiatry*, 20. doi:10.1186/s12888-020-2450-7.

Bart, O., Bar-Shalita, T., Mansour, H., & Dar, R. (2017). Relationships among sensory responsiveness, anxiety, and ritual behaviors in children with and without atypical sensory responsiveness. *Physical & occupational therapy in pediatrics*, 37(3), 322–331.

Belloch, A., Fornes, G., Carrasco, A., Lopez-Sola, C., Alonso, P., & Menchon, J. M. (2016). Incompleteness and not just right experiences in the explanation of Obsessive-Compulsive Disorder. *Psychiatry Res*, 236, 1–8. doi:10.1016/j.psychres.2016.01.012.

Bragdon, L. B. & Coles, M. E. (2017). Examining heterogeneity of obsessive-compulsive disorder: Evidence for subgroups based on motivations. *J Anxiety Disord*, 45, 64–71. doi:10.1016/j.janxdis.2016.12.002.

Brown, C., Shahab, R., Collins, K., Fleysher, L., Goodman, W. K., Burdick, K. E., & Stern, E. R. (2019). Functional neural mechanisms of sensory phenomena in obsessive-compulsive disorder. *Journal of Psychiatric Research*, 109, 68–75. doi:10.1016/j.jpsychires.2018.11.018.

Cerea, S., Lovetere, G., Bottesi, G., Sica, C., & Ghisi, M. (2022). The relationship between body dysmorphic disorder symptoms and 'not just right'experiences in a sample of individuals seeking cosmetic surgery and aesthetic medicine procedures. *Clinical psychology & psychotherapy*, 29(3), 1034–1049.

Cervin, M. (2022). *Sensory processing in children and adolescents with obsessive-compulsive and anxiety disorders Research on Child and Adolescent Psychopathology.*

Cervin, M., Miguel, E. C., Güler, A. S., Ferrão, Y. A., Erdoğdu, A. B., Lazaro, L., Gökçe, S., Geller, D. A., Yulaf, Y., Başgül, Ş. S., Özcan, Ö., Karabekiroğlu, K., Fontenelle, L. F., Yazgan, Y., Storch, E. A., Leckman, J. F., Conceição do Rosario, M., & Mataix-Cols, D. (2021). Towards a definitive symptom structure of obsessive− compulsive disorder: a factor and network analysis of 87 distinct symptoms in 1366 individuals. *Psychological medicine*, 1–13.

Cervin, M. & Perrin, S. (2019). Measuring harm avoidance, incompleteness, and disgust in youth with obsessive-compulsive disorder and anxiety disorders. *Journal of Obsessive-Compulsive & Related Disorders*, 22. doi:10.1016/j.jocrd.2019.100442.

Cervin, M. & Perrin, S. (2020). Incompleteness and disgust predict treatment outcome for pediatric obsessive-compulsive disorder. *Behavior therapy*, 52. doi:10.1016/j.beth.2020.01.007.

Cervin, M., Perrin, S., Olsson, E., Claesdotter-Knutsson, E., & Lindvall, M. (2020a). Incompleteness, harm avoidance, and disgust: A comparison of youth with OCD, anxiety disorders, and no psychiatric disorder. *Journal of Anxiety Disorders*, 69. doi:10.1016/j.janxdis.2019.102175.

Cervin, M., Perrin, S., Olsson, E., Claesdotter-Knutsson, E., & Lindvall, M. (2020b). Involvement of fear, incompleteness, and disgust during symptoms of pediatric obsessive-compulsive disorder. *European child & adolescent psychiatry*, 30(2), 271–281. doi:10.1007/s00787-020-01514-7.

Chik, H. M., Calamari, J. E., Rector, N. A., & Riemann, B. C. (2010). What do low-dysfunctional beliefs obsessive–compulsive disorder subgroups believe?

Journal of Anxiety Disorders, 24(8), 837–846. https://ac.els-cdn.com/S0887618510001325/1-s2.0-S0887618510001325-main.pdf?_tid=7361d559-7488-45b6-8602-c6a4d10a9981&acdnat=1553099167_4edfbc4967a21ea438fbd969a1f7e55b.

Coles, M. E., Frost, R. O., Heimberg, R. G., & Rhéaume, J. (2003). "Not just right experiences": perfectionism, obsessive–compulsive features and general psychopathology. *Behaviour research and therapy*, 41(6), 681–700.

Coles, M. E., Heimberg, R. G., Frost, R. O., & Steketee, G. (2005). Not just right experiences and obsessive-compulsive features: experimental and self-monitoring perspectives. *Behav Res Ther*, 43(2), 153–167. doi:10.1016/j.brat.2004.01.002.

Coles, M. E. & Ravid, A. (2016). Clinical presentation of not-just right experiences (NJREs) in individuals with OCD: Characteristics and response to treatment. *Behaviour Research and Therapy*, 87, 182–187. doi:10.1016/j.brat.2016.09.013.

Cougle, J. R. & Lee, H.-J. (2014). Pathological and non-pathological features of obsessive-compulsive disorder: Revisiting basic assumptions of cognitive models. *Journal of Obsessive-Compulsive and Related Disorders*, 3(1), 12–20.

Craske, M. G., Treanor, M., Conway, C. C., Zbozinek, T., & Vervliet, B. (2014). Maximizing exposure therapy: an inhibitory learning approach. *Behav Res Ther*, 58, 10–23. doi:10.1016/j.brat.2014.04.006.

Dar, R., Kahn, D. T., & Carmeli, R. (2012). The relationship between sensory processing, childhood rituals and obsessive–compulsive symptoms. *Journal of behavior therapy and experimental psychiatry*, 43(1), 679–684.

Dominke, C., Graham-Schmidt, K., Gentsch, A., & Schütz-Bosbach, S. (2021). Action inhibition in individuals with high obsessive-compulsive trait of incompleteness: An ERP study. *Biological Psychology*, 159, 108019.

Ecker, W. & Gonner, S. (2008). Incompleteness and harm avoidance in OCD symptom dimensions. *Behaviour research and therapy*, 46(8), 895–904. doi:10.1016/j.brat.2008.04.002.

Ecker, W., Kupfer, J., & Gönner, S. (2014). Incompleteness and harm avoidance in OCD, anxiety and depressive disorders, and non-clinical controls. *Journal of Obsessive-Compulsive and Related Disorders*, 3(1), 46–51. doi:10.1016/j.jocrd.2013.12.001.

Eisen, J. L., Sibrava, N. J., Boisseau, C. L., Mancebo, M. C., Stout, R. L., Pinto, A., & Rasmussen, S. A. (2013). Five-year course of obsessive-compulsive disorder: predictors of remission and relapse. *The Journal of Clinical Psychiatry*, 74 (3), 7286.

Ezrati, O., Friedman, J., & Dar, R. (2019). Attenuation of access to internal states in high obsessive-compulsive individuals might increase susceptibility to false feedback: Evidence from a visuo-motor hand-reaching task. *J Behav Ther Exp Psychiatry*, 65, 101445. doi:10.1016/j.jbtep.2018.12.006.

Fergus, T. A. (2014). Are "not just right experiences" (NJREs) specific to obsessive-compulsive symptoms?: evidence that NJREs span across symptoms of emotional disorders. *J Clin Psychol*, 70(4), 353–363doi:10.1002/jclp.22034.

Ferrao, Y. A., Shavitt, R. G., Prado, H., Fontenelle, L. F., Malavazzi, D. M., de Mathis, M. A., Hounie, A. G., Miguel, E. C., & do Rosario, M. C. (2012). Sensory phenomena associated with repetitive behaviors in obsessive-compulsive disorder: an exploratory study of 1001 patients. *Psychiatry Res*, 197(3), 253–258. doi:10.1016/j.psychres.2011.09.017.

Ferrão, Y. A., Shavitt, R. G., Prado, H., Fontenelle, L. F., Malavazzi, D. M., de Mathis, M. A., Hounie, A. G., Miguel, E. C., & do Rosário, M. C. (2012). Sensory phenomena associated with repetitive behaviors in obsessive-compulsive disorder: an exploratory study of 1001 patients. *Psychiatry Res*, 197(3), 253–258. doi:10.1016/j.psychres.2011.09.017.

Foa, E. B., Abramowitz, J. S., Franklin, M. E., & Kozak, M. J. (1999). Feared consequences, fixity of belief, and treatment outcome in patients with obsessive-compulsive disorder. *Behavior therapy*, 30(4), 717–724.

Foa, E. B., Coles, M., Huppert, J. D., Pasupuleti, R. V., Franklin, M. E., & March, J. (2010). Development and validation of a child version of the obsessive compulsive inventory. *Behav Ther*, 41(1), 121–132. doi:10.1016/j.beth.2009.02.001.

Foa, E. B., Huppert, J. D., & Cahill, S. P. (2006). *Emotional Processing Theory: An Update*.

Foa, E. B. & Kozak, M. J. (1995). DSM-IV field trial: obsessive-compulsive disorder. *The American journal of psychiatry*.

Foa, E. B. & McLean, C. P. (2016). The Efficacy of Exposure Therapy for Anxiety-Related Disorders and Its Underlying Mechanisms: The Case of OCD and PTSD. *Annual Review of Clinical Psychology*, 12, 1–28. doi:10.1146/annurev-clinpsy-021815-093533.

Frith, C. D., Blakemore, S.-J., & Wolpert, D. M. (2000). Abnormalities in the awareness and control of action. *Philosophical Transactions of the Royal Society of London. Series B: Biological Sciences*, 355(1404), 1771–1788.

Gentsch, A., Schütz-Bosbach, S., Endrass, T., & Kathmann, N. (2012). Dysfunctional forward model mechanisms and aberrant sense of agency in obsessive-compulsive disorder. *Biological psychiatry*, 71(7), 652–659.

Ghisi, M., Chiri, L. R., Marchetti, I., Sanavio, E., & Sica, C. (2010). In search of specificity:"Not just right experiences" and obsessive–compulsive symptoms in non-clinical and clinical Italian individuals. *Journal of Anxiety Disorders*, 24(8), 879–886. https://ac.els-cdn.com/S0887618510001374/1-s2.0-S0887618510001374-main.pdf?_tid=c7fef218-5050-40af-bb0a-42e414263353&acdnat=1553099172_8a9855045ecada251c858f9db600c2e0.

Jackson, S. R., Parkinson, A., Kim, S. Y., Schüermann, M., & Eickhoff, S. B. (2011). On the functional anatomy of the urge-for-action. *Cognitive neuroscience*, 2(3–4),227–243.

Lang, P. J. (1995). The emotion probe. Studies of motivation and attention. *Am Psychol*, 50(5), 372–385. www.ncbi.nlm.nih.gov/pubmed/7762889.

Lazarov, A., Dar, R., Liberman, N., & Oded, Y. (2012). Obsessive-compulsive tendencies may be associated with attenuated access to internal states: evidence from a biofeedback-aided muscle tensing task. *Conscious Cogn*, 21(3), 1401–1409. doi:10.1016/j.concog.2012.07.002.

Leckman, J. F., Walker, D. E., Goodman, W. K., Pauls, D. L., & Cohen, D. J. (1994). "Just right" perceptions associated with compulsive behavior in Tourette's syndrome. *Am J Psychiatry*, 151(5), 675–680. doi:10.1176/ajp.151.5.675.

Milgram, L., Sheehan, K., Cain, G., Carper, M. M., O'Connor, E. E., Freeman, J. B., Garcia, A., Case, B., & Benito, K. (2022). Comparison of patient-reported distress during harm avoidance and incompleteness exposure tasks for youth with OCD. *Journal of Obsessive-Compulsive and Related Disorders*, 35, 100760. doi:10.1016/j.jocrd.2022.100760.

Moore, J. W. (2016). What is the sense of agency and why does it matter? *Frontiers in psychology*, 7, 1272.

Moore, J. W., & Fletcher, P. C. (2012). Sense of agency in health and disease: a review of cue integration approaches. *Consciousness and cognition*, 21(1), 59–68.

Nissen, J. B., & Parner, E. (2018). The importance of insight, avoidance behavior, not-just-right perception and personality traits in pediatric obsessive-compulsive disorder (OCD): a naturalistic clinical study. *Nord J Psychiatry*, 72(7), 489–496. doi:10.1080/08039488.2018.1486454.

Pallanti, S., Barnes, J., Pittenger, C., & Eisen, J. (2017). *Incompleteness and harm avoidance in OCD. Obsessive-compulsive Disorder: Phenomenology, Pathophysiology, and Treatment*. New York: Oxford University Press.

Pietrefesa, A. S. & Coles, M. E. (2008). Moving beyond an exclusive focus on harm avoidance in obsessive compulsive disorder: considering the role of incompleteness. *Behav Ther*, 39(3), 224–231. doi:10.1016/j.beth.2007.08.004.

Pitman, R. K. (1984). Janet's Obsessions and Psychasthenia: a synopsis. *Psychiatric Quarterly*, 56(4), 291–314. www.ncbi.nlm.nih.gov/pubmed/6399751.

Poletti, M., Gebhardt, E., Pelizza, L., Preti, A., & Raballo, A. (2022). Neurodevelopmental Antecedents and Sensory Phenomena in Obsessive Compulsive Disorder: A Systematic Review Supporting a Phenomenological-Developmental Model. *Psychopathology*, 1–11.

Poletti, M., Gebhardt, E., & Raballo, A. (2022). Along the fringes of Agency: neurodevelopmental account of the obsessive mind. *CNS spectrums*, 27(5), 557–560.

Rachman, S. (1997). A cognitive theory of obsessions. *Behav Res Ther*, 35(9), 793–802. www.ncbi.nlm.nih.gov/pubmed/9299799;www.sciencedirect.com/science/article/pii/S0005796797000405.

Rasmussen, S. A. & Eisen, J. L. (1992). The epidemiology and clinical features of obsessive compulsive disorder. *Psychiatric Clinics*, 15(4), 743–758.

Reese, H. E., Scahill, L., Peterson, A. L., Crowe, K., Woods, D. W., Piacentini, J., Walkup, J. T., & Wilhelm, S. (2014). The premonitory urge to tic: measurement, characteristics, and correlates in older adolescents and adults. *Behavior therapy*, 45(2), 177–186.

Reid, J. E., Laws, K. R., Drummond, L., Vismara, M., Grancini, B., Mpavaenda, D., & Fineberg, N. A. (2021). Cognitive behavioural therapy with exposure and response prevention in the treatment of obsessive-compulsive disorder: A systematic review and meta-analysis of randomised controlled trials. *Comprehensive psychiatry*, 106, 152223.

Ricketts, E. J., Snorrason, Í., Mathew, A. S., Sigurvinsdottir, E., Ólafsson, R. P., Woods, D. W., & Lee, H.-J. (2021). Heightened Sense of Incompleteness in Excoriation (Skin-Picking) Disorder. *Cognitive Therapy and Research*, 1–8.

Rossi, S., Bartalini, S., Ulivelli, M., Mantovani, A., Di Muro, A., Goracci, A., Castrogiovanni, P., Battistini, N., & Passero, S. (2005). Hypofunctioning of sensory gating mechanisms in patients with obsessive-compulsive disorder. *Biological psychiatry*, 57(1), 16–20.

Russo, M., Naro, A., Mastroeni, C., Morgante, F., Terranova, C., Muscatello, M., Zoccali, R., Calabrò, R., & Quartarone, A. (2014). Obsessive-compulsive disorder: a "sensory-motor" problem? *International Journal of Psychophysiology*, 92(2), 74–78.

Salomon, R. (2017). The assembly of the self from sensory and motor foundations. *Social cognition*, 35(2), 87–106.

Sarah-Jayne, B., Daniel, W., & Chris, F. (2000). Why can't you tickle yourself. *Neuroreport*, 11(11), R11–R16.

Schreck, M., Georgiadis, C., Garcia, A., Benito, K., Case, B., Herren, J., Walther, M., & Freeman, J. (2021). Core motivations of childhood obsessive-compulsive disorder: the role of harm avoidance and incompleteness. *Child Psychiatry & Human Development*, 52, 957–965.

Schwartz, R. A. (2018). Treating incompleteness in obsessive-compulsive disorder: A meta-analytic review. *Journal of Obsessive-Compulsive and Related Disorders*, 19, 50–60. doi:10.1016/j.jocrd.2018.08.001.

Shephard, E., Stern, E. R., van den Heuvel, O. A., Costa, D. L., Batistuzzo, M. C., Godoy, P. B., Lopes, A. C., Brunoni, A. R., Hoexter, M. Q., & Shavitt, R. G. (2021). Toward a neurocircuit-based taxonomy to guide treatment of obsessive–compulsive disorder. *Molecular Psychiatry*, 26(9), 4583–4604.

Sibrava, N. J., Boisseau, C. L., Eisen, J. L., Mancebo, M. C., & Rasmussen, S. A. (2016). An empirical investigation of incompleteness in a large clinical sample of obsessive compulsive disorder. *J Anxiety Disord*, 42, 45–51. doi:10.1016/j.janxdis.2016.05.005.

Sica, C., Bottesi, G., Orsucci, A., Pieraccioli, C., Sighinolfi, C., & Ghisi, M. (2015). "Not Just Right Experiences" are specific to obsessive-compulsive disorder: further evidence from Italian clinical samples. *J Anxiety Disord*, 31, 73–83. doi:10.1016/j.janxdis.2015.02.002.

Sica, C., Caudek, C., Rocco Chiri, L., Ghisi, M., & Marchetti, I. (2012). "Not just right experiences" predict obsessive–compulsive symptoms in non-clinical Italian individuals: A one-year longitudinal study. *Journal of Obsessive-Compulsive and Related Disorders*, 1(3), 159–167. doi:10.1016/j.jocrd.2012.03.006.

Stein, D. J., Fineberg, N. A., Bienvenu, O. J., Denys, D., Lochner, C., Nestadt, G., Leckman, J. F., Rauch, S. L., & Phillips, K. A. (2010). Should OCD be classified as an anxiety disorder in DSM-V? *Depression and anxiety*, 27(6), 495–506.

Stern, E. R. (2014). Neural circuitry of interoception: New insights into anxiety and obsessive-compulsive disorders. *Current Treatment Options in Psychiatry*, 1, 235–247.

Stern, E. R., Brown, C., Ludlow, M., Shahab, R., Collins, K., Lieval, A., Tobe, R. H., Iosifescu, D. V., Burdick, K. E., & Fleysher, L. (2020). The buildup of an urge in obsessive–compulsive disorder: Behavioral and neuroimaging correlates. *Human brain mapping*, 41(6), 1611–1625.

Subirà, M., Sato, J. R., Alonso, P., do Rosário, M. C., Segalàs, C., Batistuzzo, M. C., Real, E., Lopes, A. C., Cerrillo, E., & Diniz, J. B. (2015). Brain structural correlates of sensory phenomena in patients with obsessive–compulsive disorder. *Journal of Psychiatry and Neuroscience*, 40(4), 232–240.

Summerfeldt, L. J., Gilbert, S. J., & Reynolds, M. (2015). Incompleteness, aesthetic sensitivity, and the obsessive-compulsive need for symmetry. *J Behav Ther Exp Psychiatry*, 49(Pt B), 141–149. doi:10.1016/j.jbtep.2015.03.006.

Summerfeldt, L. J., Kloosterman, P. H., Antony, M. M., & Swinson, R. P. (2014). Examining an obsessive-compulsive core dimensions model: Structural validity of harm avoidance and incompleteness. *Journal of Obsessive-Compulsive and Related Disorders*, 3(2), 83–94. doi:10.1016/j.jocrd.2014.01.003.

Szalai, J. (2019). The sense of agency in OCD. *Review of Philosophy and Psychology*, 10(2), 363–380.

Taylor, S., McKay, D., Crowe, K. B., Abramowitz, J. S., Conelea, C. A., Calamari, J. E., & Sica, C. (2014a). The sense of incompleteness as a motivator of obsessive-compulsive symptoms: an empirical analysis of concepts and correlates. *Behav Ther*, 45(2), 254–262. doi:10.1016/j.beth.2013.11.004.

Taylor, S., McKay, D., Crowe, K. B., Abramowitz, J. S., Conelea, C. A., Calamari, J. E., & Sica, C. (2014b). The sense of incompleteness as a motivator of obsessive-compulsive symptoms: an empirical analysis of concepts and correlates. *Behavior therapy*, 45(2), 254–262. doi:10.1016/j.beth.2013.11.004.

van den Heuvel, O. A., van Wingen, G., Soriano-Mas, C., Alonso, P., Chamberlain, S. R., Nakamae, T., Denys, D., Goudriaan, A. E., & Veltman, D. J. (2016). Brain circuitry of compulsivity. *Eur Neuropsychopharmacol*, 26(5), 810–827. doi:10.1016/j.euroneuro.2015.12.005.

Van Hulle, C. A., Esbensen, K., & Goldsmith, H. H. (2019). Co-occurrence of Sensory Overresponsivity with Obsessive-Compulsive Symptoms in Childhood and Early Adolescence. *Journal of Developmental & Behavioral Pediatrics*.

Wetterneck, C., Singh, R. S., & Woods, D. W. (2020). Hair pulling antecedents in trichotillomania: Their relationship with experiential avoidance. *Bulletin of the Menninger Clinic*, 84(1), 35–52.

World Health Organization. (2019). *International statistical classification of diseases and related health problems (11th ed.)*. https://icd.who.int.

Öst, L.-G., Enebrink, P., Finnes, A., Ghaderi, A., Havnen, A., Kvale, G., Salomonsson, S., & Wergeland, G. J. (2022). Cognitive behavior therapy for obsessive-compulsive disorder in routine clinical care: A systematic review and meta-analysis. *Behaviour research and therapy*, 104170.

Öst, L. G., Riise, E. N., Wergeland, G. J., Hansen, B., & Kvale, G. (2016). Cognitive behavioral and pharmacological treatments of OCD in children: A systematic review and meta-analysis. *Journal of Anxiety Disorders*, 43, 58–69. doi:10.1016/j.janxdis.2016.08.003.

5 Harm and Taboo Thoughts in Youth with OCD

Michelle Rozenman and Hannah Ishimuro

Some of the most common obsessions in OCD involve "taboo" or "unacceptable" thoughts. These can include: harm, aggression, violence and/or a fear that one might not be able to control impulses; intrusive sexual thoughts; and/or religious or moral scrupulosity. This symptom cluster is relatively common in pediatric OCD, and especial care should be taken when querying and treating these symptoms. We start this chapter by reviewing data that taboo thoughts in OCD are associated with stigma and misattribution of risk by families, providers, and the lay community alike. We hope this provides a context for how critical it is to thoughtfully and nonjudgmentally assess taboo thoughts, differentiate them from safety-related concerns, and provide psychoeducation to youth and care-givers to increase the likelihood of symptom disclosure. We then describe the phenomenology, prevalence, and correlates of this symptom cluster, discuss issues related to assessment with a focus on developmental tailor-ing for children and adolescents, briefly review clinician-rated, and self- and caregiver-report, measures that might be used to supplement the clin-ical interview, and finally review relevant components of exposure-based treatment for taboo thoughts in children and adolescents.

Stigma and shame associated with taboo thoughts

Before presenting the primary content of this chapter, we feel it critical to contextualize taboo thoughts and perceptions about them. We start with a comment on labels and language, review compelling survey and experi-mental data regarding stigma and misdiagnosis, with implications for inaccurate treatment, and discuss potential impacts of these on the shame and fear youth may feel about these symptoms above and beyond what they might experience with other OCD symptom domains.

Labels and language

A variety of terms have been used in the research and clinical literatures to describe aggressive, sexual, and religious obsessions. While some refer

DOI: 10.4324/9781003517429-5

to this cluster as "taboo" or "unacceptable" thoughts, others have historically referred to them as "pure" obsessions (reflecting a desire for thoughts to be pure; Brakoulias, Starcevic, Berle, Milicevic, Moses, & Hannan, 2013). The goal of researchers and treatment providers in placing labels on subgroups of OCD symptoms is to succinctly and accurately refer to the heterogeneous symptoms that make up OCD for efficient and accurate diagnosis and treatment. However, the terms "taboo" and "unacceptable" themselves may carry stigma. As we wrote this chapter, we wrestled with how to balance between using the term "taboo" to reflect that these thoughts carry high perceived social and moral burden to youth with OCD, with a concern the term itself (and our use of it in this writing) may further contribute to stigmatizing this cluster of symptoms. Even use of the words "harm", "aggressive", "violent", and "sexual" (and perhaps, to a lesser degree "religious") when referring to obsessions may connote risk, or that the youth with these symptoms have "bad" thoughts or there is something "wrong" with them.

Yet the field currently does not have better, alternate terms for describing these symptoms in an efficient way. For lack of a better term and to be consistent with the extant literature, we use the word "taboo" to refer collectively across aggressive, sexual, and religious obsessions. Individual words for aggressive, sexual, and religious obsessions are used for specificity in describing research findings or providing clinical examples. We simultaneously acknowledge that it is critical for us and others to explicitly detail to medical and mental health providers, the lay community, and families that – just like with all other obsessions – thoughts are just thoughts and there is nothing inherently "wrong" with someone for having any of these thoughts. The only actual problem with taboo thoughts, as with all other obsessions in OCD, is that they cause individuals distress and are associated with compulsions, avoidance, and reassurance-seeking that can interfere with daily functioning.

Stigma, disclosure, and misdiagnosis

Several studies highlight significant stigma associated with taboo thoughts in OCD. Surveyed adults with taboo thoughts as part of their OCD symptom profile reported more stigma and shame and reported the biggest treatment barrier as being "ashamed of my problems" compared to adults whose OCD symptoms did not include taboo thoughts (Glazier & Wetterneck, 2015). In an experimental study, adults with subclinical OCD symptoms were administered an obsession induction paradigm: when induced, harm and sexual obsessions elicited more shame and anxiety, and were considered more immoral by participants, than contamination and symmetry inductions (Visvalingam et al., 2022). Moreover, feelings of shame and anxiety related to taboo symptoms may be amplified for racial/ethnic minority youth, who may be particularly hesitant to disclose sexual or aggressive obsessions, owing to fears of racism and/or confirming stereotypes about violence or sex (Williams & Jahn, 2017).

Stigma intersects with misidentification rates for taboo obsessions, especially aggressive or sexual obsessions. When depicted in symptom vignettes, taboo thoughts were misdiagnosed at very high rates by primary care physicians (70–8 percent; Glazier et al., 2015), lay community members (60 percent; Coles, Lahey, Fawcett & Fawcett 2023), and even mental health providers (42–52 percent; Perez et al., 2022) as safety-related (e.g., suicidality) or mental health problems (e.g., psychosis), including problems with potential legal consequences (e.g., pedophilia). Mental health providers also reported being less likely to use front-line psychosocial and medical treatment to address taboo thoughts (Keleher et al., 2020; Perez et al., 2022) and were more likely to recommend inappropriate treatment (Glazier et al., 2015). In our anecdotal experience, countless youth have shared that their initial disclosures of harm-related obsessions to school personnel, primary care providers, and/or family members led to inappropriate assumptions about the youth's or others' safety, with inappropriate responses (e.g., inpatient hospitalization, being taken to the police station in the back of a police car from school).

These data and anecdotal experiences of youth with taboo thoughts highlight how difficult it may be for youth to disclose, even to expert clinicians with experience assessing and treating OCD. Based on the above-described data, youth's fears may be warranted. We ask the reader to keep these research findings in mind when reviewing this chapter, and to consider how youth with taboo thoughts (and their families) may feel fear, concern, and confusion about how these obsessions might be perceived by others above and beyond OCD-related distress that occurs for other symptoms.

What kinds of obsessions are included in taboo thoughts?

As detailed later, taboo thoughts in OCD are upsetting, distressing, anxiety-provoking, or otherwise disgusting to the youth (i.e., ego dystonic). Youth with taboo thoughts as part of their OCD presentation are unlikely to act on them. Moreover, they engage in behaviors (avoidance, compulsions, reassurance-seeking) in attempts to stop the thoughts and prevent feared events from occurring. Importantly, while some youth report these intrusive experiences as thoughts or ideas, others will describe graphic images or scenes.

Harm, aggressive, and violent obsessions

The most common set of taboo thoughts involve obsessions about harm, aggression, violence, or fears that the youth will lose control of their behavior. Some youth fear that they will be responsible for causing a catastrophic event (e.g., "if I don't say something or behave a particular way, my parent will get in a car wreck on the way home"), others fear that they may inadvertently or deliberately behave in an aggressive or violent way towards others (e.g., "if I hug my parent too tight, I'll cause them to bleed internally"; intrusive image of picking up a sharp pencil and stabbing a classmate) or themselves, or that others will behave in aggressive ways toward the youth (e.g., image that someone else harms the youth or that the youth views violence between others and cannot stop it; Mancebo et al., 2008). Some intrusive thoughts involve fears of impulsive or deliberate engagement in suicidal or self-injurious behavior (e.g., "what if I actually want to die and cut myself with razor and bleed to death?"; "I'm afraid I might accidentally swallow all the medication in the bottle when I try to take just one"), and others may involve fears of loss of impulse control (e. g., "what if I shout a curse word in the middle of class?"). The distinction between taboo obsessions and risk of harm toward self or others is that, with the former the youth feels fear, distress, or other negative emotions that result in compulsions, avoidance, and/or reassurance-seeking to prevent feared outcomes. While these thoughts can occur anytime (as with all obsessions), youth may be especially triggered by news or violent content depicted in the media, items that they perceive as weapons (e.g., knives, scissors, pens, household cleaners) and specific locations that cue danger to them (e.g., stairwell, top floor of a parking structure).

Sexual obsessions

Sexual obsessions can involve thoughts or images that the youth might inadvertently, impulsively, or deliberately engage in sex acts, kissing, or other touch with sexual intent. These thoughts may include a violent element such as assault or that the behavior is unwanted by the recipient in the thought or may be distressing to the youth because they perceive the recipient is vulnerable (e.g., younger than the youth). The youth may also fear that they wanted to engage in the behavior whether or not it was wanted by the other person or express confusion about whether the thought means they do want to engage in the behavior (e.g., "I had a thought that I wanted to engage in a sex act with my peer and that scared me because I don't actually want to"). There may be significant disgust or distress if the thought is toward the youth's family (e.g., caregiver, sibling; "that's gross, it's incest"), animals (e.g., intrusive thought of sexual behavior with family pet), or strangers (e.g., "I don't even know that person; what does it say about me that I'm thinking about a sex act with them?"). In younger children with less knowledge of intimacy, the thoughts may be described abstractly (e.g., "gross touching", "touching private parts", "kissing"). However, both younger children and adolescents may report very graphic and detailed thoughts, images, and/or impulses. Sexual intrusive thoughts differ from the attraction or sexual desire youth may feel (particularly in adolescence) because the former causes emotional and cognitive distress, rather than pleasure or enjoyment, and are associated with compulsions and avoidance, rather than approach toward sexual behavior. These symptoms may intersect with messaging from parents, school, or elsewhere about the social implications of thoughts about sex (Fernández de la Cruz et al., 2013), particularly for children, or be misinterpreted as a symptom of abuse (Veale et al., 2009). Youth may be triggered by proximity to others (e.g., "if dog sits on my lap, am I going to touch it inappropriately?"), seeing or hearing sexual content in the media or in daily life, peers discussing sexual content, or less-clothed/unclothed bodies (e.g., pool or beach; gym locker room).

Scrupulosity: religious and/or moral obsessions

Scrupulosity is a set of obsessions that include religious and/or moral intrusive thoughts, including concerns that a youth has sinned or transgressed, upset God or aligned themselves with the devil or malignant forces, violated religious dictates or social/moral norms, behaved in a way that is dishonest, immoral, wasteful, or offended others or is otherwise a "bad" person (Peris & Rozenman, 2015). Compulsions may include repetitive prayer (e.g., repeating the same line of a prayer over and over trying to perfectly understand or "mean it enough"), excessive confessing to religious leaders, caregivers, or others about even the most minor transgressions (e.g., "I used an extra paper towel to clean up a mess"), or seeking reassurance that one's behavior is not upsetting to parents, teachers, or peers (e.g., asking "are you mad at me?" many times over even though the youth did nothing or little to upset the other person). Some compulsions may appear to be entirely unrelated to scrupulosity obsessions; for example, in response to a thought that the child has upset God or behaved in conflict with some religious tenet, they may count excessively or engage in compulsions that are typically attributed to contamination concerns (e.g., washing, cleaning).

The distinction between religious scrupulosity and religious practice is that in the former the youth's behavior is agreed upon by family, community members, and religious leaders to be out of line with the faith (e.g., attempting to perfectly understand each word of a prayer, and therefore being unable to understand the gestalt of the prayer might be inconsistent with how the religious figurehead encourages prayer). It is important to query the family's value system, religious behaviors, and typical religious practice (if applicable) to understand how the youth's behavior is consistent or not with familial expectations. In our clinical experience consulting with figureheads from a variety of religions, we are consistently provided with feedback that compulsions such as repeating the same phrase of a prayer, attempting to "perfectly pray", or engagement in other compulsions is not consistent with their practice or what they encourage for members of the congregation. However, there may be occasions when a youth engages in compulsions in secrecy, and therefore the prayer, attendance at a house of worship, and so forth is initially viewed as a sign of faithfulness, and only upon detailed assessment might the family or leaders identify a youth's behavior as excessive or inconsistent. Additionally, youth can have religious obsessions in the context of a family system that either does not practice in the traditions for which the youth's symptoms present as well as in families that are non-practicing, agnostic, and atheist.

Moral scrupulosity symptoms may initially appear to reflect exceptional conscientiousness, but symptom queries may reveal that the youth's behavior is excessive and the compulsions themselves are not values-based but instead fear-based. For example, a youth with obsessions about causing drought may refuse to shower for days or weeks, despite a caregiver telling them they look unkempt. Such a youth may also "police" their family members when caregivers and/or siblings shower, wash hands, wash dishes, etc., causing significant conflict in the household. Youth may be concerned about big world matters (e.g., climate change, war) or matters that apply only to them and those around them (e.g., their own behavior in a school classroom). Youth may also have doubting obsessions, where they worry whether they are a "good" person or have upset others, and engage in excessive reassurance-seeking, apologizing, or trying to repair relationship by constantly doing good deeds for the other person.

Compulsions associated with taboo thoughts

Across aggressive, sexual, and scrupulosity obsessions, youth may feel an inflated sense of responsibility that they must respond to their taboo thoughts in order to protect themselves and others. In response, they may engage in *observable compulsions* (e.g., parent sees a youth pray; youth seeks reassurance from parent) and/or *mental compulsions* (e.g., counting up to a certain number or repeating a phrase to themselves silently to prevent a catastrophic event). Other compulsions can include checking behavior (e.g., "did I actually stab my classmate? Are they bleeding?") or attempts to neutralize thoughts, such as replacing or "undoing" a taboo thought with some "good" thought. Avoidance of people, places, media content, and objects can be significant, as youth may do everything in their power to stay away from situations where someone might be hurt, or they might engage in the feared behavior.

Familial reassurance, accommodation, and participation in compulsions

As with all OCD subtypes, depending on the youth and their symptoms, caregivers and other family members may participate in symptom management. First, family members may provide reassurance either in response to the youth asking for it or in anticipation of the youth's distress. Research finds that caregivers of OCD-affected individuals describe that they often provide reassurance because they feel unsure of how else to help their family member cope (Halldorsson et al., 2016). However, reassurance provision can leave family members feeling frustrated (Halldorsson et al., 2016). Second, family members may accommodate the youth's symptoms by either doing tasks for the youth that the youth fears doing (e.g., caregiver cuts paper for a project with sharp scissors, owing to youth's harm obsessions) and/or allowing a youth to refrain from developmentally-appropriate tasks that they would otherwise be expected to do (e.g., youth doesn't have to be in same room as sibling, owing to sexual obsessions, resulting in two different dinnertimes for the family; Peris et al., 2008). Finally, family members may actively participate in the youth's compulsions. For example, a youth may ask a caregiver to check their body for cuts or bruises after the youth has an aggressive thought, and the caregiver's checking and confirmation that they are uninjured may be the compulsion that relieves distress for the youth.

Prevalence rates and demographic features

There may be a misconception that youth, particularly young children, should not have taboo thoughts because of their developmental stage and less life experience/knowledge compared to adults. However, taboo thoughts collectively comprise one of the most common OCD clusters in youth, in some studies comparable to rates of contamination symptoms. Rates of taboo thoughts in pediatric OCD samples range from 25–80 percent (Fernández de la Cruz et al., 2013; Garcia et al., 2009; Geller et al., 2001; Mancebo et al., 2008). Rates for individual symptoms range from: 48 percent–81 percent for harm-related and aggressive obsessions (Garcia et al., 2009; Mataix-Cols et al., 2008), 11 percent–26 percent for sexual obsessions (Fernández de la Cruz et al., 2013; Geller et al., 2001), and 15 percent–38 percent for religious obsessions (Garcia et al., 2009; Geller et al., 2001). Collectively, taboo thoughts are more common in early-onset OCD than adult-onset cases (Garcia et al., 2009), with comparable rates between adolescents and adults (Butwicka & Gmitrowicz, 2010). While some studies have found sexual obsessions to occur at higher rates in adolescence compared to childhood (Fernández de la Cruz et al., 2013; Geller et al., 2001; Weidle et al., 2022), others have not (Højgaard et al., 2017). Finally, some work suggests that boys may be more likely to have sexual obsessions than girls (Mataix-Cols et al., 2008).

Taboo thoughts cluster together

Many studies support that aggressive, sexual, and scrupulosity obsessions cluster together in youth (e.g., Højgaard et al., 2017; Stewart et al., 2008) and parallel the clustering of OCD symptoms in adults (Bloch et al., 2008). Some suggest that taboo thoughts are associated with worse OCD symptom severity in youth (Storch et al., 2010) and religious symptoms in particular may be associated with worse insight into symptoms (Wu et al., 2018). Individuals with OCD broadly, and those with taboo thoughts in particular may experience thought-action fusion, or the beliefs that thinking a thought is equal to engaging in the associated behavior, and/ or will actually increase the likelihood that the feared behavior or event will occur (Rees et al., 2010). Youth may feel an inflated sense of responsibility for preventing feared events and have greater difficulty regulating emotions when they experience taboo intrusive thoughts (Berman et al., 2018). It is therefore not surprising that taboo thoughts in youth have been specifically associated with higher self-report of fear more broadly (Cervin et al., 2021; Rozenman et al., 2017). Data from youth with OCD during the COVID-19 pandemic indicated that taboo thoughts led to greater interference and distress during this global event (Nissen et al., 2020).

Clinical comorbidity

In regards to clinical comorbidity, some studies with youth have found that aggressive and sexual obsessions co-occur with tics at higher rates (Masi et al., 2010) and sexual obsessions are associated with increased depressive symptoms (Fernández de la Cruz et al., 2013; Storch et al., 2015). The latter is concerning in the context of adult OCD data, where sexual obsessions are associated with suicidal thoughts and plans, potentially because the thoughts are so distressing that people feel more hopeless (Torres et al., 2011). Additionally, harm avoidance is elevated in first degree relatives of adults with OCD (Bey et al., 2017); if this finding is replicated in youth, it may have substantial implications for family-focused treatment or modifications to how and to whom psychoeducation is provided within a family system. Careful assessment of functional impairment, associated fear, thought-action fusion, and diagnostic comorbidity are important when assessing taboo thoughts in pediatric OCD.

Assessment

Prior work suggests that youth presenting for OCD treatment may initially only disclose non-taboo obsessions, and only report taboo obsessions half-way through or near the end of treatment (Weidle et al., 2022). Progress monitoring, or continued assessment of symptoms, including for symptom domains previously denied, is crucial given how common taboo thoughts are as part of the OCD presentation. Throughout assessment (and treatment), the clinician should developmentally tailor questions to the youth's age/developmental stage and may need to infuse psychoeducation or normalization (e.g., "now we're going to talk about thoughts that lots of kids and teens have") into their queries to attempt to offset stigma and embarrassment the youth or family may feel. The interview should include information about family history, the youth's identities, and the youth and family's values in order to inform whether and how much taboo thoughts are or are not consistent with, for example, religious practice expectations. Details about prior disclosures to medical or mental health providers, school, or others may provide insights into stigma and shame that may impact assessment and treatment processes. Queries about compulsions should include both overt and mental compulsions, and clinicians may need to meet with youth and caregiver separately to increase the likelihood that youth may disclose symptoms of which caregiver may be unaware. Some youth may not describe compulsions and avoidance as irrational or unhelpful, but rather view them as protective, helpful, or morally correct.

Because of the crucial implications for treatment plan development, the clinician should be careful to assess safety (and distinguish between aggressive obsessions versus suicidal or homicidal thoughts and behaviors), distinguish between sexual thoughts and traumatic experiences, and the family's expectations for their child (Veale et al., 2009). As outlined earlier, youth with taboo thoughts are afraid of or distressed by the thoughts, do not want to harm themselves or others, and engage in compulsions or avoidance in attempts to prevent harm. That said, youth may present with both OCD including taboo thoughts and a history of suicidal thoughts and/or behaviors. During initial assessment the clinician might ask the youth if they are able to differentiate how they might feel emotionally and physically when they have taboo obsessions (e.g., scared, distressed, fight-or-flight symptoms) as compared to when they are having thoughts of not wanting to be alive (e.g., relieved, sad, hopeless), as well as differentiate between behaviors (e.g., taboo thoughts lead to compulsions, avoidance of triggering stimuli versus suicidal behaviors, plans, etc.). If the youth is able to differentiate their internal experiences and behavioral responses, this may help to fully assess the level of risk and identify appropriate treatment targets and sequencing for OCD versus safety targets. Moreover, it should be noted that adolescents may experience sexual arousal as part of pubertal development and may be further disgusted or upset because they perceive this biological response as an indication that obsessions are pleasurable to them. Physical arousal should not be taken as a firm indication that the youth enjoys or wants to engage in behavior consistent with the thought. Instead, the youth's emotional and cognitive reactions should be used to clarify whether the thoughts are part of an OCD presentation, age-appropriate sexual interest/exploration, or something else.

A variety of clinician-rated, self-report, and caregiver-report questionnaires may be used to supplement the clinical interview. It should be noted that each of these only contains one or a handful of items related to taboo thoughts, so these measures in and of themselves are insufficient to fully query taboo thoughts. The taboo thoughts most commonly covered in these measures are harm avoidance and aggressive thoughts and related compulsions. Most also include a few items related to religious or moral obsessions, and no self-/caregiver-report questionnaires include items that specifically assess sexual obsessions. Several measures also use the term "bad thoughts", which is vague and may or may not apply to any sub-group of taboo obsessions. These measures also cannot and do not attempt to distinguish between the above-described distinctions that must be made regarding safety. However, these measures may allow for youth and/or caregivers to disclose information that the clinician would then follow up on if youth and/or caregiver do not feel comfortable initially disclosing during clinical interview, owing to stigma or shame.

CYBOCS: a clinician-rated measure

The Children's Yale-Brown Obsessive Compulsive Scale (CYBOCS; Scahill et al., 1997) is a semi-structured clinical interview for caregivers and youth, including a symptom checklist and clinical severity rating of obsessive and compulsive symptoms in the past week. A benefit of the semi-structured format is that it allows interviewers to ask follow-up questions and adjust language to match the youth's developmental stage. The CYBOCS symptom checklist is used to query specific obsession and compulsion domains. Although the checklist covers aggressive, sexual, and religious/moral obsessions, the items for these domains vary in specificity and use of developmentally appropriate language and examples. The aggressive obsessions domain of the CYBOCS includes ten items, covering a range of examples such as fear of harm to self or others, impulsive aggressive or antisocial acts, and violent images. In contrast, the CYBOCS only includes three items about sexual obsessions (e.g., "content involves homosexuality") and two items about religious/moral obsessions (e.g., "excessive concern with right/wrong, morality) without specific examples. In regard to compulsions, the majority of CYBOCS items fall within the harm avoidance domain, including checking, superstitious behaviors, and other behaviors to prevent harm. However, examples of measures to prevent harm, such as removing sharp items, are not listed. Further-more, there are only two items to assess reassurance-seeking behaviors (i.e., repetitive questions, confessing), and one item queries self-harm. The CYBOCS does not include items related to thought neutralizing and praying/religious compulsions. This clinician-rated tool is currently being updated to be more consistent with current pediatric OCD research (i.e., CYBOCS Second Edition; Storch et al., 2019).

Self- and caregiver-report questionnaires

Several self-report measures mirror the structure of the CYBOCS by differentiating between symptom content via checklists and some include separate severity items. The Children's Florida Obsessive Compulsive Inventory (C-FOCI; Storch et al., 2009) is a self-report questionnaire for youth with a 17-item symptom checklist that reflects several OCD symptom clusters. While the checklist includes aggressive obsession items and associated harm avoidance and reassurance-seeking, it does not cover content related to sexual, religious, or moral thoughts. The Obsessional Compulsive Inventory – Revised (ChOCI-R; Uher et al., 2008) is a youth- and caregiver-report questionnaire that parallels the structure of the CYBOCS. In regard to taboo thoughts, the ChoCI-R has a few queries for aggressive and religious/moral obsessions, and no items specifically assess sexual thought content. Relevant compulsions assessed on the ChoCI-R are thought neutralizing, reassurance-seeking, and checking behaviors.

The Obsessive-Compulsive Inventory – Child Version – Revised (OCI-CV-R; (Abramovitch et al., 2022) is a self-report questionnaire measuring the symptom severity across five different obsessive-compulsive content domains. The questionnaire contains several items querying for "bad" thoughts, however, specific reference of sexual, aggressive, or religious/moral content is not included. Similarly, the OCI-CV-R has a subscale measuring neutralizing behaviors, but none of the items explicitly refer to content within the taboo obsessions domain.

The Multidimensional Anxiety Scale for Children Second Edition (MASC 2; March 2013) is a self- and caregiver-report measure of anxiety symptoms that also includes an obsessions and compulsions subscale. The subscale consists of ten items, three of which are related to taboo content for "bad" thoughts and aggressive and religious/moral obsessions; no items pertain to the sexual obsessions domain.

The Child Behavior Checklist (CBCL; Achenbach & Rescorla, 2001) is a broadband questionnaire completed by caregivers that provides normed information about youth behavioral and emotional problems. The CBCL has an obsessive-compulsive problems subscale, consisting of eight items of which one item asks for presence of "bad" thoughts and one related to feeling "guilty." Although not included in the obsessive-compulsive problems subscale, the CBCL includes one item querying for thinking about sex which might reflect sexual obsessions but is not included in the obsessive-compulsive problems subscale score.

Finally, while not an OCD symptom questionnaire, the Obsessive Beliefs Questionnaire – Child Version (Coles et al., 2010) assesses beliefs about OC-related thoughts, and some items in particular may provide insights into aggressive and/or morality obsessions (e.g., "I should try to prevent harmful things no matter what"; "To be a good person, I must be perfect at everything I do"). Some items may overlap with thought-action fusion for aggressive obsessions (e.g., "If a thought pops into my mind about hurting my family, it means I really want to do it"; "I always have to work hard to make sure bad things (like accidents or diseases) don't happen"; I have to make sure others don't get into serious trouble because of things I do"; "If I'm not super careful, I will have a bad accident or cause a bad accident"; "having violent thoughts means I will lose control and become violent"). A few items may overlap with scrupulosity (i.e., "Just thinking about swearing at God is as bad as actually doing it"; "If I have an evil idea, that means I really want to do it"; "having an evil thought is just like doing it"). And a few more items may reflect thought-action fusion more broadly and/or appear to have ecological validity as potential correlates of taboo thoughts (e.g., "I am a terrible person if I have nasty thoughts"; "I should not have weird or gross thoughts"). As a result, the OBQ-CV may be a useful supplement for assessment of thought-action fusion associated with taboo thoughts and/or possibly assessment of the thoughts themselves.

Treatment

As with other OCD subtypes and described in detail later in this book, exposure-based intervention is currently the evidence-based psychosocial treatment with most scientific support for pediatric OCD (Geller et al., 2012). Despite clinician fears that exposures may be difficult, owing to sensitive content (e.g., "exposure tasks feel inappropriate"; Keleher et al., 2020), youth with aggressive (Højgaard et al., 2017), sexual (Fernández de la Cruz et al., 2013; Weidle et al., 2022), and religious (Wu et al., 2018) obsessions respond to exposure-based cognitive behavioral therapy (CBT) at comparable rates to youth with other OCD symptoms (Storch et al., 2007). Nonetheless, developmental considerations may shape how clinicians apply treatment to taboo symptoms.

First, clinicians may need to be especially sensitive to stage of development, and tailor their language to the youth's age and cognitive functioning. The clinician might use gentler language earlier in the treatment process when planning exposures (e.g., "do you ever have thoughts about people getting hurt?") and then use open-ended queries to determine how graphic the thoughts are and what kind of language the youth uses to describe symptoms to determine core fears and exposure targets. Knowledge of the family's context, caregiver expectations and values, and youth's developmental stage is critical so that the clinician can work with the family to determine what exposures may be consistent versus inconsistent. The clinician might also need to query what comprises youth and/or family values versus what is fear-based for the youth (or for caregivers who have difficulty watching their child be distressed).

For example, a five-year-old child who has not received sex education and whose sexual obsessions involve a fear of kissing family members and peers but no other sexual behavior, can engage in exposures related to being near family members and peers, holding hands with family members, and kissing family members on the cheek. Such a child would likely not need sex education or discussion of sex as part of the treatment. In contrast, an older adolescent who has had sex education at school or elsewhere, and whose symptoms include intrusive thoughts about sex with resulting avoidance of being in the same room with their sibling, might ultimately do exposures (near the end of treatment and after lots of slow, graded approach) that involve sitting next to sibling on the couch holdings hands or hugging. In some families, it might even be viewed as acceptable to do exposures where the target teen and their sibling lay in bed or on the couch together to watch a movie or sleep as an exposure at the top of the teen's hierarchy. In a family that is not often physically affectionate, the therapist may work with youth and parent to identify whether physical touch such as hand-holding or hugging is a true violation of morals or values (e.g., religious family where members of opposite genders do not touch) and/or provide psychoeducation about why such exposures might be important to the youth's core obsessions. Without providing reassurance, psychoeducation about what does versus does not constitute sex may also be relevant. All of this might be done without violating a caregiver's belief that their teen should not be sexually active.

More broadly, psychoeducation and rationale for exposures may need to be reviewed frequently throughout treatment, and potentially as frequently as each session. Ideally, in treatment both the youth and caregiver(s) would have a clear understanding about why specific exposures that appear strange or dangerous (e.g., holding knife to therapist's neck allows youth to practice distress tolerance associated with obsessions about stabbing people) are important to long-term functioning (e.g., ultimately, youth could enter the family's kitchen and help with meal preparation). Throughout, the clinician should be aware and regularly assess whether the psychoeducation provided is a form of reassurance-provision and reduces exposure-associated distress for the youth and use removal of reassurance to titrate difficulty of exposures over time.

The clinician should also discuss with youth and family any additional cultural or community factors that might intersect with the content of obsessions, religious and otherwise. As part of these discussions, the clinician should solicit from youth and caregivers their reactions to discussing symptoms, and then use this information to sensitively provide treatment that is consistent with or helps to compromise between the exposure-based approach and the family's values. The clinician may need to seek consultation from religious figureheads that practice in a consistent way with the family's practice, experts in providing gender-affirming care to disentangle taboo thoughts about gender identity and sexual orientation versus a youth exploring or who identifies as gender expansive or sexual minority, and/or experts in racism and microaggressions when the youth is either from a racial/ethnic minority background and/or has intrusive thoughts related to experiences with or fears of racism.

Next, in addition to specific exposure and response prevention for observable/overt compulsions, the clinician should regularly discuss potential neutralizing and other mental compulsions with the youth. The youth should have a firm understanding of how these mental acts only strengthen negative reinforcement of compulsions removing distress, and ultimately may contribute to symptom maintenance and even worsening. Similarly, regular assessment with both youth and family members can reveal reassurance-seeking by the youth and/or reassurance provision and/or accommodation by family members. Some families may have been participating in compulsions or avoidance (e.g., not touching their child because of child's fears of incest) to the point where family participation in compulsions, reassurance-seeking, and other accommodation may have become a "new normal" that inadvertently contributes to symptom maintenance. Distinctions can be made between shame reduction versus reassurance-provision (Visvalingam et al., 2022), where the former aims to increase the youth's disclosure of symptoms but not reduce OCD-related distress and the latter either aims to or secondarily reduces immediate distress associated with obsessions.

Third wave approaches that focus on mindfulness (e.g., mindfulness practice; mindfulness-based stress reduction), acceptance (e.g., acceptance and commitment therapy), and distress tolerance strategies in the context of emotion regulation (e.g., dialectical behavior therapy) may also accompany exposure-based treatment (Guo et al., 2020). In contrast, or perhaps in addition to cognitive strategies, the goal from the third wave perspective is to examine thoughts more objectively and without judging the thoughts or oneself. For example, the mindfulness approach in responding to thoughts might be "a thought is just a thought, and I sometimes have upsetting thoughts. I don't need to respond to every thought I have", which is consistent with classic exposure treatment whereby thoughts might be externalized. Indeed, in our clinical experience, we often find that talking to kids and teens about trying to control, manage, or otherwise mentally respond to thoughts may actually be unnecessary. Instead, the clinician might focus on how the goal of treatment is to support the youth in reducing compulsions and avoidance, which interfere with their ability to legitimately make choices about their behavior that are not based exclusively on fear, distress, or disgust. Said differently, when youth engage in compulsions, or attempt to negotiate with obsessions using neutralizing or other mental techniques, they are responding with fear rather than a true choice about how their behavior might be consistent with their values or people, places, and things that matter to them.

The clinician who is new to treating taboo thoughts or OCD more generally might seek expert consultation from the point of initial assessment and throughout the course of treatment. Clinicians can also review materials prepared by experts, including best practices in CBT for taboo thoughts broadly (Williams et al., 2022), as well as the distinction between sexual obsessions and pedophilia (Bonagura et al., 2022), use of imaginal exposures (Lau-Zhu et al., 2022), and treatment of aggressive obsessions (Milliner-Oar et al., 2015) and scrupulosity (Peris & Rozenman, 2015).

Summary

Taboo thoughts in OCD can include aggressive, sexual, and religious or moral obsessions. These are common in pediatric OCD, with higher rates in adolescence than childhood. Taboo thoughts are often misdiagnosed by medical and mental health providers, and can be associated with shame, fear, and embarrassment for youth and their caregivers. These obsessions can be accompanied by both observable and mental compulsions, as well as significant attempts to avoid, neutralize, or seek reassurance by youth. A range of self- and caregiver-report questionnaires can be administered to supplement the initial clinical interview and for progress monitoring throughout treatment. Assessment and treatment require an understanding of how the family's value system may intersect with symptoms, developmental tailoring of both queries and exposure tasks, and psychoeducation for the family that the taboo thoughts in and of themselves do not signify risk for the youth or others.

References

Abramovitch, A., Abramowitz, J. S., McKay, D., Cham, H., Anderson, K. S., Farrell, L., Geller, D. A., Hanna, G. L., Mathieu, S., McGuire, J. F., Rosenberg, D. R., Stewart, S. E., Storch, E. A., & Wilhelm, S. (2022). The OCI-CV-R: A Revision of the Obsessive-Compulsive Inventory – Child Version. *Journal of Anxiety Disorders*, 86. https://doi.org/10.1016/j.janxdis.2022.102532.

Achenbach, T.M., & Rescorla, L.A. (2001). Manual for the ASEBA School-Age Forms & Profiles. Burlington, VT: University of Vermont, Research Center for Children, Youth, & Families.

Berman, N. C., Shaw, A. M., & Wilhelm, S. (2018). Emotion Regulation in Patients with Obsessive Compulsive Disorder: Unique Effects for Those with "Taboo Thoughts." *Cognitive Therapy and Research*, 42(5). doi:10.1007/s10608-018-9911-z.

Bey, K., Lennertz, L., Riesel, A., Klawohn, J., Kaufmann, C., Heinzel, S., Grützmann, R., Kathmann, N., & Wagner, M. (2017). Harm avoidance and childhood adversities in patients with obsessive–compulsive disorder and their unaffected first-degree relatives. *Acta Psychiatrica Scandinavica*, 135(4). doi:10.1111/acps.12707.

Bloch, M. H., Landeros-Weisenberger, A., Rosario, M. C., Pittenger, C., & Leckman, J. F. (2008). Meta-analysis of the symptom structure of obsessive-compulsive disorder. *The American Journal of Psychiatry*, 165(12), 1532–1542. doi:10.1176/appi.ajp.2008.08020320.

Bonagura, A., Abrams, D., & Teller, J. (2022). Diagnostic Differential Between Pedophilic-OCD and Pedophilic Disorder: An Illustration with Two Vignettes. *Archives of Sexual Behavior*, 51(4). doi:10.1007/s10508-021-02273-5.

Brakoulias, V., Starcevic, V., Berle, D., Milicevic, D., Moses, K., & Hannan, A. (2013). "Pure obsessions" are not so "pure" after all: A description of the characteristics of unacceptable/taboo thoughts in obsessivecompulsive disorder. *Australian and New Zealand Journal of Psychiatry*, 47.

Butwicka, A. & Gmitrowicz, A. (2010). Symptom clusters in obsessive-compulsive disorder (OCD): Influence of age and age of onset. *European Child and Adolescent Psychiatry*, 19(4). doi:10.1007/s00787-009-0055-2.

Cervin, M., Perrin, S., Olsson, E., Claesdotter-Knutsson, E., & Lindvall, M. (2021). Involvement of fear, incompleteness, and disgust during symptoms of pediatric obsessive–compulsive disorder. *European Child and Adolescent Psychiatry*, 30(2). https://doi.org/10.1007/s00787-020-01514-7.

Coles, A. R., Lahey, C. A., Fawcett, E. J., & Fawcett, J. M. (2023). *Overcoming the forbidden: Identification and stigma of unacceptable thoughts in obsessive–compulsive disorder. Stigma and Health.* Advance online publication. https://doi.org/10.1037/sah0000490

Coles, M. E., Wolters, L. H., Sochting, I., De Haan, E., Pietrefesa, A. S., & Whiteside, S. P. (2010). Development and initial validation of the Obsessive Belief Questionnaire-Child Version (OBQ-CV). *Depression and Anxiety*, 27(10). https://doi.org/10.1002/da.20702.

Fernández de la Cruz, L., Barrow, F., Bolhuis, K., Krebs, G., Volz, C., Nakatani, E., Heyman, I., & Mataix-Cols, D. (2013). Sexual obsessions in pediatric obsessive-compulsive disorder: Clinical characteristics and treatment outcomes. *Depression and Anxiety*, 30(8). doi:10.1002/da.22097.

Garcia, A. M., Freeman, J. B., Himle, M. B., Berman, N. C., Ogata, A. K., Ng, J., Choate-Summers, M. L., & Leonard, H. (2009). Phenomenology of early childhood onset obsessive compulsive disorder. *Journal of Psychopathology and Behavioral Assessment*, 31(2). doi:10.1007/s10862-008-9094-0.

Geller, D. A., Biederman, J., Faraone, S., Agranat, A., Cradock, K., Hagermoser, L., Kim, G., Frazier, J., & Coffey, B. J. (2001). Developmental aspects of obsessive compulsive disorder: Findings in children, adolescents, and adults. *Journal of Nervous and Mental Disease*, 189(7). doi:10.1097/00005053-200107000-00009.

Geller, D. A., March, J., Psychiatry, Flament, M., Whitaker, A., Rapoport, J., al., et, Apter, A., Fallon, T. J., King, R. A., al., et, Heyman, I., Fombonne, E., Simmons, H., Ford, T., Meltzer, H., Goodman, R., Geller, D., Biederman, J., … Tolin, D. F., American Academy of Child & Adolescent Psychiatry (2012). Practice Parameter for the Assessment and Treatment of Children and Adolescents With Obsessive-Compulsive Disorder. *Journal of the American Academy of Child & Adolescent Psychiatry*, 51(1), 98–113. doi:10.1016/j.jaac.2011.09.019.

Glazier, K., Swing, M., & McGinn, L. K. (2015). Half of obsessive-compulsive disorder cases misdiagnosed: Vignette-based survey of primary care physicians. *Journal of Clinical Psychiatry*, 76(6). doi:10.4088/JCP.14m09110.

Glazier, K. & Wetterneck, C. (2015). Stigma and Shame as Barriers to Treatment for Obsessive-Compulsive and Related Disorders. *Journal of Depression and Anxiety*, 04(03). https://doi.org/10.4172/2167-1044.1000191.

Guo, S., Rozenman, M., Bennett, S. M., Peris, T. S., & Bergman, R. L. (2020). Flexible Adaptation of Evidence-based Treatment Principles and Practices in an Intensive Outpatient Setting for Pediatric OCD. *Https://Doi.Org/10.1080/23794925.2020.1784061*, 5(3), 301–321. doi:10.1080/23794925.2020.1784061.

Halldorsson, B., Salkovskis, P. M., Kobori, O., & Pagdin, R. (2016). I do not know what else to do: Caregivers' perspective on reassurance seeking in OCD. *Journal of Obsessive-Compulsive and Related Disorders*, 8. doi:10.1016/j.jocrd.2015.11.003.

Højgaard, D. R. M. A., Mortensen, E. L., Ivarsson, T., Hybel, K., Skarphedinsson, G., Nissen, J. B., Valderhaug, R., Dahl, K., Weidle, B., Torp, N. C., Grados, M., Lewin, A. B., Melin, K. H., Storch, E. A., Wolters, L. H., Murphy, T. K., Sonuga-Barke, E. J. S., & Thomsen, P. H. (2017). Structure and clinical correlates of obsessive–compulsive symptoms in a large sample of children and adolescents: a factor analytic study across five nations. *European Child and Adolescent Psychiatry*, 26(3). doi:10.1007/s00787-016-0887-5.

Keleher, J., Jassi, A., & Krebs, G. (2020). Clinician-reported barriers to using exposure with response prevention in the treatment of paediatric obsessive-compulsive disorder. *Journal of Obsessive-Compulsive and Related Disorders*, 24. doi:10.1016/j.jocrd.2019.100498.

Lau-Zhu, A., Farrington, A., & Bissessar, C. (2022). Boosting exposure and response prevention with imagery-based techniques: A case study tackling sexual obsessions in an adolescent. *Cognitive Behaviour Therapist*, 15. doi:10.1017/S1754470X22000058.

Mancebo, M. C., Garcia, A. M., Pinto, A., Freeman, J. B., Przeworski, A., Stout, R., Kane, J. S., Eisen, J. L., & Rasmussen, S. A. (2008). Juvenile-onset OCD: clinical features in children, adolescents and adults. *Acta Psychiatrica Scandinavica*, 118(2), 149–159. doi:10.1111/j.1600-0447.2008.01224.x.

Masi, G., Millepiedi, S., Perugi, G., Pfanner, C., Berloffa, S., Pari, C., Mucci, M., & Akiskal, H. S. (2010). A naturalistic exploratory study of the impact of demographic, phenotypic and comorbid features in pediatric obsessive-compulsive disorder. *Psychopathology*, 43(2), 69–78. doi:10.1159/000274175.

Mataix-Cols, D., Nakatani, E., Micali, N., & Heyman, I. (2008). Structure of Obsessive-Compulsive Symptoms in Pediatric OCD. *Journal of the American Academy of Child & Adolescent Psychiatry*, 47(7), 773–778. doi:10.1097/CHI.0B013E31816B73C0.

Milliner-Oar, E. L., Cadman, J. H., & Farrell, L. J. (2015). Treatment of aggressive obsessions in childhood obsessive-compulsive disorder. In *Clinical Handbook of Obsessive-Compulsive and Related Disorders: A Case-Based Approach to Treating Pediatric and Adult Populations*. doi:10.1007/978-3-319-17139-5_11.

Nissen, J. B., Højgaard, D. R. M. A., & Thomsen, P. H. (2020). The immediate effect of COVID-19 pandemic on children and adolescents with obsessive compulsive disorder. *BMC Psychiatry*, 20(1). doi:10.1186/s12888-020-02905-5.

Perez, M. I., Limon, D. L., Candelari, A. E., Cepeda, S. L., Ramirez, A. C., Guzick, A. G., Kook, M., La Buissonniere Ariza, V., Schneider, S. C., Goodman, W. K., & Storch, E. A. (2022). Obsessive-compulsive disorder misdiagnosis among mental healthcare providers in Latin America. *Journal of*

Obsessive-Compulsive and Related Disorders, 32. doi:10.1016/j. jocrd.2021.100693.

Peris, T. S., Bergman, R. L., Langley, A., Chang, S., McCracken, J. T., & Piacentini, J. (2008). Correlates of accommodation of pediatric obsessive-compulsive disorder: parent, child, and family characteristics. *Journal of the American Academy of Child and Adolescent Psychiatry*, 47, 1173–1181. doi:10.1016/S0084-3954(09)79526-0.

Peris, T. S. & Rozenman, M. (2015). Treatment of scrupulosity in childhood obsessive-compulsive disorder. In *Clinical Handbook of Obsessive-Compulsive and Related Disorders: A Case-Based Approach to Treating Pediatric and Adult Populations*. doi:10.1007/978-3-319-17139-5_10.

Rees, C. S., Draper, M., & Davis, M. C. (2010). The Relationship Between Magical Thinking, Thought-Action Fusion and Obsessive-Compulsive Symptoms. *International Journal of Cognitive Therapy*, 3(3), 304–311. https://doi.org/10.1521/ijct. 2010.3.3.304.

Rozenman, M., Peris, T., Bergman, R. L., Chang, S., O'Neill, J., McCracken, J. T., & Piacentini, J. (2017). Distinguishing Fear Versus Distress Symptomatology in Pediatric OCD. *Child Psychiatry and Human Development*, 48(1). doi:10.1007/ s10578-016-0653-4.

Scahill, L., Riddle, M. A., McSwiggin-Hardin, M., Ort, S. I., King, R. A., Goodman, W. K., Cicchetti, D., & Leckman, J. F. (1997). Children's Yale-Brown Obsessive Compulsive Scale: reliability and validity. *Journal of the American Academy of Child and Adolescent Psychiatry*, 36(6), 844–852. doi:10.1097/ 00004583-199706000-00023.

Stewart, S. E., Rosario, M. C., Baer, L., Carter, A. S., Brown, T. A., Scharf, J. M., Illmann, C., Leckman, J. F., Sukhodolsky, D., Katsovich, L., Rasmussen, S., Goodman, W., Delorme, R., Leboyer, M., Chabane, N., Jenike, M. A., Geller, D. A., & Pauls, D. L. (2008). Four-factor structure of obsessive-compulsive disorder symptoms in children, adolescents, and adults. *Journal of the American Academy of Child and Adolescent Psychiatry*, 47(7), 763–772. doi:10.1097/ CHI.0b013e318172ef1e.

Storch, E. A., Bussing, R., Jacob, M. L., Nadeau, J. M., Crawford, E., Mutch, P. J., Mason, D., Lewin, A. B., & Murphy, T. K. (2015). Frequency and Correlates of Suicidal Ideation in Pediatric Obsessive–Compulsive Disorder. *Child Psychiatry and Human Development*, 46(1). doi:10.1007/s10578-014-0453-7.

Storch, E. A., Khanna, M., Merlo, L. J., Loew, B. A., Franklin, M., Reid, J. M., Goodman, W. K., & Murphy, T. K. (2009). Children's Florida obsessive compulsive inventory: Psychometric properties and feasibility of a self-report measure of obsessive-compulsive symptoms in youth. *Child Psychiatry and Human Development*, 40(3). doi:10.1007/s10578-009-0138-9.

Storch, E. A., Larson, M. J., Muroff, J., Caporino, N., Geller, D., Reid, J. M., Morgan, J., Jordan, P., & Murphy, T. K. (2010). Predictors of functional impairment in pediatric obsessive-compulsive disorder. *Journal of Anxiety Disorders*, 24(2), 275–283. doi:10.1016/j.janxdis.2009.12.004.

Storch, E. A., McGuire, J. F., Wu, M. S., Hamblin, R., McIngvale, E., Cepeda, S. L., Schneider, S. C., Rufino, K. A., Rasmussen, S. A., Price, L. H., & Goodman, W. K. (2019). Development and Psychometric Evaluation of the Children's Yale-Brown Obsessive-Compulsive Scale Second Edition. *Journal of the*

American Academy of Child and Adolescent Psychiatry, 58(1). doi:10.1016/j. jaac.2018.05.029.

Storch, E. A., Merlo, L. J., Larson, M. J., Bloss, C. S., Geffken, G. R., Jacob, M. L., Murphy, T. K., & Goodman, W. K. (2007). Symptom dimensions and cognitive-behavioural therapy outcome for pediatric obsessive-compulsive disorder. *Acta Psychiatrica Scandinavica*, 0(0), 071106215000001-?. doi:10.1111/j.1600-0447.2007.01113.x.

Torres, A. R., Ramos-Cerqueira, A. T. A., Ferrão, Y. A., Fontenelle, L. F., Do Rosário, M. C., & Miguel, E. C. (2011). Suicidality in obsessive-compulsive disorder: Prevalence and relation to symptom dimensions and comorbid conditions. *Journal of Clinical Psychiatry*, 72(1). doi:10.4088/JCP.09m05651blu.

Uher, R., Heyman, I., Turner, C. M., & Shafran, R. (2008). Self-, parent-report and interview measures of obsessive-compulsive disorder in children and adolescents. *Journal of Anxiety Disorders*, 22(6). doi:10.1016/j.janxdis.2007.10.001.

Veale, D., Freeston, M., Krebs, G., Heyman, I., & Salkovskis, P. (2009). Risk assessment and management in obsessive-compulsive disorder. In *Advances in Psychiatric Treatment*, 15(5). doi:10.1192/apt.bp.107.004705.

Visvalingam, S., Crone, C., Street, S., Oar, E. L., Gilchrist, P., & Norberg, M. M. (2022). The causes and consequences of shame in obsessive-compulsive disorder. *Behaviour Research and Therapy*, 151. doi:10.1016/j.brat.2022.104064.

Weidle, B., Skarphedinsson, G., Højgaard, D. R. M. A., Thomsen, P. H., Torp, N. C., Melin, K., & Ivarsson, T. (2022). Sexual obsessions in children and adolescents: Prevalence, clinical correlates, response to cognitive-behavior therapy and long-term follow up. *Journal of Obsessive-Compulsive and Related Disorders*, 32. doi:10.1016/j.jocrd.2022.100708.

Williams, M. T. & Jahn, M. E. (2017). Obsessive-compulsive disorder in African American children and adolescents: Risks, resiliency, and barriers to treatment. *American Journal of Orthopsychiatry*, 87(3). doi:10.1037/ort0000188.

Williams, M. T., Whittal, M. L., & La Torre, J. (2022). Best practices for CBT treatment of taboo and unacceptable thoughts in OCD. *Cognitive Behaviour Therapist*, 15(5). doi:10.1017/S1754470X22000113.

Wu, M. S., Rozenman, M., Peris, T. S., O'Neill, J., Bergman, R. L., Chang, S., & Piacentini, J. (2018). Comparing OCD-affected youth with and without religious symptoms: Clinical profiles and treatment response. *Comprehensive Psychiatry*. doi:10.1016/j.comppsych.2018.07.009.

6 Sensory Dysregulation in Obsessive-Compulsive-Related Disorders

David C. Houghton

Introduction

Obsessive-compulsive related disorders (OCRDs) are generally conceptualized as fear-based and impulse-control disorders, in which the
pathology is attributed to maladaptive cognitions, difficulty regulating
emotions, and impaired self-control. These "top-down" conceptualizations
dominate most theoretical models of OCD. However, potentially important "bottom-up" processes have been identified, which may help inform
neurodevelopmental models of OCD. From as far back as 1903, Pierre
Janet's early account of obsessive-compulsive disorder (OCD) described
the foundation of the illness as a psychasthenic state characterized by
feelings of 'incompleteness' (Pitman, 1987). Janet depicted incompleteness
as a chronic sense of perceptual unease in which the imperfections of the
world feel intolerable and states of uniformity and order are constantly
sought. While Janet's model fell out of favor among theorists for nearly a
century, findings from recent research warrant reconsideration. A growing
body of research has indeed documented abnormal sensory phenomena in
OCRDs including OCD as well as chronic tic disorder (CTD), body-
focused repetitive behaviors (BFRBs) (e.g., trichotillomania, excoriation
disorder), body dysmorphic disorder (BDD), and health anxiety disorder
(HAD). Evidence suggests these experiences are not epi-phenomenal, but
rather that dysregulation of sensory and perceptual processes may precede
the clinical onset of OCRDs, have significant influence on symptom
expression, and therefore may represent a key neurodevelopmental component of OCRD etiology.

Premonitory urges

Although many compulsive behavior symptoms of OCRDs are preceded
by cognitive or affective events, some are completed without any explicit
reason or justification. This is especially the case in children and adolescents, who are still developing insight and meta-cognition (Lewin et al.,
2010), or the ability to identify and describe their own thoughts. Instead,

DOI: 10.4324/9781003517429-6

affected persons describe a vague somatic "urge", "craving", or "desire" to engage in the compulsion, which is often difficult to tolerate or resist. This is most clearly seen in CTD, as tics are purposeless behaviors that lack obsessional precursors. Persons with CTDs frequently describe "premonitory urges" that precede tics and are temporarily alleviated upon tic execution (Banaschewski et al., 2003; Leckman et al., 1993). Accordingly, theorists posited that premonitory urges may act as negative reinforcers and represent a key factor maintaining tic symptoms. Since the identification of premonitory urges as potentially important aspects of CTDs, research has likewise identified similar premonitory urge phenomena in other OCRDs. These will be discussed in the following sections.

Obsessive-Compulsive Disorder (OCD)

Many individuals with OCD report experiencing abnormal sensory phenomena and premonitory urges that instigate symptoms. In fact, even "cognitive" obsessions in OCD are known to often contain rich sensory features (Porth & Geller, 2018), such as in cases where contamination fears and washing compulsions are brought on, owing to physical sensations that one's hands are "dirty" or "greasy" (Lapidus et al., 2014; Olatunji et al., 2007; Shapira et al., 2003; Stein et al., 2001). Explicit sensory experiences and urges that occur outside of cognitive obsessions are described in a variety of ways, including "not just right" experiences (Coles et al., 2003; Diniz et al., 2006; Ecker & Gönner, 2008; Ghisi et al., 2010; Leckman et al., 1994; Lee et al., 2009; Moretz & McKay, 2009; Summers et al., 2014), feelings of "incompleteness" (Ecker & Gönner, 2008; Ghisi et al., 2010; Pietrefesa & Coles, 2009; Pitman, 1987; Summerfeldt, 2004), and somatic urges for action (da Silva Prado et al., 2008; Ferrao et al., 2012; Miguel et al., 2000). "Not just right" experiences (NJREs) reflect an inner feeling that something is wrong, uncertain, or not under control, which must be corrected. "Incompleteness" experiences are similar to NJREs, often reflecting an inner feeling that something is wrong and that one must perform a compulsion or ritual until achieving a sense of completion (Pietrefesa & Coles, 2009; Pitman, 1987). Premonitory urges in OCD come in many forms and resemble those from CTDs, having been described as aversive bodily sensations (e.g., tension) or energy surges (da Silva Prado et al., 2008; Ferrao et al., 2012; Miguel et al., 2000; Rosario et al., 2009). These different types of sensory and/or urge phenomena are often referred to interchangeably. Although NJREs are common among non-clinical, healthy individuals (Coles et al., 2003; Ghisi et al., 2010) and are found in non-OCRD pathologies such as anxiety disorders (Fergus, 2014), most evidence suggests a strong relationship between NJREs and OCD (Cervin et al., 2020; Coles et al., 2003; Sica et al., 2015; Summers et al., 2014). Indeed, one study found that NJREs were the strongest feature differentiating youth with OCD from youth with anxiety disorders (Cervin et al., 2021). There is mixed data regarding the prevalence of NJREs and similar sensory phenomena in adult OCD patients (Ghisi et al., 2010; Leckman et al., 1994; Shavitt et al., 2014; Sibrava et al., 2016). However, some evidence suggests NJREs are more common in childhood OCD than adult-onset OCD (Ferrao et al., 2012). It is important to note that OCD patients are significantly bothered by sensory-related obsessions and premonitory urges, as many report greater distress and impairment from these experiences as compared to cognitive obsessions and compulsive behaviors (da Silva Prado et al., 2008; Ferrao et al., 2012).

Chronic Tic Disorders (CTD)

As previously mentioned, premonitory urges are widely recognized as important contributors to CTDs. Evidence shows that most CTD patients (~90 percent) report some type of premonitory urge experience, however children report urges less frequently (Leckman et al., 1993) and the prevalence of urges increases with age (Sambrani et al., 2016) (discussed later in Chapter). The urge often occurs in the same body area as the tic it precedes, but they can be felt as generalized across the whole body (Miguel et al., 1995). A significant portion of persons with CTDs also report NJREs and feelings of incompleteness, with estimates ranging between 30–90 percent (Leckman et al., 1994; Miguel et al., 2000; Neal & Cavanna, 2013).

Body-Focused Repetitive Behaviors (BFRBs)

Tracing back to early behavior analytic studies in youth, BFRBs have long been understood to be triggered by sensory experiences and maintained by sensory feedback (Miltenberger et al., 1998; Rapp et al., 1999; Williams et al., 2007). Sensory cues for hair pulling and skin picking include visual and tactile sensations, such as undesired colors (e.g., coarse hairs, blemishes) or other aesthetic qualities (e.g., rough skin imperfections or "out of place" hair) (Grant et al., 2007; Mansueto et al., 1997; Snorrason et al., 2015; Snorrason et al., 2019; Snorrason et al., 2010; Wilhelm & Margraf, 1993). Additionally, a recent study documented heightened incompleteness experiences in persons with skin picking disorder (Ricketts et al., 2021). Upon symptom completion, most individuals report experiencing a sense of pleasure, gratification, or relief (Bohne et al., 2005; Christenson et al., 1991; Keuthen et al., 2000; Meunier et al., 2009; Tucker et al., 2011; Woods et al., 2006). Our understanding of premonitory urge phenomena in BFRBs is limited, particularly in children. However, case reports show that affected youth experience urge phenomena (Pinto et al., 2017; Swedo & Rapoport, 1991), and the incidence of affected youth reporting urge phenomena appears to increase with age (Panza et al., 2013; Schumer et al., 2015) until the experience is nearly universal (~80 percent) in affected adults (Dieringer et al., 2019).

Body Dysmorphic Disorder (BDD)

BDD is a characterized by a disruption of healthy body image wherein affected individuals obsess over a perceived flaw in their physical appearance and engage in compulsive rituals designed to disguise or eliminate the perceived flaw (e.g., mirror checking, excessive grooming, make-up application, reassurance seeking). BDD typically onsets during early adolescence (Phillips et al., 2005), coinciding with developmentally appropriate increases in interest toward sexual attraction and body aesthetics. Urges to engage in appearance checking or modification have not been identified in BDD, but persons with BDD do exhibit visual abnormalities related to distortions of self-perception (Li et al., 2013). BDD has also been associated with NJREs and feelings of incompleteness. A study by Summers and colleagues found that (a) persons with BDD experience more severe NJREs than healthy individuals; (b) there is a positive correlation between severity of incompleteness/NJREs and BDD symptoms; and (c) physiological reactivity in response to a task designed to elicit body concerns was positively correlated with incompleteness severity (Summers et al., 2017). Furthermore, that research group found that individuals with BDD exhibit greater discomfort than healthy controls when exposed to appearance-related (i.e., drawing of a man with crooked facial features) and non-appearance-related visual NJRE stimuli (i.e., a cluttered table).

Health Anxiety Disorder

Health anxiety disorder (HAD) is characterized by persistent preoccupation with bodily sensations, which are deemed abnormal or pathogenic, and a resulting conviction that one has or might have a serious medical problem. Very little research has been conducted on HAD in youth, but the disorder certainly affects persons across the lifespan (Wright & Asmundson, 2003). Urge phenomena have not been documented in HAD. However, studies have consistently linked HAD to excessive focus on and misinterpretation of bodily sensations, with affected persons experiencing normal body sensations as more intense or more aversive than healthy individuals (Barsky & Klerman, 1983). Theorists have speculated that the somatic amplification of body signals in BDD is due to misattribution (i. e., stomach tension being misinterpreted as pain), or cognitive biases toward illness. However, there may also be some perceptual abnormality that supports amplification of body signals in HAD.

Altered Sensation and Perception in OCRDs

Interoception

Interoception refers to the process by which one detects, integrates, and interprets internal body sensations (Craig, 2002; Khalsa et al., 2018; Tsakiris & Critchley, 2016). Appropriate awareness of body sensations is critical for maintaining homeostasis as well as selecting and executing adaptive behaviors. Indeed, interoceptive dysfunction is thought to exert widespread negative effects on a variety of psychological processes such as attention, decision-making, and emotion (Craig, 2002). In children, abnormally increased cardiac sensitivity has been linked to anxiety symptoms (Eley et al., 2004), while decreased cardiac sensitivity has been linked to obesity and picky eating (Koch & Pollatos, 2014; Mata et al., 2015). Research has furthermore documented a range of abnormal interoceptive processes across psychiatric populations that overlap and co-occur with OCRDs, including autism spectrum disorder, attention-deficit/hyperactivity disorder, feeding and eating disorders, and oppositional defiant disorder (Brewer et al., 2021; Gourley et al., 2013; Pollatos et al., 2008).

In OCRDs, a vast majority of research has been conducted in adults, but interoceptive abnormalities have been reported consistently. Objective investigations using heartbeat detection tasks and similar methods have consistently found reduced interoceptive accuracy across OCRDs (Barsky et al., 1995; Demartini et al., 2021; Ganos et al., 2015; Krautwurst et al., 2014; Krautwurst et al., 2016; Kunstman et al., 2016; Lazarov et al., 2014; Pile et al., 2018; Pratt, 2014; Rae et al., 2019; Schultchen et al., 2019; Tyrer et al., 1980). Obsessive-compulsive traits in non-clinical populations have also been linked to reduced propensity to utilize interoceptive signals to gauge arousal (Lazarov et al., 2010), suggesting OCRDs may be associated with deficient interoceptive accuracy and increased reliance on external proxies. In contrast, research generally indicates that persons with OCRDs appraise bodily sensations as overly intense or threatening (Deacon & Abramowitz, 2006; Eng et al., 2020), with self-report studies documenting perceived increases in interoceptive sensitivity in OCD (Eng et al., 2020; Jokić & Purić, 2021), CTD (Eddy et al., 2014; Rae et al., 2019), BFRBs (Teng et al., 2002; Woods et al., 1996), BDD (Grunewald et al., 2023), and HAD (Krautwurst et al., 2016). These findings suggest that certain, danger-related interoceptive signals may be exaggerated in OCRDs, owing possibly to hyperarousal and/or fear-related attentional bias.

Exteroception

The perception of environmental stimuli, or exteroception, has received less attention than interoception for its role in OCRDs and other child psychopathologies. Still, extant data generally indicate that some children exhibit markedly elevated reactivity to and avoidance of benign environ-mental stimuli (e.g., sock seams, perfumes) (Dunn & Westman, 1997). Children who exhibit sensory hypersensitivity appear to have elevated risk for psychiatric disorders, particularly anxiety disorders, attentional dis-orders, and disruptive behavior disorders (Andersson et al., 2008; Bar-Shalita et al., 2008; Conelea et al., 2014; Gourley et al., 2013; Gouze et al., 2009; Keuler et al., 2011; Perez-Robles et al., 2013). However, there is at least one conflicting report showing no association between childhood sensory abnormalities and psychopathology (Van Hulle et al., 2012).

Similar to findings related to self-reported interoception, research has consistently revealed self-reported increases in sensitivity to external sti-muli in OCRDs including OCD (Ben-Sasson & Podoly, 2017; Cervin, 2023; Dar et al., 2012; Lewin et al., 2015; Rieke & Anderson, 2009), CTDs (Cohen & Leckman, 1992; Isaacs et al., 2020; Ludlow & Wilkins, 2016; Soler et al., 2019), BFRBs (Falkenstein et al., 2018; Houghton et al., 2018), and HAD (Barsky & Wyshak, 1990; Barsky et al., 1990). To my knowledge, no study has examined external sensory sensitivity in BDD, but there is evidence of enhanced aesthetic sensitivity and atten-tion to detail (Kaplan et al., 2013; Madsen et al., 2013). There also appears to be a high degree of overlap between emergent conditions characterized by sensory intolerance (e.g., Misophonia, "Sensory Proces-sing Disorder") and OCRDs, as studies have documented elevated rates of OCRDs among samples of patients with sensory intolerance (Smith et al., 2022; Taylor et al., 2014; Wu et al., 2014), including among child-hood samples (Van Hulle et al., 2019). Yet, investigations of external sensory sensitivity utilizing objective measurement tools largely mirror those from investigations of interoceptive sensitivity. Several studies found no evidence of abnormal sensory thresholds in OCRDs (Barsky et al., 1995; Belluscio et al., 2011; Güçlü et al., 2015; Haenen et al., 2010; Puts et al., 2015) or altered pain thresholds/tolerance (Blum et al., 2017; Grant et al., 2017; Lautenbacher et al., 1998). However, a minority of studies have reported anomalous findings such as decreased tactile detection thresholds in BFRBs (Houghton et al., 2019) and HAD (Rodic et al., 2016), poor olfaction in OCD (Segalas et al., 2011) and CTD (Kronenbuerger et al., 2018), as well as increased physiologic reactivity and slow habituation to aversive external stimulation in OCD (Janik et al., 2018; Podoly et al., 2022).

Models of sensory dysregulation in OCRDs

Currently available evidence shows that symptoms of OCRDs are fre-quently maintained by sensory phenomena such as premonitory urges, that persons with OCRDs perceive themselves to be abnormally sensitive to interoceptive and exteroceptive signals, but that there is little evidence for objective physiological sensory abnormalities. Given these mixed findings, it is presently unclear whether abnormal sensory experiences in OCRDs are functionally significant and related to a causal etiologic mechanism. However, there are several promising explanations for various sensory phenomena in OCRDs, which collectively point to disruptions in sensory processing and integration between top-down cognitive influences and bottom-up sensory afferents.

Sensory Gating

Although few studies have identified objective sensory abnormalities in OCRDs such as reduced detection thresholds or heightened interoceptive awareness, research has consistently identified one objective sensory deficit among OCRDs. Sensory gating is an adaptive process in which some sensory information is selectively inhibited before reaching conscious awareness, which is believed to sharpen perception, conserve attentional resources, and enhance focus on relevant sensory information while mitigating background noise. Indeed, the peripheral nervous system has an immense sum of sensory receptors that are rarely, if ever, at complete rest, meaning they are constantly conveying afferent sensory messages to the brain. The brain then must decipher information from torrents of afferent sensory inputs that occur in complex temporal patterns. If some filtering of sensory inputs did not occur, one would be overwhelmed with cascades of mostly irrelevant information, which would likely impede perception, attention, cognitive operations, and adaptive behavior. Furthermore, adaptive sensory gating appears to mature as children age (Davies et al., 2009), suggesting that developmental adversities may hinder gating efficiency and increase risk for psychopathology.

Faulty sensory gating has been closely tied to psychotic-spectrum disorders (McGhie & Chapman, 1961; Patterson et al., 2008), attentional disorders (Micoulaud-Franchi et al., 2019; Micoulaud-Franchi et al., 2015), as well as "sensory processing disorders" (SPDs) (Davies et al., 2009). SPDs are a purported childhood-onset disorder characterized by excessive (or reduced) exteroceptive sensitivity (Houghton et al., 2020) (discussed below). Reduced gating has also been documented in OCRDs, including OCD (Hashimoto et al., 2008; Rossi et al., 2005; Xiao et al., 2010), CTDs (Castellanos et al., 1996; Swerdlow et al., 2001; Zebardast et al., 2013), BFRBs (Houghton et al., 2019), and BDD (Giannopoulos et al., 2021; Kapsali et al., 2020). No research has yet linked sensory gating to HAD, but experts have posited a role for deficient gating among persons with HAD and similar somatoform disorders (Boutros & Peters, 2012). Impaired sensory gating may contribute to symptoms of OCRDs by allowing excessive irrelevant sensory afferent information to reach conscious awareness, which results in feelings of over-inundation (i. e., hypersensitivity) and difficulty habituating to stimulation. Over-stimulation does tend to elicit compensatory behaviors designed to distract from aversive inputs and replace such discomforts with more pleasurable stimuli (Dunn, 2001), and others have suggested that faulty sensory gating could disrupt action selection and suppression of unwanted behaviors (Koziol et al., 2011).

Models of premonitory urges

Substantial evidence indicates that premonitory urges are governed by activity in limbic sensory and motor areas, specifically the insular and cingulate cortices (Jackson et al., 2011). Indeed, Jackson and colleagues demonstrated that neural substrates of premonitory urges in CTDs align closely with those of normal urges for action from our everyday lives (e.g., urge to yawn). The role of the insula in generating urges for action, as well as pathological urges to engage in compulsive behavior, was most clearly demonstrated in a study that found insula lesions among nicotine addicts were associated with a complete elimination of the urge to smoke (Naqvi & Bechara, 2009; Naqvi et al., 2007). Unfortunately, this neurobiological account for premonitory urges fails to explain the development of premonitory urges in OCRDs.

Behavioral models of the development of premonitory urges are generally based on the notion that tension reduction, or negative reinforcement, maintains the urge-tic relationship. This is generally supported by reinforced tic suppression studies in which tic rate increases when urges are strong, urge strength increases during tic suppression, and urge strength attenuates during free-to-tic conditions (Brandt et al., 2016; Houghton et al., 2014; Langelage et al., 2022). However, the negative reinforcement hypothesis does not account for the fact that premonitory urges are not always present when tics first emerge in childhood (Sambrani et al., 2016; Woods et al., 2005). Tic typically onset around ages 6–7, whereas awareness of premonitory urges can emerge up to three years after tic onset (Banaschewski et al., 2003; Leckman et al., 1993). Woods and colleagues proposed that urges may be present in young children with CTDs, but that younger children cannot reliably notice and describe the urge experience (Woods et al., 2005). This is supported by research showing that interoceptive abilities typically do not fully develop until the ages of 5.8–7.8 years (Sigmundsson et al., 2000). Indeed, recent findings suggest that 80–95 percent of children with CTDs experience some degree of a premonitory urge experience (Openneer et al., 2020). Because sensory experiences can be made conscious or more salient through learning (Cameron, 2001), perhaps the sequelae of tics (e.g., change in proprioception, distraction, pain, teasing) provide the feedback necessary to increase awareness toward private sensations that precede tics. Upon becoming aware that some internal sensation exists prior to the tic, the urge then transitions from a benign experience with no functional significance to one that is functionally linked to the tic and tic-related consequences (e.g., discomfort, distraction, teasing). Finally, just as other benign stimuli can acquire aversive valence when such stimuli predict a negative outcome (Kamin et al., 1963; Rescorla & Solomon, 1967), the urge then acquires an aversive valence, and escape from the urge becomes reinforcing. This conceptualization is supported by studies showing that premonitory urges are associated with neural activation of regions involved in negative affect and punishment-based learning (Wang et al., 2011), as well as data showing that urge severity is associated with indices of functional and social impairment (Woods et al., 2005) and peer victimization (Zinner et al., 2012).

Taken together, premonitory urges for compulsive behaviors may be universally present as signals of impending action, but as compulsive behavior symptoms become intrusive and individuals attempt to predict and suppress such actions, urges acquire aversive valence and become functionally tied to symptoms. Premonitory urges can thus be considered "normal", in that they mirror common urges for action, but only because they signal the emergence of undesired symptoms do they acquire aversive valence. In the next section, the process through which benign interoceptive signals can intensify and become aversive is discussed.

The "alliesthesia" and somatosensory amplification models

Some have suggested that abnormal sensory experiences in OCRDs could be caused by a pathogenic integration between higher-order cognitive processes and lower-order perceptual afferents (Paulus & Stein, 2010). Specifically, Paulus and Stein argued that fear-based disorders (e.g., anxiety, OCD, BDD, HAD) are characterized by negatively biased internal cognitive models that facilitate hypervigilance to potential threats (Stein & Nesse, 2011), translating to hyper-attention toward sensory stimuli that may signal danger. Similarly, persistent hypervigilance to threat appears to be tied to evolutionary processes related to early threat detection and precautionary responses. By means of a process known as alliesthesia (Cabanac, 1971), the internal condition of an individual is intertwined with external stimuli that impact the internal environment, causing stimuli to acquire an emotional significance based on their perceived pleasantness or unpleasantness. The central and peripheral nervous systems of the body continuously transmit a stream of noisy and unclear sensory inputs that require integration and interpretation. Individuals who are vigilant for threats tend to perceive stimuli with negative emotional impact as more intense, as these stimuli could potentially indicate danger. Coupled with faulty sensory gating and an increase in the amount of irrelevant information reaching conscious awareness, affected persons may constantly struggle to interpret the threat relevance of various ambiguous suprathreshold stimuli. Consequently, ambiguous stimuli have the potential to trigger anxious catastrophizing, whereby a seemingly harmless sensory encounter (e.g., a buzzing noise) is perceived as unusually intense or even catastrophic (e.g., "There might be a swarm of bees in this room!").

Perhaps this model could be extended beyond the mischaracterization of threat-related stimuli in anxiety/OCD/HAD/BDD and into other OCRDs such as BFRBs and CTDs. Indeed, arguments have been made for the role of alliesthesia, threat prediction, and reward anticipation in similar compulsive behavior disorders, drug addiction. Paulus and Stewart (Paulus & Stewart, 2014) argued that persons with substance use disorders encounter an "embodied" experience, similar to craving, that is subserved by frequent errors between their predicted versus actual body state (e.g., "elated" versus "tense"). Furthermore, an innovative study utilizing a bayesian computational model of neurophysiological data from individuals with various psychopathologies (i.e., anxiety, depression, substance use disorders, and eating disorders) found increased interoceptive error rates across all pathologies as compared to controls during interoceptive challenge (a combined breath-holding and heartbeat-counting task) (Smith et al., 2020). It could therefore be that compulsive tics and BFRBs are associated with a similar interoceptive reward-prediction error, specifically related to proprioceptive, visceral, and dermatological sensations.

Unfortunately, the models proposed by Paulus and colleagues have been concerned with interoception and do not deliver an account of exteroceptive hypersensitivity. Yet, from the perspective of health anxiety and similar unexplained medical symptom disorders (i.e., conversion disorder, somatization disorders, psychogenic non-epileptic seizures), experts have explored how the intensity of both internal and external sensory experiences can be amplified, even in the absence of objective differences in sensory thresholds (Barsky & Wyshak, 1990; Köteles & Witthöft, 2017). Somatosensory amplification refers to the notion that a combination of body hypervigilance and strong emotional reactivity to sensation can result in the intensification of certain sensory experiences. This concept shares many similarities with other models of medically unexplained symptoms such as central sensitization in chronic pain. Because external stimuli can affect the internal milieu, it stands to reason that certain environmental exposures (i.e., a strange smell) can trigger health worries and undergo amplification. This has important theoretical implications for emerging conditions that overlap with OCRDs, namely SPDs and "idiopathic environmental intolerances" (IEI). As has been discussed in other reviews (Houghton et al., 2020), children with sensory processing disorders almost universally express elevated symptoms of OCRDs and anxiety, thus suggesting that environmental hypersensitivity in sensory processing disorders could result from top-down amplification of sensory inputs. Likewise, controversial conditions characterized by IEI such as misophonia (selective sound sensitivity), multiple chemical (olfactory) sensitivity, and electromagnetic sensitivity share many characteristics with OCRDs and could potentially be conceptualized under this model. Support for this notion comes from data indicating that top-down belief systems significantly influence IEI symptom expression. For example, in persons with purported electromagnetic sensitivity, their actual exposure to electromagnetism does not influence symptom severity (Rubin et al., 2010), but perceived electromagnetism exposure does influence symptoms (Szemerszky et al., 2015; Witthöft & Rubin, 2013)

Issues for further investigation

This chapter has provided evidence for premonitory urge phenomena as well as subjective increases in sensitivity to interoceptive and exteroceptive stimuli. I also discussed several preliminary models for sensory dysregulation in OCRDs. Yet, this area of research is still early stages, with many unanswered questions and untested assumptions. The following sections will detail several important avenues for further research.

Sensory processing disorders?

As discussed previously and in other reports (Houghton et al., 2020), researchers and clinicians have increasingly argued for the existence of SPDs. These conditions are not recognized by DSM-5 and ICD-11, and it is presently unclear whether these conditions represent valid diagnoses or are best conceptualized as symptom clusters that often co-occur with anxiety-related pathologies and autistic traits. For instance, many children exhibit select hypersensitivities and strong responses to certain stimuli (e. g., food textures, smells, clothing material), which do not necessarily impair functioning and may vanish with age. However, there is some evidence that children with SPDs have objective sensory abnormalities (Bar-Shalita et al., 2009; McIntosh et al., 1999; Schaaf et al., 2003), potentially supporting the validity of SPD as a unique pathology. However, other research points to symptoms of SPDs in children as representing early risk factors for anxiety disorders and related pathologies (Carpenter et al., 2019). For example, a longitudinal twin study in 1,613 children found that the number of tactile or auditory sensory over-responsivity symptoms was positively correlated with likelihood of OCD diagnoses (Van Hulle et al., 2019).

In order to significantly advance research on SPDs and their relationships with OCRDs, future studies ought to take certain steps to maximize impact and interpretability. First, it is crucial that scientists establish consensus in defining the core constructs of sensory psychopathology. Once clear definitions of pathological sensory constructs (e.g., "sensory over-responsivity") and the diagnostic validity of sensory processing disorders have been established, researchers can develop psychometrically valid assessment strategies. Relatedly, future studies ought to utilize both subjective and objective assessment methods and clearly differentiate between the two processes. Objective measures of sensory function sometimes align with self-reported perception (Bar-Shalita et al., 2009), but this is not always the case (Kozak & Miller, 1982). Careful attention to both components of the large sensory processes apparatus should enable more precise conclusions regarding the interplay between conscious feeling states, beliefs, physiological responses to stimulation, and behavior. Finally, the neurophysiological deficits that purportedly underlie SPDs may interact significantly with various environmental factors and comorbidities, such as physical health (e.g., nutrition), neuroendocrine/hormonal processes, motor development, and cognitive and social experiences (i.e., exposure to diverse, highly stimulating environments).

Treatment

While sensory dysregulation has garnered attention as a potential OCRD mechanism, there is little empirical guidance on effective treatments, and the limited but existing evidence suggests the need for further refinement of existing treatments. There are behavioral treatment strategies aimed at children with purported sensory processing disorders, such as "sensory integration therapy". Unfortunately, sensory integration therapy has not undergone rigorous clinical trials, and existing evidence points to questionable efficacy (Complementary et al., 2012). Cognitive-behavioral therapies for OCRDs, which boast considerable empirical support, have been investigated regarding effects on patients who exhibit sensory dysregulation. A meta-analysis of CBT for incompleteness symptoms in OCD found that incompleteness was modestly improved over the course of treatment, with stronger effect sizes noted for treatments that explicitly targeted incompleteness (Schwartz, 2018). In contrast, other studies have shown that NJREs and incompleteness symptoms are associated with poor OCD treatment outcomes (Cervin & Perrin, 2021; Nissen & Parner, 2018). Given these data, there is a clear need to further investigate the efficacy of CBT-based interventions for sensory components of OCRDs.

There is perhaps room for innovative new treatment methodologies that are agnostic to diagnosis but instead aim directly at sensory dysregulation. One example of such an approach is known as Flotation-REST (Reduced Environmental Stimulation Therapy), which involves using sensory deprivation in a saltwater floatation chamber to encourage mindfulness meditation and relaxation. Early data point to robust anxiolytic effects of Flotation-REST (Feinstein et al., 2018), as well as improvements in interoceptive awareness (Feinstein et al., 2018) and decreased functional connectivity within somatomotor and default mode networks (Al Zoubi et al., 2021). Other potential treatment avenues include non-invasive neuromodulation, particularly targeting the insula

(Ibrahim et al., 2019). However, preliminary investigation of insular neuromodulation via transcranial magnetic stimuli showed treatment-related decreases in interoceptive accuracy but increases in perceptual confidence (Pollatos et al., 2016). It is currently unclear how such treatment effects would translate into OCRD patients and whether approaches that are suitable for adults would exhibit similar efficacy in youth.

Summary

Research reviewed in the current chapter demonstrates that symptoms of many OCRDs are instigated by sensory phenomena, affected individuals exhibit subjective sensory abnormalities, but that sensory abnormalities are not necessarily caused by objective sensory deficits. However, there is evidence for more subtle sensory gating abnormalities and disrupted sensory integration processes in OCRDs. Taken together, this evidence shows that sensory dysregulation is a potentially important component of OCRD psychopathology. It is therefore unsurprising that research in this area is growing at a rapid pace, and hopefully we will receive significant new insights that will help develop a more comprehensive understanding of how sensory dysregulation interacts with other risk factors and etiological mechanisms. Within these efforts, there is a clear need for additional research on targeted and innovative treatment approaches for sensory aspects of OCRDs. Such research would significantly advance our ability to provide comprehensive care for individuals with OCRDs and may also have significant implications for conditions similar to OCRDs that also exhibit similar sensory abnormalities (Khalsa et al., 2018).

References

Al Zoubi, O., Misaki, M., Bodurka, J., Kuplicki, R., Wohlrab, C., Schoenhals, W. A., Refai, H. H., Khalsa, S. S., Stein, M. B., & Paulus, M. P. (2021). Taking the body off the mind: Decreased functional connectivity between somatomotor and default-mode networks following Floatation-REST. *Human brain mapping*, 42 (10), 3216–3227.

Andersson, L., Johansson, A., Millqvist, E., Nordin, S., & Bende, M. (2008). Prevalence and risk factors for chemical sensitivity and sensory hyperreactivity in teenagers. *Int J Hyg Environ Health*, 211(5–6),690–697. doi:10.1016/j.ijheh.2008.02.002.

Banaschewski, T., Woerner, W., & Rothenberger, A. (2003). Premonitory sensory phenomena and suppressibility of tics in Tourette syndrome: developmental aspects in children and adolescents. *Developmental medicine and child neurology*, 45(10), 700–703.

Bar-Shalita, T., Vatine, J. J., & Parush, S. (2008). Sensory modulation disorder: a risk factor for participation in daily life activities. *Dev Med Child Neurol*, 50(12), 932–937. doi:10.1111/j.1469-8749.2008.03095.x.

Bar-Shalita, T., Vatine, J.-J., Seltzer, Z., & Parush, S. (2009). Psychophysical correlates in children with sensory modulation disorder (SMD). *Physiology & behavior*, 98(5), 631–639.

Barsky, A. J., Brener, J., Coeytaux, R. R., & Cleary, P. D. (1995). Accurate awareness of heartbeat in hypochondriacal and non-hypochondriacal patients. *J Psychosom Res*, 39(4), 489–497. doi:10.1016/0022-3999(94)00166–00163.

Barsky, A. J. & Klerman, G. L. (1983). Overview: hypochondriasis, bodily complaints, and somatic styles. *American journal of psychiatry*, 140(3), 273–283. doi:10.1176/ajp.140.3.273.

Barsky, A. J. & Wyshak, G. (1990). Hypochondriasis and somatosensory amplification. *Br J Psychiatry*, 157, 404–409. doi:10.1192/bjp.157.3.404.

Barsky, A. J., Wyshak, G., & Klerman, G. L. (1990). The somatosensory amplification scale and its relationship to hypochondriasis. *J Psychiatr Res*, 24(4), 323–334. doi:10.1016/0022-3956(90)90004-a.

Belluscio, B. A., Jin, L., Watters, V., Lee, T. H., & Hallett, M. (2011). Sensory sensitivity to external stimuli in Tourette syndrome patients. *Mov Disord*, 26(14), 2538–2543. doi:10.1002/mds.23977.

Ben-Sasson, A. & Podoly, T. Y. (2017). Sensory over responsivity and obsessive compulsive symptoms: A cluster analysis. *Compr Psychiatry*, 73, 151–159. doi:10.1016/j.comppsych.2016.10.013.

Blum, A. W., Redden, S. A., & Grant, J. E. (2017). Sensory and physiological dimensions of cold pressor pain in trichotillomania. *Journal of Obsessive-Compulsive and Related Disorders*, 12, 29–33. doi:10.1016/j.jocrd.2016.12.001.

Bohne, A., Keuthen, N., & Wilhelm, S. (2005). Pathologic hairpulling, skin picking, and nail biting. *Annals of Clinical Psychiatry*, 17(4), 227–232.

Boutros, N. N. & Peters, R. (2012). Internal gating and somatization disorders: Proposing a yet un-described neural system. *Medical Hypotheses*, 78(1), 174–178. doi:10.1016/j.mehy.2011.10.020.

Brandt, V. C., Beck, C., Sajin, V., Baaske, M. K., Bäumer, T., Beste, C., Anders, S., & Münchau, A. (2016). Temporal relationship between premonitory urges and tics in Gilles de la Tourette syndrome. *Cortex*, 77, 24–37.

Brewer, R., Murphy, J., & Bird, G. (2021). Atypical interoception as a common risk factor for psychopathology: A review. *Neuroscience & Biobehavioral Reviews*, 130, 470–508. doi:10.1016/j.neubiorev.2021.07.036.

Cabanac, M. (1971). Physiological Role of Pleasure: A stimulus can feel pleasant or unpleasant depending upon its usefulness as determined by internal signals. *Science*, 173(4002), 1103–1107.

Cameron, O. G. (2001). Interoception: the inside story—a model for psychosomatic processes. *Psychosomatic Medicine*, 63(5), 697–710.

Carpenter, K. L., Baranek, G. T., Copeland, W. E., Compton, S., Zucker, N., Dawson, G., & Egger, H. L. (2019). Sensory over-responsivity: an early risk factor for anxiety and behavioral challenges in young children. *Journal of abnormal child psychology*, 47, 1075–1088.

Castellanos, F. X., Fine, E. J., Kaysen, D., Marsh, W. L., Rapoport, J. L., & Hallett, M. (1996). Sensorimotor gating in boys with Tourette's syndrome and ADHD: preliminary results. *Biological psychiatry*, 39(1), 33–41.

Cervin, M. (2023). Sensory Processing Difficulties in Children and Adolescents with Obsessive-Compulsive and Anxiety Disorders. *Research on Child and Adolescent Psychopathology*, 51(2), 223–232. doi:10.1007/s10802-022-00962-w.

Cervin, M. & Perrin, S. (2021). Incompleteness and Disgust Predict Treatment Outcome in Pediatric Obsessive-Compulsive Disorder. *Behavior therapy*, 52(1), 53–63. doi:10.1016/j.beth.2020.01.007.

Cervin, M., Perrin, S., Olsson, E., Claesdotter-Knutsson, E., & Lindvall, M. (2020). Incompleteness, harm avoidance, and disgust: a comparison of youth with OCD, anxiety disorders, and no psychiatric disorder. *Journal of anxiety disorders*, 69, 102175.

Cervin, M., Perrin, S., Olsson, E., Claesdotter-Knutsson, E., & Lindvall, M. (2021). Involvement of fear, incompleteness, and disgust during symptoms of pediatric obsessive-compulsive disorder. *Eur Child Adolesc Psychiatry*, 30(2), 271–281. doi:10.1007/s00787-020-01514-7.

Christenson, G. A., Mackenzie, T. B., & Mitchell, J. E. (1991). Characteristics of 60 adult hair pullers. *The American journal of psychiatry*.

Cohen, A. J. & Leckman, J. F. (1992). Sensory phenomena associated with Gilles de la Tourette's syndrome. *The Journal of clinical psychiatry*, 53, 319–323.

Coles, M. E., Frost, R. O., Heimberg, R. G., & Rheaume, J. (2003). "Not just right experiences": perfectionism, obsessive-compulsive features and general psychopathology. *Behav Res Ther*, 41(6), 681–700. doi:10.1016/s0005-7967(02)00044-x.

Complementary, S. O., Medicine, I., Disabilities, C. o. C. w., Zimmer, M., Desch, L., Rosen, L. D., Bailey, M. L., Becker, D., Culbert, T. P., McClafferty, H., & Sahler, O. J. Z. (2012). Sensory integration therapies for children with developmental and behavioral disorders. *Pediatrics*, 129(6), 1186–1189.

Conelea, C. A., Carter, A. C., & Freeman, J. B. (2014). Sensory over-responsivity in a sample of children seeking treatment for anxiety. *J Dev Behav Pediatr*, 35(8), 510–521. doi:10.1097/DBP.0000000000000092.

Craig, A. D. (2002). How do you feel? Interoception: the sense of the physiological condition of the body. *Nat Rev Neurosci*, 3(8), 655–666. doi:10.1038/nrn894.

da Silva Prado, H., do Rosário, M. C., Lee, J., Hounie, A. G., Shavitt, R. G., & Miguel, E. C. (2008). Sensory phenomena in obsessive-compulsive disorder and tic disorders: a review of the literature. *CNS Spectrums*, 13(5), 425–432.

Dar, R., Kahn, D. T., & Carmeli, R. (2012). The relationship between sensory processing, childhood rituals and obsessive-compulsive symptoms. *J Behav Ther Exp Psychiatry*, 43(1), 679–684. doi:10.1016/j.jbtep.2011.09.008.

Davies, P. L., Chang, W. P., & Gavin, W. J. (2009). Maturation of sensory gating performance in children with and without sensory processing disorders. *Int J Psychophysiol*, 72(2), 187–197. doi:10.1016/j.ijpsycho.2008.12.007.

Deacon, B. & Abramowitz, J. (2006). Anxiety sensitivity and its dimensions across the anxiety disorders. *Journal of anxiety disorders*, 20(7), 837–857.

Demartini, B., Nisticò, V., Ranieri, R., Scattolini, C., Fior, G., Priori, A., Gambini, O., & Ricciardi, L. (2021). Reduced interoceptive accuracy in patients with obsessive–compulsive disorder: A case-control study. *Journal of Clinical Neuroscience*, 90, 152–154.

Dieringer, M., Beck, C., Verrel, J., Münchau, A., Zurowski, B., & Brandt, V. (2019). Quality and temporal properties of premonitory urges in patients with skin picking disorder. *Cortex*, 121, 125–134. doi:10.1016/j.cortex.2019.08.015.

Diniz, J. B., Rosario-Campos, M. C., Hounie, A. G., Curi, M., Shavitt, R. G., Lopes, A. C., & Miguel, E. C. (2006). Chronic tics and Tourette syndrome in patients with obsessive–compulsive disorder. *Journal of psychiatric research*, 40 (6), 487–493.

Dunn, W. (2001). The sensations of everyday life: Empirical, theoretical, and pragmatic considerations. *The American Journal of Occupational Therapy*, 55(6), 608–620.

Dunn, W. & Westman, K. (1997). The sensory profile: the performance of a national sample of children without disabilities. *The American Journal of Occupational Therapy*, 51(1), 25–34.

Ecker, W. & Gönner, S. (2008). Incompleteness and harm avoidance in OCD symptom dimensions. *Behaviour research and therapy*, 46(8), 895–904.

Eddy, C. M., Rickards, H. E., & Cavanna, A. E. (2014). Physiological awareness is negatively related to inhibitory functioning in Tourette syndrome. *Behavior modification*, 38(2), 319–335.

Eley, T. C., Stirling, L., Ehlers, A., Gregory, A. M., & Clark, D. M. (2004). Heartbeat perception, panic/somatic symptoms and anxiety sensitivity in children. *Behav Res Ther*, 42(4), 439–448. doi:10.1016/S0005-7967(03)00152–00159.

Eng, G. K., Collins, K. A., Brown, C., Ludlow, M., Tobe, R. H., Iosifescu, D. V., & Stern, E. R. (2020). Dimensions of interoception in obsessive-compulsive disorder. *Journal of Obsessive-Compulsive and Related Disorders*, 27, 100584.

Falkenstein, M. J., Conelea, C. A., Garner, L. E., & Haaga, D. A. F. (2018). Sensory over-responsivity in trichotillomania (hair-pulling disorder). *Psychiatry research*, 260, 207–218. doi:10.1016/j.psychres.2017.11.034.

Feinstein, J. S., Khalsa, S. S., Yeh, H.-w., Wohlrab, C., Simmons, W. K., Stein, M. B., & Paulus, M. P. (2018). Examining the short-term anxiolytic and antidepressant effect of Floatation-REST. *PLoS One*, 13(2), e0190292.

Feinstein, J. S., Khalsa, S. S., Yeh, H., Al Zoubi, O., Arevian, A. C., Wohlrab, C., Pantino, M. K., Cartmell, L. J., Simmons, W. K., Stein, M. B., & Paulus, M. P. (2018). The Elicitation of Relaxation and Interoceptive Awareness Using Floatation Therapy in Individuals With High Anxiety Sensitivity. *Biological psychiatry: cognitive neuroscience and neuroimaging*, 3(6), 555–562. doi:10.1016/j.bpsc.2018.02.005.

Fergus, T. A. (2014). Are "not just right experiences" (NJREs) specific to obsessive-compulsive symptoms?: evidence that NJREs span across symptoms of emotional disorders. *J Clin Psychol*, 70(4), 353–363. doi:10.1002/jclp.22034.

Ferrao, Y. A., Shavitt, R. G., Prado, H., Fontenelle, L. F., Malavazzi, D. M., de Mathis, M. A., Hounie, A. G., Miguel, E. C., & do Rosario, M. C. (2012). Sensory phenomena associated with repetitive behaviors in obsessive-compulsive disorder: an exploratory study of 1001 patients. *Psychiatry Res*, 197(3), 253–258. doi:10.1016/j.psychres.2011.09.017.

Ganos, C., Garrido, A., Navalpotro-Gómez, I., Ricciardi, L., Martino, D., Edwards, M. J., Tsakiris, M., Haggard, P., & Bhatia, K. P. (2015). Premonitory urge to tic in Tourette's is associated with interoceptive awareness. *Movement Disorders*, 30(9), 1198–1202.

Ghisi, M., Chiri, L. R., Marchetti, I., Sanavio, E., & Sica, C. (2010). In search of specificity:"Not just right experiences" and obsessive–compulsive symptoms in non-clinical and clinical Italian individuals. *Journal of anxiety disorders*, 24(8), 879–886.

Giannopoulos, A. E., Spantideas, S. T., Capsalis, C., Papageorgiou, P., Kapsalis, N., Kontoangelos, K., & Papageorgiou, C. (2021). Instantaneous radiated power of brain activity: application to prepulse inhibition and facilitation for body dysmorphic disorder. *BioMedical Engineering OnLine*, 20(1), 1–21.

Gourley, L., Wind, C., Henninger, E. M., & Chinitz, S. (2013). Sensory Processing Difficulties, Behavioral Problems, and Parental Stress in a Clinical Population of Young Children. *J Child Fam Stud*, 22(7), 912–921. doi:10.1007/s10826-012-9650-9.

Gouze, K. R., Hopkins, J., LeBailly, S. A., & Lavigne, J. V. (2009). Re-examining the epidemiology of sensory regulation dysfunction and comorbid psychopathology. *J Abnorm Child Psychol*, 37(8), 1077–1087. doi:10.1007/s10802-009-9333-1.

Grant, J. E., Odlaug, B. L., & Potenza, M. N. (2007). Addicted to Hair Pulling? How an Alternate Model of Trichotillomania May Improve Treatment Outcome. *Harvard Review of Psychiatry*, 15(2), 80–85. doi:10.1080/10673220701298407.

Grant, J. E., Redden, S. A., & Chamberlain, S. R. (2017). Cold pressor pain in skin picking disorder. *Psychiatry research*, 249, 35–38. doi:10.1016/j.psychres.2016.12.050.

Grunewald, W., Fogelberg, S., Ferguson, W., Hines, S., Fortenberry, B., & Smith, A. R. (2023). Longitudinal relationships between specific domains of interoception and muscle dysmorphia symptoms. *Eat Behav*, 48, 101686. doi:10.1016/j.eatbeh.2022.101686.

Güçlü, B., Tanıdır, C., Çanayaz, E., Güner, B., İpek Toz, H., Üneri, Ö. Ş., & Tommerdahl, M. (2015). Tactile processing in children and adolescents with obsessive–compulsive disorder. *Somatosensory & Motor Research*, 32(3), 163–171. doi:10.3109/08990220.2015.1023950.

Haenen, M.-A., Schmidt, A. J. M., Schoenmakers, M., & van den Hout, M. A. (2010). Tactual Sensitivity in Hypochondriasis. *Psychotherapy and Psychosomatics*, 66(3), 128–132. doi:10.1159/000289122.

Hashimoto, T., Shimizu, E., Koike, K., Orita, Y., Suzuki, T., Kanahara, N., Matsuzawa, D., Fukami, G., Miyatake, R., Shinoda, N., Fujisaki, M., Shirayama, Y., Hashimoto, K., & Iyo, M. (2008). Deficits in auditory P50 inhibition in obsessive-compulsive disorder. *Prog Neuropsychopharmacol Biol Psychiatry*, 32 (1), 288–296. doi:10.1016/j.pnpbp.2007.08.021.

Houghton, D. C., Alexander, J. R., Bauer, C. C., & Woods, D. W. (2018). Abnormal perceptual sensitivity in body-focused repetitive behaviors. *Comprehensive psychiatry*, 82, 45–52. doi:10.1016/j.comppsych.2017.12.005.

Houghton, D. C., Capriotti, M. R., Conelea, C. A., & Woods, D. W. (2014). Sensory Phenomena in Tourette Syndrome: Their Role in Symptom Formation and Treatment. *Current Developmental Disorders Reports*, 1(4), 245–251. doi:10.1007/s40474-014-0026-2.

Houghton, D. C., Stein, D. J., & Cortese, B. M. (2020). Review: Exteroceptive Sensory Abnormalities in Childhood and Adolescent Anxiety and Obsessive-Compulsive Disorder: A Critical Review. *J Am Acad Child Adolesc Psychiatry*, 59(1), 78–87. doi:10.1016/j.jaac.2019.06.007.

Houghton, D. C., Tommerdahl, M., & Woods, D. W. (2019). Increased tactile sensitivity and deficient feed-forward inhibition in pathological hair pulling and skin picking. *Behav Res Ther*, 120, 103433. doi:10.1016/j.brat.2019.103433.

Ibrahim, C., Rubin-Kahana, D. S., Pushparaj, A., Musiol, M., Blumberger, D. M., Daskalakis, Z. J., Zangen, A., & Le Foll, B. (2019). The insula: a brain stimulation target for the treatment of addiction. *Frontiers in pharmacology*, 10, 720.

Isaacs, D., Key, A. P., Cascio, C. J., Conley, A. C., Walker, H. C., Wallace, M. T., & Claassen, D. O. (2020). Sensory Hypersensitivity Severity and Association with Obsessive-Compulsive Symptoms in Adults with Tic Disorder. *Neuropsychiatr Dis Treat*, 16, 2591–2601. doi:10.2147/NDT.S274165.

Jackson, S. R., Parkinson, A., Kim, S. Y., Schüermann, M., & Eickhoff, S. B. (2011). On the functional anatomy of the urge-for-action. *Cognitive neuroscience*, 2(3–4), 227–243.

Janik, P., Milanowski, L., & Szejko, N. (2018). Phenomenology and Clinical Correlates of Stimulus-Bound Tics in Gilles de la Tourette Syndrome. *Front Neurol*, 9, 477. doi:10.3389/fneur.2018.00477.

Jokić, B. & Purić, D. (2021). Seeking proxies for internal states as a possible alternative for rationality and experientiality. *Sage Open*, 11(1), 2158244020986533.

Kamin, L., Brimer, C., & Black, A. (1963). Conditioned suppression as a monitor of fear of the CS in the course of avoidance training. *Journal of comparative and physiological psychology*, 56(3), 497.

Kaplan, R. A., Rossell, S. L., Enticott, P. G., & Castle, D. J. (2013). Own-body perception in body dysmorphic disorder. *Cognitive Neuropsychiatry*, 18(6), 594–614. doi:10.1080/13546805.2012.758878.

Kapsali, F., Zioga, I., Papageorgiou, P., Smyrnis, N., Chrousos, G. P., & Papageorgiou, C. (2020). Event-related EEG oscillations in body dysmorphic disorder. *European Journal of Clinical Investigation*, 50(3), e13208.

Keuler, M. M., Schmidt, N. L., Van Hulle, C. A., Lemery-Chalfant, K., & Goldsmith, H. H. (2011). Sensory overresponsivity: prenatal risk factors and temperamental contributions. *J Dev Behav Pediatr*, 32(7), 533–541. doi:10.1097/DBP.0b013e3182245c05.

Keuthen, N. J., Deckersbach, T., Wilhelm, S., Hale, E., Fraim, C., Baer, L., O'sullivan, R. L., & Jenike, M. A. (2000). Repetitive skin-picking in a student population and comparison with a sample of self-injurious skin-pickers. *Psychosomatics*, 41(3), 210–215.

Khalsa, S. S., Adolphs, R., Cameron, O. G., Critchley, H. D., Davenport, P. W., Feinstein, J. S., Feusner, J. D., Garfinkel, S. N., Lane, R. D., & Mehling, W. E. (2018). Interoception and mental health: a roadmap. *Biological psychiatry: cognitive neuroscience and neuroimaging*, 3(6), 501–513.

Koch, A. & Pollatos, O. (2014). Interoceptive sensitivity, body weight and eating behavior in children: a prospective study. *Front Psychol*, 5, 1003. doi:10.3389/fpsyg.2014.01003.

Köteles, F. & Witthöft, M. (2017). Somatosensory amplification–An old construct from a new perspective. *Journal of Psychosomatic Research*, 101, 1–9.

Kozak, M. J. & Miller, G. A. (1982). Hypothetical constructs versus intervening variables: A re-appraisal of the three-systems model of anxiety assessment. *Behavioral assessment*.

Koziol, L. F., Budding, D. E., & Chidekel, D. (2011). Sensory integration, sensory processing, and sensory modulation disorders: Putative functional neuroanatomic underpinnings. *The Cerebellum*, 10(4), 770–792.

Krautwurst, S., Gerlach, A. L., Gomille, L., Hiller, W., & Witthoft, M. (2014). Health anxiety–an indicator of higher interoceptive sensitivity? *J Behav Ther Exp Psychiatry*, 45(2), 303–309. doi:10.1016/j.jbtep.2014.02.001.

Krautwurst, S., Gerlach, A. L., & Witthoft, M. (2016). Interoception in pathological health anxiety. *J Abnorm Psychol*, 125(8), 1179–1184. doi:10.1037/abn0000210.

Kronenbuerger, M., Belenghi, P., Ilgner, J., Freiherr, J., Hummel, T., & Neuner, I. (2018). Olfactory functioning in adults with Tourette syndrome. *PLoS One*, 13 (6), e0197598. doi:10.1371/journal.pone.0197598.

Kunstman, J. W., Clerkin, E. M., Palmer, K., Peters, M. T., Dodd, D. R., & Smith, A. R. (2016). The power within: The experimental manipulation of power interacts with trait BDD symptoms to predict interoceptive accuracy. *J Behav Ther Exp Psychiatry*, 50, 178–186. doi:10.1016/j.jbtep.2015.08.003.

Langelage, J., Verrel, J., Friedrich, J., Siekmann, A., Schappert, R., Bluschke, A., Roessner, V., Paulus, T., Bäumer, T., Frings, C., Beste, C., & Münchau, A. (2022). Urge-tic associations in children and adolescents with Tourette syndrome. *Scientific Reports*, 12(1), 16008. doi:10.1038/s41598-022-19685-5.

Lapidus, K. A., Stern, E. R., Berlin, H. A., & Goodman, W. K. (2014). Functional neuroimaging and models for obsessive-compulsive disorder and obsessive compulsive spectrum disorders.

Lautenbacher, S., Pauli, P., Zaudig, M., & Birbaumer, N. (1998). Attentional control of pain perception: the role of hypochondriasis. *Journal of Psychosomatic Research*, 44(2), 251–259.

Lazarov, A., Dar, R., Oded, Y., & Liberman, N. (2010). Are obsessive-compulsive tendencies related to reliance on external proxies for internal states? Evidence from biofeedback-aided relaxation studies. *Behav Res Ther*, 48(6), 516–523. doi:10.1016/j.brat.2010.02.007.

Lazarov, A., Liberman, N., Hermesh, H., & Dar, R. (2014). Seeking proxies for internal states in obsessive–compulsive disorder. *Journal of abnormal psychology*, 123(4), 695.

Leckman, J. F., Walker, D. E., & Cohen, D. J. (1993). Premonitory urges in Tourette's syndrome. *The American journal of psychiatry*.

Leckman, J. F., Walker, D. E., Goodman, W. K., Pauls, D. L., & Cohen, D. J. (1994). "Just right" perceptions associated with compulsive behavior in Tourette's syndrome. *The American journal of psychiatry*.

Lee, J. C., Prado, H. S., Diniz, J. B., Borcato, S., da Silva, C. B., Hounie, A. G., Miguel, E. C., Leckman, J. F., & do Rosário, M. C. (2009). Perfectionism and sensory phenomena: phenotypic components of obsessive-compulsive disorder. *Comprehensive psychiatry*, 50(5), 431–436.

Lewin, A. B., Bergman, R. L., Peris, T. S., Chang, S., McCracken, J. T., & Piacentini, J. (2010). Correlates of insight among youth with obsessive-compulsive disorder. *J Child Psychol Psychiatry*, 51(5), 603–611. doi:10.1111/j.1469-7610.2009.02181.x.

Lewin, A. B., Wu, M. S., Murphy, T. K., & Storch, E. A. (2015). Sensory Over-Responsivity in Pediatric Obsessive Compulsive Disorder. *Journal of psychopathology and behavioral assessment*, 37(1), 134–143. doi:10.1007/s10862-014-9442-1.

Li, W., Arienzo, D., & Feusner, J. D. (2013). Body dysmorphic disorder: neuro-biological features and an updated model. *Zeitschrift Für Klinische Psychologie Und Psychotherapie.*

Ludlow, A. K. & Wilkins, A. J. (2016). Atypical Sensory behaviours in children with Tourette's Syndrome and in children with Autism Spectrum Disorders. *Research in Developmental Disabilities*, 56, 108–116. doi:10.1016/j.ridd.2016.05.019.

Madsen, S. K., Bohon, C., & Feusner, J. D. (2013). Visual processing in anorexia nervosa and body dysmorphic disorder: Similarities, differences, and future research directions. *Journal of psychiatric research*, 47(10), 1483–1491.

Mansueto, C. S., Stemberger, R. M. T., Thomas, A. M., & Golomb, R. G. (1997). Trichotillomania: A comprehensive behavioral model. *Clinical Psychology Review*, 17(5), 567–577.

Mata, F., Verdejo-Roman, J., Soriano-Mas, C., & Verdejo-Garcia, A. (2015). Insula tuning towards external eating versus interoceptive input in adolescents with overweight and obesity. *Appetite*, 93, 24–30. doi:10.1016/j.appet.2015.03.024.

McGhie, A. & Chapman, J. (1961). Disorders of attention and perception in early schizophrenia. *Br J Med Psychol*, 34, 103–116. doi:10.1111/j.2044-8341.1961.tb00936.x.

McIntosh, D. N., Miller, L. J., Shyu, V., & Hagerman, R. J. (1999). Sensory-modulation disruption, electrodermal responses, and functional behaviors. *Developmental medicine and child neurology*, 41(9), 608–615.

Meunier, S. A., Tolin, D. F., & Franklin, M. (2009). Affective and sensory correlates of hair pulling in pediatric trichotillomania. *Behavior modification*, 33(3), 396–407.

Micoulaud-Franchi, J.-A., Lopez, R., Cermolacce, M., Vaillant, F., Péri, P., Boyer, L., Richieri, R., Bioulac, S., Sagaspe, P., & Philip, P. (2019). Sensory gating capacity and attentional function in adults with ADHD: a preliminary neurophysiological and neuropsychological study. *Journal of Attention Disorders*, 23 (10), 1199–1209.

Micoulaud-Franchi, J.-A., Lopez, R., Vaillant, F., Richieri, R., El-Kaim, A., Bioulac, S., Philip, P., Boyer, L., & Lancon, C. (2015). Perceptual abnormalities related to sensory gating deficit are core symptoms in adults with ADHD. *Psychiatry research*, 230(2), 357–363.

Miguel, E. C., Coffey, B. J., Baer, L., Savage, C. R., Rauch, S. L., & Jenike, M. A. (1995). Phenomenology of intentional repetitive behaviors in obsessive-compulsive disorder and Tourette's disorder. *The Journal of clinical psychiatry.*

Miguel, E. C., do Rosário-Campos, M. C., da Silva Prado, H., Do Valle, R., Rauch, S. L., Coffey, B. J., Baer, L., Savage, C. R., O'Sullivan, R. L., & Leckman, J. F. (2000). Sensory phenomena in obsessive-compulsive disorder and Tourette's disorder. *The Journal of clinical psychiatry*, 61(2), 19253.

Miltenberger, R. G., Long, E. S., Rapp, J. T., Lumley, V., & Elliott, A. J. (1998). Evaluating the function of hair pulling: A preliminary investigation. *Behavior therapy*, 29(2), 211–219.

Moretz, M. W. & McKay, D. (2009). The role of perfectionism in obsessive–compulsive symptoms:"Not just right" experiences and checking compulsions. *Journal of anxiety disorders*, 23(5), 640–644.

Naqvi, N. H. & Bechara, A. (2009). The hidden island of addiction: the insula. *Trends Neurosci*, 32(1), 56–67. doi:10.1016/j.tins.2008.09.009.

Naqvi, N. H., Rudrauf, D., Damasio, H., & Bechara, A. (2007). Damage to the insula disrupts addiction to cigarette smoking. *Science*, 315(5811), 531–534.

Neal, M. & Cavanna, A. E. (2013). "Not just right experiences" in patients with Tourette syndrome: complex motor tics or compulsions? *Psychiatry research*, 210(2), 559–563.

Nissen, J. B. & Parner, E. (2018). The importance of insight, avoidance behavior, not-just-right perception and personality traits in pediatric obsessive-compulsive disorder (OCD): a naturalistic clinical study. *Nordic journal of psychiatry*, 72(7), 489–496.

Olatunji, B. O., Lohr, J. M., Sawchuk, C. N., & Tolin, D. F. (2007). Multimodal assessment of disgust in contamination-related obsessive-compulsive disorder. *Behaviour research and therapy*, 45(2), 263–276.

Openneer, T. J. C., Tárnok, Z., Bognar, E., Benaroya-Milshtein, N., Garcia-Delgar, B., Morer, A., Steinberg, T., Hoekstra, P. J., Dietrich, A., Apter, A., Baglioni, V., Ball, J., Benaroya-Milshtein, N., Bodmer, B., Bognar, E., Burger, B., Buse, J., Cardona, F., Correa Vela, M., ... & EMTICS Collaborative Group. (2020). The Premonitory Urge for Tics Scale in a large sample of children and adolescents: psychometric properties in a developmental context. An EMTICS study. *European Child & Adolescent Psychiatry*, 29(10), 1411–1424. doi:10.1007/s00787-019-01450-1.

Panza, K. E., Pittenger, C., & Bloch, M. H. (2013). Age and gender correlates of pulling in pediatric trichotillomania. *J Am Acad Child Adolesc Psychiatry*, 52(3), 241–249. doi:10.1016/j.jaac.2012.12.019.

Patterson, J. V., Hetrick, W. P., Boutros, N. N., Jin, Y., Sandman, C., Stern, H., Potkin, S., & Bunney, W. E., Jr. (2008). P50 sensory gating ratios in schizophrenics and controls: a review and data analysis. *Psychiatry Res*, 158(2), 226–247. doi:10.1016/j.psychres.2007.02.009.

Paulus, M. P. & Stein, M. B. (2010). Interoception in anxiety and depression. *Brain structure and Function*, 214, 451–463.

Paulus, M. P. & Stewart, J. L. (2014). Interoception and drug addiction. *Neuropharmacology*, 76, 342–350.

Perez-Robles, R., Doval, E., Jane, M. C., Caldeira da Silva, P., Papoila, A. L., & Virella, D. (2013). The role of sensory modulation deficits and behavioral symptoms in a diagnosis for early childhood. *Child Psychiatry Hum Dev*, 44(3), 400–411. doi:10.1007/s10578-012-0334-x.

Phillips, K. A., Menard, W., Fay, C., & Weisberg, R. (2005). Demographic characteristics, phenomenology, comorbidity, and family history in 200 individuals with body dysmorphic disorder. *Psychosomatics*, 46(4), 317–325. doi:10.1176/appi.psy.46.4.317.

Pietrefesa, A. S. & Coles, M. E. (2009). Moving beyond an exclusive focus on harm avoidance in obsessive-compulsive disorder: behavioral validation for the separability of harm avoidance and incompleteness. *Behavior therapy*, 40(3), 251–259.

Pile, V., Lau, J. Y. F., Topor, M., Hedderly, T., & Robinson, S. (2018). Interoceptive Accuracy in Youth with Tic Disorders: Exploring Links with Premonitory Urge, Anxiety and Quality of Life. *Journal of Autism and Developmental Disorders*, 48 (10), 3474–3482. doi:10.1007/s10803-018-3608-8.

Pinto, A. C., Andrade, T. C., Brito, F. F., Silva, G. V., Cavalcante, M. L., & Martelli, A. C. (2017). Trichotillomania: a case report with clinical and dermatoscopic differential diagnosis with alopecia areata. *An Bras Dermatol*, 92(1), 118–120. doi:10.1590/abd1806-4841.20175136.

Pitman, R. K. (1987). Pierre Janet on obsessive-compulsive disorder (1903). Review and commentary. *Arch Gen Psychiatry*, 44(3), 226–232. doi:10.1001/archpsyc.1987.01800150032005.

Podoly, T. Y., Derby, D. S., & Ben-Sasson, A. (2022). Sensory over-responsivity and obsessive-compulsive disorder: Measuring habituation and sensitivity through self-report, physiological and behavioral indices. *Journal of psychiatric research*, 149, 266–273. doi:10.1016/j.jpsychires.2022.02.037.

Pollatos, O., Herbert, B. M., Mai, S., & Kammer, T. (2016). Changes in interoceptive processes following brain stimulation. *Philosophical Transactions of the Royal Society B: Biological Sciences*, 371(1708), 20160016. doi:10.1098/rstb.2016.0016.

Pollatos, O., Kurz, A. L., Albrecht, J., Schreder, T., Kleemann, A. M., Schopf, V., Kopietz, R., Wiesmann, M., & Schandry, R. (2008). Reduced perception of bodily signals in anorexia nervosa. *Eat Behav*, 9(4), 381–388. doi:10.1016/j.eatbeh.2008.02.001.

Porth, R. & Geller, D. (2018). Atypical symptom presentations in children and adolescents with obsessive compulsive disorder. *Comprehensive psychiatry*, 86, 25–30.

Pratt, M. (2014). *Interoceptive awareness and self-objectification in body dysmorphic disorder*. Royal Holloway, University of London.

Puts, N. A. J., Harris, A. D., Crocetti, D., Nettles, C., Singer, H. S., Tommerdahl, M., Edden, R. A. E., & Mostofsky, S. H. (2015). Reduced GABAergic inhibition and abnormal sensory symptoms in children with Tourette syndrome. *Journal of Neurophysiology*, 114(2), 808–817. doi:10.1152/jn.00060.2015.

Rae, C. L., Larsson, D. E. O., Garfinkel, S. N., & Critchley, H. D. (2019). Dimensions of interoception predict premonitory urges and tic severity in Tourette syndrome. *Psychiatry research*, 271, 469–475. doi:10.1016/j.psychres.2018.12.036.

Rapp, J. T., Miltenberger, R. G., Galensky, T. L., Ellingson, S. A., & Long, E. S. (1999). A functional analysis of hair pulling. *Journal of Applied Behavior Analysis*, 32(3), 329–337.

Rescorla, R. A. & Solomon, R. L. (1967). Two-process learning theory: Relationships between Pavlovian conditioning and instrumental learning. *Psychological review*, 74(3), 151.

Ricketts, E. J., Snorrason, Í., Mathew, A. S., Sigurvinsdottir, E., Ólafsson, R. P., Woods, D. W., & Lee, H.-J. (2021). Heightened Sense of Incompleteness in Excoriation (Skin-Picking) Disorder. *Cognitive Therapy and Research*, 1–8.

Rieke, E. F. & Anderson, D. (2009). Adolescent/Adult Sensory Profile and obsessive–compulsive disorder. *The American Journal of Occupational Therapy*, 63(2), 138–145.

Rodic, D., Meyer, A. H., Lieb, R., & Meinlschmidt, G. (2016). The association of sensory responsiveness with somatic symptoms and illness anxiety. *International journal of behavioral medicine*, 23, 39–48.

Rosario, M. C., Prado, H. S., Borcato, S., Diniz, J. B., Shavitt, R. G., Hounie, A. G., Mathis, M. E., Mastrorosa, R. S., Velloso, P., & Perin, E. A. (2009).

Validation of the University of São Paulo sensory phenomena scale: Initial psychometric properties. *CNS Spectrums*, 14(6), 315–323.

Rossi, S., Bartalini, S., Ulivelli, M., Mantovani, A., Di Muro, A., Goracci, A., Castrogiovanni, P., Battistini, N., & Passero, S. (2005). Hypofunctioning of sensory gating mechanisms in patients with obsessive-compulsive disorder. *Biol Psychiatry*, 57(1), 16–20. doi:10.1016/j.biopsych.2004.09.023.

Rubin, G. J., Nieto-Hernandez, R., & Wessely, S. (2010). Idiopathic environmental intolerance attributed to electromagnetic fields (formerly 'electromagnetic hypersensitivity'): an updated systematic review of provocation studies. *Bioelectromagnetics: Journal of the Bioelectromagnetics Society, The Society for Physical Regulation in Biology and Medicine, The European Bioelectromagnetics Association*, 31(1), 1–11.

Sambrani, T., Jakubovski, E., & Muller-Vahl, K. R. (2016). New Insights into Clinical Characteristics of Gilles de la Tourette Syndrome: Findings in 1032 Patients from a Single German Center. *Front Neurosci*, 10, 415. doi:10.3389/fnins.2016.00415.

Schaaf, R. C., Miller, L. J., Seawell, D., & O'Keefe, S. (2003). Children with disturbances in sensory processing: A pilot study examining the role of the parasympathetic nervous system. *The American Journal of Occupational Therapy*, 57 (4), 442–449.

Schultchen, D., Zaudig, M., Krauseneck, T., Berberich, G., & Pollatos, O. (2019). Interoceptive deficits in patients with obsessive-compulsive disorder in the time course of cognitive-behavioral therapy. *PLoS One*, 14(5), e0217237.

Schumer, M. C., Panza, K. E., Mulqueen, J. M., Jakubovski, E., & Bloch, M. H. (2015). Long-Term Outcome in Pediatric Trichotillomania. *Depress Anxiety*, 32 (10), 737–743. doi:10.1002/da.22390.

Schwartz, R. A. (2018). Treating incompleteness in obsessive-compulsive disorder: A meta-analytic review. *Journal of Obsessive-Compulsive and Related Disorders*, 19, 50–60.

Segalas, C., Labad, J., Alonso, P., Real, E., Subira, M., Bueno, B., Jimenez-Murcia, S., & Menchon, J. M. (2011). Olfactory identification and discrimination in obsessive-compulsive disorder. *Depress Anxiety*, 28(10), 932–940. doi:10.1002/da.20836.

Shapira, N. A., Liu, Y., He, A. G., Bradley, M. M., Lessig, M. C., James, G. A., Stein, D. J., Lang, P. J., & Goodman, W. K. (2003). Brain activation by disgust-inducing pictures in obsessive-compulsive disorder. *Biological psychiatry*, 54(7), 751–756.

Shavitt, R. G., de Mathis, M. A., Oki, F., Ferrao, Y. A., Fontenelle, L. F., Torres, A. R., Diniz, J. B., Costa, D. L., do Rosário, M. C., & Hoexter, M. Q. (2014). Phenomenology of OCD: lessons from a large multicenter study and implications for ICD-11. *Journal of psychiatric research*, 57, 141–148.

Sibrava, N. J., Boisseau, C. L., Eisen, J. L., Mancebo, M. C., & Rasmussen, S. A. (2016). An empirical investigation of incompleteness in a large clinical sample of obsessive compulsive disorder. *J Anxiety Disord*, 42, 45–51. doi:10.1016/j.janxdis.2016.05.005.

Sica, C., Bottesi, G., Orsucci, A., Pieraccioli, C., Sighinolfi, C., & Ghisi, M. (2015). "Not Just Right Experiences" are specific to obsessive–compulsive disorder: Further evidence from Italian clinical samples. *Journal of anxiety disorders*, 31, 73–83.

Sigmundsson, H., Whiting, H., & Loftesnes, J. (2000). Development of proprioceptive sensitivity. *Experimental Brain Research*, 135, 348–352.

Smith, B. L., Gutierrez, R., & Ludlow, A. K. (2022). A comparison of food avoidant behaviours and sensory sensitivity in adults with and without Tourette syndrome. *Appetite*, 168, 105713. doi:10.1016/j.appet.2021.105713.

Smith, R., Kuplicki, R., Feinstein, J., Forthman, K. L., Stewart, J. L., Paulus, M. P., Tulsa, i., & Khalsa, S. S. (2020). A Bayesian computational model reveals a failure to adapt interoceptive precision estimates across depression, anxiety, eating, and substance use disorders. *PLOS Computational Biology*, 16(12), e1008484. doi:10.1371/journal.pcbi.1008484.

Snorrason, I., Olafsson, R. P., Houghton, D. C., Woods, D. W., & Lee, H.-J. (2015). 'Wanting'and 'liking'skin picking: A validation of the Skin Picking Reward Scale. *Journal of Behavioral Addictions*, 4(4), 250–260.

Snorrason, I., Ricketts, E. J., Olafsson, R. P., Rozenman, M., Colwell, C. S., & Piacentini, J. (2019). Disentangling reward processing in trichotillomania:'-Wanting'and 'liking'hair pulling have distinct clinical correlates. *Journal of psychopathology and behavioral assessment*, 41, 271–279.

Snorrason, Í., Smári, J., & Olafsson, R. P. (2010). Emotion regulation in pathological skin picking: Findings from a non-treatment seeking sample. *Journal of Behavior Therapy and Experimental Psychiatry*, 41(3), 238–245.

Soler, N., Hardwick, C., Perkes, I. E., Mohammad, S. S., Dossetor, D., Nunn, K., Bray, P., & Dale, R. C. (2019). Sensory dysregulation in tic disorders is associated with executive dysfunction and comorbidities. *Mov Disord*, 34(12), 1901–1909. doi:10.1002/mds.27817.

Stein, D. J., Liu, Y., Shapira, N. A., & Goodman, W. K. (2001). The psychobiology of obsessive-compulsive disorder: how important is the role of disgust? *Current Psychiatry Reports*, 3(4), 281–287.

Stein, D. J. & Nesse, R. M. (2011). Threat detection, precautionary responses, and anxiety disorders. *Neuroscience & Biobehavioral Reviews*, 35(4), 1075–1079.

Summerfeldt, L. J. (2004). Understanding and treating incompleteness in obsessive-compulsive disorder. *J Clin Psychol*, 60(11), 1155–1168. doi:10.1002/jclp.20080.

Summers, B. J., Fitch, K. E., & Cougle, J. R. (2014). Visual, tactile, and auditory "not just right" experiences: associations with obsessive-compulsive symptoms and perfectionism. *Behavior therapy*, 45(5), 678–689.

Summers, B. J., Matheny, N. L., & Cougle, J. R. (2017). 'Not just right' experiences and incompleteness in body dysmorphic disorder. *Psychiatry research*, 247, 200–207.

Swedo, S. E. & Rapoport, J. L. (1991). Annotation: trichotillomania. *J Child Psychol Psychiatry*, 32(3), 401–409. doi:10.1111/j.1469-7610.1991.tb00319.x.

Swerdlow, N. R., Karban, B., Ploum, Y., Sharp, R., Geyer, M. A., & Eastvold, A. (2001). Tactile prepuff inhibition of startle in children with Tourette's syndrome: in search of an "fMRI-friendly" startle paradigm. *Biological psychiatry*, 50(8), 578–585.

Szemerszky, R., Gubányi, M., Árvai, D., Dömötör, Z., & Köteles, F. (2015). Is there a connection between electrosensitivity and electrosensibility? A replication study. *International journal of behavioral medicine*, 22, 755–763.

Taylor, S., Conelea, C. A., McKay, D., Crowe, K. B., & Abramowitz, J. S. (2014). Sensory intolerance: latent structure and psychopathologic correlates. *Compr Psychiatry*, 55(5), 1279–1284. doi:10.1016/j.comppsych.2014.03.007.

Teng, E. J., Woods, D. W., Twohig, M. P., & Marcks, B. A. (2002). Body-focused repetitive behavior problems: Prevalence in a nonreferred population and differences in perceived somatic activity. *Behavior modification*, 26(3), 340–360.

Tsakiris, M. & Critchley, H. (2016). Interoception beyond homeostasis: affect, cognition and mental health. 371, 20160002. The Royal Society.

Tucker, B. T., Woods, D. W., Flessner, C. A., Franklin, S. A., & Franklin, M. E. (2011). The skin picking impact project: phenomenology, interference, and treatment utilization of pathological skin picking in a population-based sample. *Journal of anxiety disorders*, 25(1), 88–95.

Tyrer, P., Lee, I., & Alexander, J. (1980). Awareness of cardiac function in anxious, phobic and hypochondriacal patients. *Psychol Med*, 10(1), 171–174. doi:10.1017/s0033291700039726.

Van Hulle, C. A., Esbensen, K., & Goldsmith, H. H. (2019). Co-occurrence of sensory over-responsivity with obsessive-compulsive symptoms in childhood and early adolescence. *Journal of developmental and behavioral pediatrics: JDBP*, 40 (5), 377.

Van Hulle, C. A., Schmidt, N. L., & Goldsmith, H. H. (2012). Is sensory over-responsivity distinguishable from childhood behavior problems? A phenotypic and genetic analysis. *Journal of Child Psychology and Psychiatry*, 53(1), 64–72.

Wang, Z., Maia, T. V., Marsh, R., Colibazzi, T., Gerber, A., & Peterson, B. S. (2011). The neural circuits that generate tics in Tourette's syndrome. *American journal of psychiatry*, 168(12), 1326–1337.

Wilhelm, F. & Margraf, J. (1993). Nail-biting: Description, etiological models, and treatment. *Verhaltenstherapie*, 3(3), 176–196.

Williams, T. I., Rose, R., & Chisholm, S. (2007). What is the function of nail biting: an analog assessment study. *Behaviour research and therapy*, 45(5), 989–995.

Witthöft, M. & Rubin, G. J. (2013). Are media warnings about the adverse health effects of modern life self-fulfilling? An experimental study on idiopathic environmental intolerance attributed to electromagnetic fields (IEI-EMF). *Journal of Psychosomatic Research*, 74(3), 206–212.

Woods, D. W., Flessner, C. A., Franklin, M. E., Keuthen, N. J., Goodwin, R. D., Stein, D. J., & Walther, M. R. (2006). The Trichotillomania Impact Project (TIP): exploring phenomenology, functional impairment, and treatment utilization. *Journal of Clinical Psychiatry*, 67(12), 1877.

Woods, D. W., Miltenberger, R. G., & Flach, A. D. (1996). Habits, tics, and stuttering. Prevalence and relation to anxiety and somatic awareness. *Behav Modif*, 20(2), 216–225. doi:10.1177/01454455960202005.

Woods, D. W., Piacentini, J., Himle, M. B., & Chang, S. (2005). Premonitory Urge for Tics Scale (PUTS): Initial Psychometric Results and Examination of the Premonitory Urge Phenomenon in Youths with Tic Disorders. *Journal of Developmental & Behavioral Pediatrics*, 26(6). https://journals.lww.com/jrnldbp/ Fulltext/2005/12000/Premonitory_Urge_for_Tics_Scale__PUTS___Initial.1.asp x.

Wright, K. D. & Asmundson, G. J. (2003). Health anxiety in children: development and psychometric properties of the Childhood Illness Attitude Scales. *Cogn Behav Ther*, 32(4), 194–202. doi:10.1080/16506070310014691.

Wu, M. S., Lewin, A. B., Murphy, T. K., & Storch, E. A. (2014). Misophonia: Incidence, Phenomenology, and Clinical Correlates in an Undergraduate Student Sample [https://doi.org/10.1002/jclp.22098]. *Journal of clinical psychology*, 70(10), 994–1007. doi:10.1002/jclp.22098.

Xiao, Z. P., Chen, X. S., Wang, J. J., Tang, Y. X., Zhang, T. H., Zhang, M. D., Fan, Q., Lou, F. Y., & Chen, C. (2010). Experimental study on sensory gating in generalized anxiety and obsessive compulsive disorders. *Zhonghua Yi Xue Za Zhi*, 90(3), 169–172. www.ncbi.nlm.nih.gov/pubmed/20356551.

Zebardast, N., Crowley, M. J., Bloch, M. H., Mayes, L. C., Vander Wyk, B., Leckman, J. F., Pelphrey, K. A., & Swain, J. E. (2013). Brain mechanisms for prepulse inhibition in adults with Tourette syndrome: initial findings. *Psychiatry Research: Neuroimaging*, 214(1), 33–41.

Zinner, S. H., Conelea, C. A., Glew, G. M., Woods, D. W., & Budman, C. L. (2012). Peer victimization in youth with Tourette syndrome and other chronic tic disorders. *Child Psychiatry & Human Development*, 43, 124–136.

7 Health Anxiety in Children

Kelly N. Banneyer, Liza Bonin, Victoria R. Bacon, Karina Silva, Lindsay T. Ives and Aditi Sabhlok

Diagnostic criteria and prevalence of health anxiety-related disorders in youth

Best practice for assessment, especially in children and adolescents, involves multi-informant and multi-method assessment. While there have been some specific measures of health anxiety that have been adapted for use with children (either self-report or parent-report), primarily in research settings, it is important to note that psychometric properties are not currently available (see Haig-Ferguson et al., 2021). Because of this, relying on diagnostic interviews is important, as is a thorough understanding of the diagnoses associated with health anxiety symptoms, particularly illness anxiety disorder and somatic symptom disorder.

When discussing the prevalence rate of health anxiety among youth, it is important to consider the inconsistency in defining health anxiety and changes in the diagnostic criteria in the past decade. Some researchers over the years have suggested that the true prevalence rate for severe health anxiety in children is unknown (Delparte et al., 2015; Wright & Asmundson, 2003). It has previously been believed that clinical levels of health anxiety do not present until early or middle adulthood (American Psychiatric Association, 2013; Rask et al., 2012). However, developing research suggests that children and adolescents do worry about their health and the health of others, and that "health anxiety" is much more prevalent (Delparte et al., 2015; Koteles et al., 2015 Rask et al., 2012). A study by Rask and colleagues (2012) explored parent-reported HA symptoms and their associations with physical and mental health among a sample of 5–7-year-old who were recruited to participate in a longitudinal study from a birth cohort (Rask et al., 2012). Findings demonstrated that HA symptoms were present in 17.6 percent of the sample, with 2.4 percent of children demonstrating considerable (present "a lot" of the time) symptoms. Rask and colleagues (2016) recently published a follow-up study assessing health anxiety symptoms using the same birth cohort sample with children now aged 11–12 years (Rask et al., 2012). Findings demonstrated that health anxiety symptoms at ages 5–7 were

DOI: 10.4324/9781003517429-7

significantly associated with health anxiety symptoms at ages 11–12 years old (Rask et al., 2012). These results suggest that health anxiety common in preadolescents and may continue from early childhood. Additionally, a study by Sirri and colleagues (2015) found that 15.7 percent of a sample of 14- to 19-year-olds reported elevated health anxiety concerns.

Historically, the DSM-IV classified individuals with preoccupation about having a serious disease as having hypochondriasis. This diagnosis consisted of "preoccupation with having, or the idea that one has, a serious disease based on the person's misinterpretation of bodily symptoms" (American Psychiatric Association, 1994, p. 465). "Hypochondriasis" was replaced by "illness anxiety disorder" and "somatic symptom disorder" in the *Diagnostic and Statistical Manual, 5th Edition* (American Psychiatric Association, 2013). These categories were maintained in the most recent text revision of the DSM (DSM-5-TR; APA, 2022) and are defined below.

Illness Anxiety Disorder

Illness anxiety disorder (IAD) is classified under Somatic Symptom and Related Disorders in the DSM-5-TR (American Psychiatric Association, 2022). The core diagnostic criteria for IAD include "preoccupation with having or acquiring a serious illness" without the presence of significant somatic symptoms (American Psychiatric Association, 2022, p. 357). Criteria further outline that if an individual does have a medical condition, or elevated risk for developing one, their preoccupation must be disproportionate to what would be expected. Additional criteria include exhibiting an elevated level of anxiety about health and becoming easily distressed about one's health status. Behavioral symptoms of IAD include "excessive health-related behaviors," such as repeatedly checking the body for signs of illness or maladaptive avoidance of health-related situations including medical appointments or hospitals (American Psychiatric Association, 2022, p. 357). Excessive concern about illness must be present for a minimum of six months, although the specific illness feared does not need to remain the same over time. Finally, this anxiety should not be better explained by another mental disorder, such as somatic symptom disorder, an anxiety disorder, or an obsessive-compulsive or related disorder. The following are two specifiers for IAD: *Care-seeking type* includes excessive engagement in medical care (e.g., physician appointments, testing, procedures), while *care-avoidant type* is characterized by avoidance of medical care.

It is estimated that one-third of individuals who would have been diagnosed with hypochondriasis using DSM-IV would now be diagnosed with IAD. According to the DSM-5-TR, IAD is thought to be rare in children (American Psychiatric Association, 2022, p. 358). However, it is noted that health-related anxieties can onset during childhood or adolescence, and as described above, emerging research indicated IAD may be more common in youth than previously identified.

Somatic Symptom Disorder

Somatic symptom disorder (SSD) is classified in the same diagnostic category as IAD within the DSM-5-TR (American Psychiatric Association, 2022). Both disorders are characterized by anxiety about health and related excessive and maladaptive behavioral symptoms. However, whereas individuals with IAD endorse no to mild somatic symptoms, SSD diagnostic criteria require the presence of significantly distressing or impairing somatic symptoms (American Psychiatric Association, 2022, p. 359). Criterion B for SSD entails at least one of the following: (1) the presence of disproportionate or recurring thoughts regarding the significance of somatic symptoms; (2) a consistently high level of anxiety regarding symptoms or health; and/or (3) excessive time and effort spent related to the symptoms or concerns (American Psychiatric Association, 2022, p. 351). Symptoms must be "persistent," (i.e., last longer than six months) but may vary in the type of somatic symptom that is present. SSD includes three specifiers. *With predominant pain* specifies that symptoms are primarily pain-related. Persistent should be used if severe symptoms and notable impairment have been present for longer than six months. Finally, there is a severity specifier. *Mild* specifies that only one of the symptoms in Criterion B is present; *moderate* that two or more Criterion B symptoms are present; and *severe* that there are multiple somatic symptoms, or one very severe symptom, in addition to the presence of two or more items in Criterion B. Approximately two-thirds of individuals who would have previously received the diagnosis of hypochondriasis in DSM-IV would now be considered to have SSD (American Psychiatric Association, 2022, p. 357).

Regarding developmental considerations, children with SSD most frequently endorse abdominal pain, headache, fatigue, and nausea (American Psychiatric Association, 2022, p. 353). Additionally, they usually endorse only one somatic symptom. Somatic symptom disorder has been associated with 8 percent to 12.5 percent of children and adolescents (Campo, 2012; Cozzi et al., 2017; Jackson & Kroenke, 2008). Early investigations by Offord and colleagues (1987) assessed the six-month prevalence of four psychiatric disorders in 2,674 children (Offord et al., 1987). Findings indicated that approximately 8 percent of the 12- to 16-year-olds suffered from somatic symptoms disorder. Similarly, during the 1990s, Eminson and colleagues (1996) examined the lifetime prevalence of physical symptoms and illness attitudes in a school population of 805 students (ages 11–16 years) (Eminson et al., 1996). Findings demonstrated that 8.3 percent of their sample met criteria for a diagnosis of somatization disorder based on the DSM III-R threshold, with 9.5

percent of girls and 7.1 percent of boys meeting criteria (Eminson et al., 1996). Furthermore, a recent investigation conducted by Cozzi and colleagues (2017) found that 8.6 percent of the children suffered from somatic pain, while functional pain had a prevalence of 13.4 percent in a sample of children ages 7–17 who arrived at an emergency room, owing to complaints of pain (Cozzi et al., 2017).

Underlying Theory

Some degree of health-related anxiety is adaptive if it functions as a motivator to take constructive measures to promote health and seek medical attention when warranted. Problematic or maladaptive health anxiety involves excessive or unproductive fears based on misappraisals of benign internal cues or other triggering stimuli. The critical mechanisms for the development and maintenance of pediatric health anxiety include maladaptive cognitive and behavioral processes occurring at both child/adolescent and family system levels (Abramowitz, et al., 2002; Warwick & Salkovskis, 1990; Rask, 2019). This cycle is similar to that which occurs with obsessive-compulsive disorder, and association between the two conditions has been longstanding (Barsky, 1992).

Our cognitive behavioral model of pediatric health anxiety is delineated below (Refer to Figure 1, Bonin & Banneyer); it includes core health anxiety mechanisms that are present in both pediatric and adult populations and is augmented to include the developmentally important role of caregivers in pediatric populations. The model outlines how predisposing or risk factors and fear cues can both contribute to an anxiety cycle of specific thoughts, feelings, and behaviors that maintain health anxiety. Proposed maintaining factors for health anxiety include cognitive biases, experiences and interpretations of physiological stimuli, and behavioral responses to health information.

Predisposing (risk) factors

Research identifying individual risk factors for health anxiety is sparse. Existing studies examining demographic factors, including gender, age, and ethnicity, find either inconsistent results or do not suggest differences in risk (Noyes et al., 2002; Parker et al., 2023; Weck et al., 2014). Demographic factors that are consistently related to higher levels of health anxiety include lower socioeconomic status and fewer years of education (Weck et al., 2014), but it is worth noting that social inequities in health broadly may offer some explanation of this relationship (Barbek et al., 2022). Beyond demographics, additional risk factors for developing health anxiety may include personality and temperament, psychosocial comorbidities, experiences with illness or injury, and parent behaviors.

Regarding personality and temperament, high levels of neuroticism within the "Big Five" model of personality is an established correlate of health anxiety (Ferguson, 2004). Neuroticism includes a predisposition to experience aversive mood states such as anger, disgust, guilt, and fearfulness (Watson & Pennebaker, 1989). The higher-order domain of neuroticism and a lower-order facet of anxiety are most strongly associated with a fear of illness and death core to health anxiety (Cox et al., 2000). Neuroticism is further associated with vulnerabilities to anxiety, depression, and other psychopathology.

The hereditary component of anxiety is well-documented, including a genetic vulnerability to developing anxiety and parental modeling of anxiety-maintaining behaviors (Drake & Ginsburg, 2012; Gouze et al., 2017). Parental beliefs and attitudes about health and illness are specifically related to health anxiety in children (Koteles et al., 2015; Marshall et al., 2007). Regarding comorbidities with other anxiety disorders, health anxiety is associated with separation anxiety and generalized anxiety disorder (Gureje et al., 1997; Noyes et al., 2002). Beyond anxiety disorders, health anxiety has also been associated with depressive symptoms and major depressive disorder (Noyes et al., 2002; Robbins & Kirkmayer, 1996). Although early research points to childhood adversity or trauma playing a role in developing health anxiety (Barksky et al., 1994), more recent research suggests that adverse childhood experiences broadly do not differ between individuals with health anxiety and typical controls (Gehrt et al., 2022). Additionally, health anxiety and obsessive-compulsive disorder often overlap, with studies finding that the lifetime prevalence of obsessive-compulsive disorder in a sample of hypochondriacal patients was four times higher (8 percent) than in a comparison group (2 percent) (Barsky, 1992; Villadsen et al., 2017).

However, adverse childhood experiences related explicitly to significant illness or injury to oneself, family, or close friends may be a risk factor for future development of health anxiety (Noyes et al., 2002). Relatedly, individuals with active health conditions, including those associated with chronic pain and fatigue, may experience higher levels of health anxiety (Daniels et al., 2020; Parker et al., 2023). Interactions likely exist between experiencing prior or current health concerns and interpersonal processes that contribute to maintaining health anxiety. The literature base includes a more considerable emphasis on these interpersonal processes than individual and contextual risk factors in the role of health anxiety (Williams, 2004).

Finally, it should be noted that caregiver modeling of and response to children's health concerns are important to consider as a risk factor. A caregiver may potentially reinforce or change a child's beliefs about their health through their own response to the child's concerns. For example, if they talk to great extent about the child's worries, or they model checking behaviors related to their own health, they may perpetuate their child's anxiety. Alternatively, if they redirect a child's attention rather than reinforcing worry, or model confidence in managing their own health, they may lessen a child's anxiety. This is also true concerning parental responses and behaviors to somatic symptoms, as caregivers are positioned to make decisions about scheduling doctor's appointments and attending school when their child is endorsing symptoms. Additionally, their interpretation of and response to symptoms is important to consider. For example, caregivers may give varying levels of attention to symptoms, encourage active or passive coping strategies, and convey an attitude that their child's symptoms are benign or catastrophize them. A caregiver may amplify a child's anxiety by bringing them to the emergency room whenever they experience somatic symptoms; conversely, they may alleviate a child's anxiety by modeling a confident attitude about the child's ability to manage symptoms and engage in age-appropriate activities. In conclusion, caregiver behaviors concerning health concerns and somatic symptoms may predispose a child to interpret fear cues in a specific way as well as maintain the cycle of health anxiety.

Triggers/fear cues

There are a broad range of internal cues that can trigger health anxiety. These include benign body sensations (e.g., racing heart, shortness of breath, nausea or other sensations associated with emotional arousal or substances such as caffeine), innocuous body variations (e.g., form or color of stool, skin appearance), and minor physical symptoms (e.g., headache, rash, muscle pain, sore throat) (Rachman, 2012; Warwick & Salkovskis, 1990). In addition to physical experiences, intrusive thoughts, images, or doubts about illness can serve as an internal cue for health anxiety episodes (Rachman, 2012). There also exist external cues, such as exposure to illness-relevant situations or stimuli in the environment (e.g., hospitals, viewing illness content on internet or TV shows, news coverage about threat of disease, experience of family member or friend with illness, caregiver guidance about prevention of illness) (Rachman, 2012; Warwick & Salkovskis, 1990). When conceptualizing health anxiety in pediatric populations, it is important to not only consider internal and external triggers for the child/adolescent, but also the experience and management of fear cues within the family and their contributions to fear learning (Ingerman et al., 2022).

Maintaining factors

Various cognitive and behavioral processes have been proposed as maintaining factors in models of health anxiety (Warwick & Salkovskis, 1990). A recent systematic review (Leonidou & Panayiotou, 2018) examined studies related to the central tenants of the cognitive-behavioral model

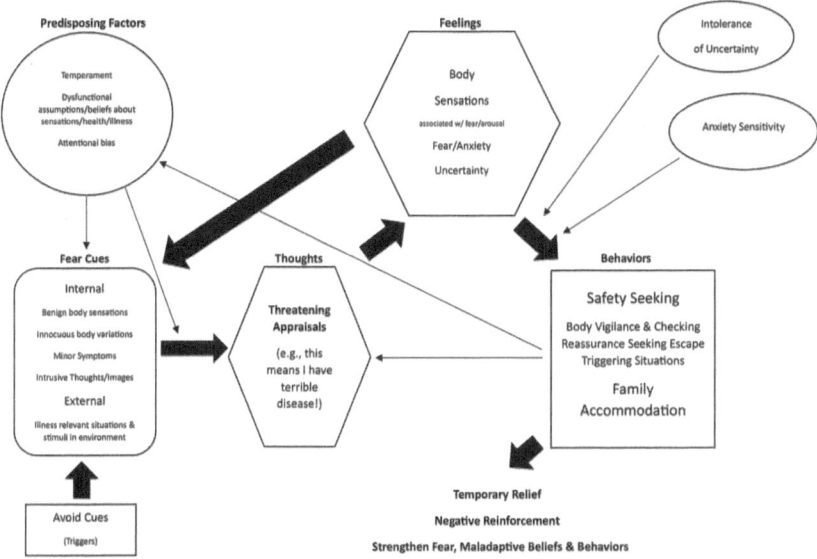

Figure 7.1 Model of Health Anxiety Theory.

and derived supported domains including: attentional biases, memory and interpretation biases, awareness and perception of physiological sensations, negativity bias, emotional processing of health information, and behavioral avoidance. These domains may be more broadly characterized as cognitive, physiological, and behavioral interpretations and responses to health information. This follows the cognitive behavioral model that incorporates thoughts, feelings, and behaviors as depicted in Figure 7.1.

Thoughts (Cognitions)

Once an individual appraises stimuli such as benign sensations as highly significant or threatening (i.e., "This means I have a terrible disease"), these triggers take on a negative valence, and health anxiety results (Warwick & Salkovskis, 1990; Abramowitz, Schwartz, & Whiteside, 2002). Dysfunctional core beliefs, attentional biases, and other cognitive processes (e.g., intolerance of uncertainty) play important role in the development and maintenance of maladaptive health anxiety (Abramowitz et al., 2002; Rachman, 2012; Warwick & Salkovskis, 1990; Wright et al., 2016).

Dysfunctional Core Beliefs. In keeping with Warwick and Salkovskis (1990) cognitive behavioral model, children and adolescents who struggle with health anxiety often maintain dysfunctional assumptions or beliefs about illness, the meaning of symptoms, health care, and their vulnerability and/or inability to cope with illness (Rask et al., 2012; Wright &

Asmundson, 2003). These beliefs are conceptualized as developed in context of experiences or learning history (e.g., illness in self, family, experiences with health care, caregiver modeling; Salkvovskis, 1996). Catastrophic misinterpretation of physiological stimuli could include attributing symptoms of benign illness with catastrophic causes (Bailey & Wells, 2015). For example, "I have a sore throat," might lead to, "I have throat cancer." Youth with health anxiety may also have difficulty tolerating uncertainty related to ambiguous somatic stimuli (i.e., increased heart rate). Researchers suggest that intolerance of uncertainty is associated with health anxiety, although mediated by anxiety sensitivity (Wright et al., 2016).

In pediatric populations, caregiver assumptions or core beliefs about health and illness, including their willingness to tolerate symptoms in their child, is an important contributing and maintaining mechanism (Thorgaard et al., 2018; Rask, 2019). Similarly, trait-like beliefs that limit a child or caregiver's tolerance for aversive states or ambiguity (i.e., anxiety sensitivity, intolerance of uncertainty) set the stage for unproductive avoidance, safety-seeking, and family accommodation (Wright et al., 2016, Bredemeier et al., 2023).

Attentional Bias. Attentional biases refer to automatic and intentional processes of favoring or attending to threatening, rather than neutral, stimuli (Cisler & Koster, 2010; Derryberry & Reed, 2002). Individuals with health anxiety may be more vigilant towards health-threat information or have difficulty disengaging from illness information once they have attended (Rogers et al., 2022; Shi et al., 2022). Further, they are more likely to interpret even ambiguous or non-threatening information as threatening (Du et al., 2023). Then, when an individual does experience pain or negative physiological stimuli, they are more likely to get stuck in maladaptive thinking traps such as catastrophizing (Parker et al., 2023).

Within the cognitive-behavioral model of health anxiety, once a trigger has been identified as threatening, it potentially becomes target of preoccupation. This preoccupation involves attentional bias and hypervigilance to one's body, physical sensations, and/or other illness-related information (Abramowitz et al., 2002, Warwick & Salkovskis, 1990). Ironically, attending to sensations has the potential to amplify these experiences (Barends et. al., 2020; Marcus et al., 2007) and their importance. From a developmental perspective, children are primed to be attuned to safety messages (both verbal and nonverbal) from their caregivers. Excessive caregiver attention and engagement in their child's preoccupation as well caregiver over-concern about their child's symptoms is likely to reinforce and strengthen the child's appraisals of threat and preoccupation with bodily sensations or variations (Thorgaard et al., 2018; Ingeman et al., 2022; Rapee, 2012).

Threatening Appraisals. The essential cognitive process experienced by individuals with health anxiety is appraisal of bodily sensations, symptoms or other health-related stimuli as threatening (Warwick & Salkovskis, 1990, Marcus et al., 2007; Leonidou & Panayioutou, 2018). Individuals with problematic health anxiety tend to overestimate the significance and seriousness of bodily sensations, variations, symptoms, and medical information as well as the probability of being affected by a dreaded illness (Salkovskis, 1996; Rachman, 2012). In children and adolescents, these negative appraisals are similar to those seen in adults (Rask et al., 2012; Sirri et al., 2015), albeit with more diffuse less well-developed cognitions in younger children (Rask, 2019; Rask et al., 2012; Sirri et al., 2015). One threat appraisal variation commonly seen in pediatric populations involves overly rule-governed concern about others in their environment violating "safety rules."

Feelings (emotions and sensations)

Threatening appraisals about health yield a range of uncomfortable experiences such as fear, anxiety, dread, uncertainty, and bodily sensations associated with emotional arousal/fear (i.e., the flight-or-fight response). Some also experience disturbing intrusive thoughts and images. In turn, these negative emotions, sensations, and/or intrusive thoughts are appraised as unacceptable and/or threatening. In particular, the benign physical sensations associated with emotional arousal and fear often cue more fear in context of health anxiety, yielding a vicious "fear of fear" cycle (Marcus et al., 2007; Rachman, 2012). Individuals with health anxiety often report amplified somatosensory experiences; however, little evidence exists to suggest that physiological stimuli are truly experienced in a heightened sense (Barsky & Wyshak, 1990; Barsky et al., 1990). Instead, increased sensitivity and over-interpretation of stimuli likely better explain these amplified feelings (Marcus et al., 2007). This may be due partly to anxiety sensitivity, a fear of arousal-related bodily sensations owing to beliefs that they are a sign of danger (Taylor, 1995). For example, an individual may believe that a fast heartbeat means they are having a heart attack (Reiss, 1991). Although often associated with panic disorder, anxiety sensitivity is documented as a correlate of health anxiety in both adults and children (Gerolimatos & Edelstein, 2012; Muris et al., 2001; Tsao et al., 2009; Wheaton et al., 2010). Further, anxiety sensitivity is related to attentional biases and maladaptive cognitions, thus contributing to the complex interactions between physiological stimuli and cognitive processes (Fergus & Bardeen, 2013; Lees et al., 2005).

Behaviors

When individuals with health anxiety perceive threat and the associated uncomfortable emotions, sensations, and doubt are activated, they naturally experience the urge to engage in safety behaviors. Individuals with health anxiety may engage in a variety of safety behaviors with the perception of protecting health and reducing distress, which leads to immediate relief in the short-term (Abramowitz & Moore, 2007). Although engagement in safety behaviors provides short-term relief, they ultimately lead to maintenance and exacerbation of symptoms (Olatunji et al., 2011). Key differences exist in the presentation of health anxiety in children, particularly related to parental reassurance, accommodation, and participation in safety behaviors that likely serve as additional maintaining factors (Haig-Ferguson et al., 2021). Common safety-seeking behaviors which maintain health anxiety include body checking, health-related reassurance seeking, and escape and avoidance of triggers, and in children, family accommodation results when family members help children engage in these safety behaviors (Halldorsson & Salkovskis, 2023; Lebowitz et al., 2013; Taylor & Asmundson, 2004; Wright & Asmundson, 2003, Warwick & Salkovskis, 1990).

Body Checking and Reassurance Seeking. Body checking involves assessing for health utilizing a wide variety of methods including heart rate monitors, blood pressure monitors, or examining skin for lumps or abnormalities (Abramowitz & Moore, 2007). Increased hypervigilance to body sensations yields a range of behavioral responses aimed at avoiding or reducing perceived threat (Abramowitz, et al., 2002; Rachman, 2012). These behaviors might include monitoring of symptoms (e.g., pulse, temperature), body inspections (e.g., skin, throat), internet searches related to illness or body symptoms, and/or visits to doctor to check on symptoms (Warwick & Salkovskis, 1990). Reassurance seeking includes asking about health status from other individuals such as friends or family (Goetz et al., 2013). Further, individuals may seek reassurance through internet searches or utilizing healthcare services (Baumgartner & Hartmann, 2011; Muse et al., 2012). In pediatric populations, seeking reassurance about illness, body status, or the environment is a frequent safety behavior and typically sought from caregivers, rather than predominantly health-care professionals (Rask, 2019).

Family accommodation, either through participation or facilitation of safety seeking behaviors or avoidance, is common response to anxiety among caregivers and is a key maintaining factor in pediatric health anxiety (Abramowitz et al., 2002; Benito et al., 2015; Halldorsson & Salkovskis, 2023; Lebowitz et al., 2013). Common examples of caregiver accommodation to their child's health anxiety include providing repeated verbal reassurances about safety and health status, participating in body checks (e.g., taking temperature, inspecting skin), providing items needed for checks (e.g., access to blood pressure monitor), and arranging for repeated doctor visits.

Escape, Avoidance, and other Preventative Measures. In context of health anxiety, seeking to escape or avoid potentially triggering situations and fear cues is a central maintaining factor (Warwick & Salkovskis,

1990; Rachman, 2012). Some individuals with health anxiety may avoid healthcare services (Starcevic, 2013). Additional avoidance extends to situations or stimuli that are perceived as health threatening or avoidance of negative affectivity associated with such stimuli (Brady & Lohr, 2014; Karimi et al., 2019). Commonly avoided situations include the following: TV shows, movies, internet sites, stories, or conversation that involve illness, bodily symptoms, or death; places or activities where individual might have contact with sick people or that have been associated with illness; and activities that might trigger bodily symptoms (e. g., eating certain foods, drinking caffeinated soda, exercise). Avoidance in pediatric health anxiety might also involve taking extra precautions to support safety such as maintaining proximity to one's caregiver in case of illness, always keeping cell phone or water bottle on hand "just in case," maintaining an extra healthy diet, or checking food expiration dates. Caregivers often facilitate escape, avoidance, or excessively cautious behaviors (Benito et al., 2015), often without recognizing of the role of such accommodation on maintenance of their child's fear and associated behaviors.

Unfortunately, these heath anxiety avoidance and safety seeking behaviors serve to maintain behavioral symptoms, underlying beliefs, and (mis) interpretations (Warwick & Salkovskis, 1990; Abramowitz et al., 2002). One key maintaining mechanism for how this occurs is through negative reinforcement (Abramowitz et al., 2007). Specifically, the unproductive safety seeking behavioral response (including accommodation) are negatively reinforced by the immediate reduction in distress as temporary relief they engender (Abramowitz & Moore, 2007). Avoidance, escape, and safety seeking begets more avoidance, escape, and safety seeking. This yields an unproductive negative reinforcement cycle that includes the child and important others who engage in accommodation (Lebowitz et al., 2013).

Moreover, and highly important from a maintenance perspective, engaging in avoidance/escape and safety seeking behaviors (i.e., checking, reassurance seeking, or other preventative measures) functionally prevents disconfirmation of threat related beliefs (Abramowitz et al., 2007; Rachman 2012; Halldorsson & Salkovskis, 2023). These are missed opportunities for youth to learn more adaptive, or non-threat responses through inhibitory learning (Craske et al., 2022). Instead of learning that one (or one's child) is capable of managing the distress, doubt, and discomfort and that such behaviors are not necessary or functional, fear learning is strengthened; the child (and caregiver's), cognitive biases, misinterpretation of bodily cues, and misappraisals of threat, including perceived inability to manage the potential threat, have been maintained and potentially amplified (Warwick & Salkovskis, 1990; Abramowitz et al., 2002; Craske et al., 2022).

The COVID-19 pandemic brought about heightened avoidance behaviors. Even though early reports indicated that children were either asymptomatic or experience mild symptoms to COVID-19 (Lu et al., 2020), anxiety surrounding health and safety became omnipresent. The COVID-19 pandemic has been associated with increased clinginess, distraction, irritability, and persistent fear and reassurance-seeking behaviors surrounding illness. This was demonstrated among 320 children and adolescents (168 girls and 142 boys) aged 3–18 at the onset of the pandemic (Jiao et al., 2020). Furthermore, a study by Kim and colleagues (2022) found a higher mean number of medical visits for health anxiety symptoms among children and adolescents (ages 0–19) in Korea after the onset of the pandemic (Kim et al., 2022). Although epidemiological studies are scarce surrounding health anxiety among youth after COVID-19, the literature further supports overall increased in anxiety symptoms among youth (Kim et al., 2022; Gamonal Limcaoco et al., 2020).

Prior to the COVID-19 pandemic, if an individual were to report that they took their temperature each morning before going to the office, they used hand sanitizer after interacting with each person they met, they stayed six feet away from others, and they wore masks in all public space to avoid illness, this would have been considered diagnostic. However, during the height of the pandemic, this was considered appropriate practice. It is crucial to take cultural and family variables into account when assessing whether health anxiety is excessive. For instance, for someone who has an immunocompromised family member living in the home, hygiene behaviors may look different and be expected in that context compared to other family units. Additionally, a child with chronic illness may have specific medical procedures or checks they are required to do for their condition, and this is important to understand.

Case examples

Below are two case examples of different developmental periods of childhood to provide an overview of how health anxiety symptoms can in different symptom clusters. Each example incorporates aspects of the symptomatology described above, in addition to giving concrete examples of precipitating and maintaining factors that resulted in clinically elevated presentations of symptoms. While individual factors of culture and diversity are crucial within conceptualization and treatment planning, these aspects are intentionally left as vague and undefined in the following case examples as specific individual cultural factors are not directly related to onset of health anxiety symptoms.

A school-age child with illness anxiety disorder

"Luis" was a 7-year-old boy initially referred by his family for a diagnostic evaluation of anxiety after having significant difficulty adapting to a classroom environment. He was in preschool at the onset of the

COVID-19 pandemic and completed virtual school for the entire year of kindergarten. Upon returning to in-person school in 1st grade, Luis was very distressed about being in close contact with others for fear of contracting COVID-19 or another illness, including the flu or monkey pox. Luis's anxiety was triggered when asked to enter the classroom or indoor, crowded such as restaurants and stores.

Luis' anxiety symptoms primarily presented as avoidance, reassurance-seeking, and checking behaviors. When a family outing was suggested, Luis would request for the family to stay home. On school days, he demonstrated school avoidant behaviors, such as requesting to stay home, crying on the way to school, and clinging to a parent when it was time for him to enter the school building. Once in the classroom, Luis would not sit close to classmates and would instead stand at the side of the classroom to ensure he was socially distanced from others. In public settings, Luis sometimes hid himself in the bathroom or asked to go outside to avoid breathing air that "may contain germs." Luis also frequently sought reassurance from his family. He frequently asked about whether he had been exposed to different illnesses and if he would become sick. Luis also requested for his parent to take his temperature several times per day to "check" an be sure he did not have a fever. These safety behaviors served to maintain health anxiety.

The family described that the onset of the COVID-19 pandemic was a significant precipitating event for Luis's anxiety. The family made the decision to socially isolate for close to 18 months after the onset of the pandemic, owing to a family member with health concerns. During this time, Luis only interacted with others outside his immediate family through phone and video calls. The family reported they frequently discussed the pandemic, and Luis was often exposed to news stations which maintained his fear of the illness. However, the family described that once all family members had been vaccinated, they were ready to stop socially isolating. However, the family perceived that Luis did not understand why family routines and practices were changing. They described Luis as perceiving himself to be in significant danger and fear of becoming ill. Earlier in the pandemic, Luis's level of social isolation and safety behaviors seemed in line with his family's. However, he had difficulty adapting and shifting with his family's practices.

Luis' presentation was marked by significant health anxiety, and he was given a diagnosis of Illness Anxiety Disorder. Although there were multiple factors that had precipitated and maintained Luis's anxiety during the beginning of the pandemic, he also demonstrated multiple strengths. For instance, he has a strong family support system with common family goals for Luis to be able to attend and engage in school appropriately. Additionally, Luis had a desire to make friends and start to play sports, even though proximity to others was still anxiety-provoking for him. Luis was also very motivated by concrete rewards. All of these factors will benefit Luis as he and his family engage in behavioral intervention.

An adolescent with somatic symptom disorder

"Emma" was a 14-year-old girl referred to an outpatient psychology service for diagnostic evaluation for anxiety by her pediatrician. Specifically, Emma presented with significant distress and preoccupation about recurrent headaches and abdominal pain, which she attributed may be due to significant health concerns. Emma's somatic symptoms have been recurring for the past six months, and she has started to avoid sports team practices owing to preoccupation with these concerns.

Emma's anxiety regarding somatic symptoms also manifested as emotional outbursts and overanalyzing or checking her bodily sensations (e.g. "Am I starting to get a stomach ache?"), leading to hypervigilance for symptoms. Notably, Emma engaged in frequent checking behaviors, including body scanning for pain and monitoring pain levels of headaches and abdominal pain. The somatic discomfort and pain were misinterpreted as high severity, which led to increased anxiety. To attempt to extinguish these negative thoughts and feelings of anxiety, Emma sought reassurance from her parents about the symptoms so as not to exacerbate them. Additionally, she began to avoid sports practices, owing to perceived association that increased physical activity would exacerbate the symptoms. Time spent asking questions or engaging in checking behaviors interfered with Emma's routine and schedule, most significantly at home, and affected her relationship with family members. These behaviors emerged several years ago, although exacerbated following the onset of the COVID-19 pandemic.

Family culture, practices, and values regarding health and responsibility intersected with and precipitated Emma's anxiety and checking behaviors. It was hypothesized that her anxiety was maintained, in part, by parental accommodation, via parents' attention to her anxiety responses and reassurance. Her family also used different parenting approaches to respond to Emma's anxiety at times; her father typically provided positive attention and reassurance, while her mother alternated between reassurance, reprimands, and ignoring Emma's behavior, consistent with the way she was parented as a child. The inconsistent cycle of positive and negative reinforcement may have also contributed to the maintenance of her symptoms.

Emma's constellation of symptoms was indicative of Somatic Symptom Disorder, with predominant pain, persistent, moderate, owing to the longstanding presence of somatic complaints primarily related to pain and involving excessive concern and checking behaviors. However, it should be noted Emma demonstrated many strengths and notable protective factors. She was intelligent, had a strong family and peer support system, and was highly motivated by positive interpersonal relationships. Emma was forthcoming and expressed openness to seeking and receiving help with her anxiety, and she demonstrated insight regarding the interference of her symptoms with daily functioning, particularly at home. Moreover, she noted less interference of her symptoms in contexts that closely aligned with her values regarding education, respect, and performance, such as school, where she described her focus on class activities helps to minimize time engaged in ruminating about or engaging in behaviors that reinforced her anxiety surrounding somatic symptoms. These factors would be incorporated into treatment.

Summary

Health anxiety is a cluster of anxiety symptoms that is increasingly common in children and adolescents. Youth with health anxiety often present with significant fears about contracting an illness or disease. This fear is often accompanied by avoidance or checking behaviors related to health. Diagnostically, youth with these symptoms may be diagnosed with illness anxiety disorder or somatic symptom disorder, although health anxiety symptoms can be present within other anxiety or obsessive-compulsive categories. Health anxiety symptoms follow a pattern of negative reinforcement consistent with obsessive-compulsive disorder and is often considered as an obsessive-compulsive-related disorder because of this presentation. It is important to take contextual factors into account when determining if health-related anxiety and safety behaviors are appropriate or indicative of a clinical presentation and need for intervention.

References

Abramowitz, J. S. & Moore, E. L. (2007). An experimental analysis of hypochondriasis. *Behaviour Research and Therapy*, 45(3), 413–424. doi:10.1016/j.brat.2006.04.005.

Abramowitz, J. S., Schwartz, S. A., & Whiteside, S. P. (2002). A contemporary conceptual model of hypochondriasis. *Mayo Clinic Proceedings*, 77(12), 1323–1330. doi:10.4065/77.12.1323.

American Psychiatric Association. (1994). Somatoform disorders. In *Diagnostic and Statistical Manual of Mental Disorders* (4th Ed.).

American Psychiatric Association. (2022). Somatic symptom and related disorders. In *Diagnostic and Statistical Manual of Mental Disorders* (5th Ed., rev. text). doi:10.1176/appi.books.9780890425787.

Asmundson, G. J. G., Taylor, S., & Cox, B. J. (2001). Health anxiety: Clinical and research perspectives on hypochondriasis and related conditions. West Sussex.

Barsky, A. J. (1992). Hypochondriasis and obsessive compulsive disorder. *Psychiatric Clinics of North America*.

Barbek, R. M., Makowski, A. C., & von dem Knesebeck, O. (2022). Social inequalities in health anxiety: A systematic review and meta-analysis. *Journal of Psychosomatic Research*, 153, 110706.

Bailey, R. & Wells, A. (2015). Metacognitive beliefs moderate the relationship between catastrophic misinterpretation and health anxiety. *Journal of Anxiety Disorders*, 34, 8–14. doi:10.1016/j.janxdis.2015.05.005.

Barends, H., Claassen-van Dessel, N., van der Wouden, J. C., Twisk, J. W. R., Terluin, B., van der Horst, H. E., & Dekker, J. (2020). Impact of symptom focusing and somatosensory amplification on persistent physical symptoms: A three-year follow-up study. *Journal of Psychosomatic Research*, 135, 110131. doi:10.1016/j.jpsychores.2020.110131.

Barsky, A. J., Wool, C., Barnett, M. C., & Cleary, P. D. (1994). Histories of childhood trauma in adult hypochondriacal patients. *The American Journal of Psychiatry*, 151(3), 397–401. doi:10.1176/ajp.151.3.397.

Barsky, A. J. & Wyshak, G. (1990). Hypochondriasis and somatosensory amplification. *The British Journal of Psychiatry*, 157, 404–409. doi:10.1192/bjp.157.3.404.

Baumgartner, S. E. & Hartmann, T. (2011). The role of health anxiety in online health information search. *Cyberpsychology, Behavior, and Social Networking*, 14(10), 613–618.

Benito, K. G., Caporino, N. E., Frank, H. E., Ramanujam, K., Garcia, A., Freeman, J., Kendall, P. C., Geffken, G., & Storch, E. A. (2015). Development of the pediatric accommodation scale: Reliability and validity of clinician- and parent-report measures. *Journal of Anxiety Disorders*, 29, 14–24. doi:10.1016/j.janxdis.2014.10.004.

Brady, R. E. & Lohr, J. M. (2014). A behavioral test of contamination fear in excessive health anxiety. *Journal of Behavior Therapy and Experimental Psychiatry*, 45(1), 122–127. doi:10.1016/j.jbtep.2013.09.011.

Bredemeier, K., Church, L. D., Bounoua, N., Feler, B., & Spielberg, J. M. (2023). Intolerance of uncertainty, anxiety sensitivity, and health anxiety during the COVID-19 pandemic: Exploring temporal relationships using cross-lag analysis. *Journal of Anxiety Disorders*, 93, 102660. doi:10.1016/j.janxdis.2022.102660.

Campo, J. V. (2012). Annual Research Review: Functional somatic symptoms and associated anxiety and depression–developmental psychopathology in pediatric practice. *Journal of Child Psychology and Psychiatry*, 53(5), 575–592.

Cisler, J. M. & Koster, E. H. (2010). Mechanisms of attentional biases towards threat in anxiety disorders: An integrative review. *Clinical Psychology Review*, 30(2), 203–216.

Cox, B. J., Borger, S. C., Asmundson, G. J. G., & Taylor, S. (2000). Dimensions of hypochondriasis and the five-factor model of personality. *Personality and Individual Differences*, 29(1), 99–108. doi:10.1016/S0191-8869(99)00180-00184.

Cozzi, G., Minute, M., Skabar, A., Pirrone, A., Jaber, M., Neri, E., … & Barbi, E. (2017). Somatic symptom disorder was common in children and adolescents attending an emergency department complaining of pain. *Acta Paediatrica*, 106(4), 586–593.

Craske, M. G., Treanor, M., Zbozinek, T. D., & Vervliet, B. (2022). Optimizing exposure therapy with an inhibitory retrieval approach and the OptEx Nexus. *Behaviour research and therapy*, 152, 104069doi:10.1016/j.brat.2022.104069.

Delparte, C. A., Wright, K. D., Walker, J. R., Feldgaier, S., Furer, P., Reiser, S. J., & Sharpe, D. (2015). Confirmatory factor analysis of the childhood illness attitude scales. *Children's Health Care*, 44(4), 322–340.

Daniels, J., Parker, H., & Salkovskis, P. M. (2020). Prevalence and treatment of Chronic Fatigue Syndrome/Myalgic Encephalomyelitis and co-morbid severe health anxiety. *International Journal of Clinical and Health Psychology*, 20(1), 10–19. doi:10.1016/j.ijchp.2019.11.003.

Derryberry, D. & Reed, M. A. (2002). Anxiety-related attentional biases and their regulation by attentional control. *Journal of Abnormal Psychology*, 111(2), 225.

Drake, K. L. & Ginsburg, G. S. (2012). Family factors in the development, treatment, and prevention of childhood anxiety disorders. *Clinical Child and Family Psychology Review*, 15, 144–162.

Du, X., Witthöft, M., Zhang, T., Shi, C., & Ren, Z. (2023). Interpretation bias in health anxiety: A systematic review and meta-analysis. *Psychological Medicine*, 53(1), 34–45. doi:10.1017/S0033291722003427.

Eminson, M., Benjamin, S., Shortall, A., Woods, T., & Faragher, B. (1996). Physical symptoms and illness attitudes in adolescents: an epidemiological study. *Journal of Child Psychology and Psychiatry*, 37(5), 519–528.

Fergus, T. A. & Bardeen, J. R. (2013). Anxiety sensitivity and intolerance of uncertainty: Evidence of incremental specificity in relation to health anxiety. *Personality and Individual Differences*, 55(6), 640–644.

Ferguson, E. (2004). Personality as a predictor of hypochondriacal concerns: Results from two longitudinal studies. *Journal of Psychosomatic Research*, 56(3), 307–312.

Fritz, G. K., Fritsch, S., & Hagino, O. (1997). Somatoform disorders in children and adolescents: A review of the past 10 years. *Journal of the American Academy of Child and Adolescent Psychiatry*, 36(10), 1329–1338. doi:10.1097/00004583-199710000-00014.

Gamonal Limcaoco, R. S., Mateos, E. M., Fernández, J. M., & Roncero, C. (2020). Anxiety, worry and perceived stress in the world due to the COVID-19 pandemic, March 2020. Preliminary results. *MedRxiv*, 2020–2004.

Gehrt, T. B., Obermann, M., Toth, F. E., & Frostholm, L. (2022). Adverse childhood experiences in patients with severe health anxiety: No evidence for an increased frequency compared to patients with obsessive–compulsive disorder. *Scandinavian Journal of Psychology*, 63(6), 565–572. doi:10.1111/sjop.12856.

Gerolimatos, L. A. & Edelstein, B. A. (2012). Predictors of health anxiety among older and young adults. *International Psychogeriatrics*, 24(12), 1998–2008.

Goetz, A. R., Lee, H.-J., & Cougle, J. R. (2013). The association between health anxiety and disgust reactions in a contamination-based behavioral approach task. *Anxiety, Stress & Coping: An International Journal*, 26(4), 431–446. doi:10.1080/10615806.2012.684241.

Gouze, K. R., Hopkins, J., Bryant, F. B., & Lavigne, J. V. (2017). Parenting and anxiety: Bi-directional relations in young children. *Journal of Abnormal Child Psychology*, 45, 1169–1180.

Gureje, O., Simon, G. E., Ustun, T. B., & Goldberg, D. P. (1997). Somatization in cross-cultural perspective: A World Health Organization study in primary care. *American Journal of Psychiatry*, 154(7), 989–995.

Haig-Ferguson, A., Cooper, K., Cartwright, E., Loades, M., & Daniels, J. (2021). Practitioner review: Health anxiety in children and young people in the context of the COVID-19 pandemic. *Behavioural and Cognitive Psychotherapy*, 49(2), 129–143. doi:10.1017/S1352465820000636.

Halldorsson, B. & Salkovskis, P.M. (2023). Reassurance and its alternatives: Overview and cognitive behavioral conceptualisation. *Journal of Obsessive-Compulsive and Related Disorders*, 36. doi:10.1016/j.jocrd.2023.10078.

Ingeman, K., Hulgaard, D. R., & Rask, C. U. (2022). Health anxiety by proxy – through the eyes of the parents. *Journal of child health care: for professionals working with children in the hospital and community.* doi:10.1177/13674935221095648.

Jackson, J. L. & Kroenke, K. (2008). Prevalence, impact, and prognosis of multi-somatoform disorder in primary care: a 5-year follow-up study. *Psychosomatic Medicine*, 70(4), 430–434.

Jiao, W. Y., Wang, L. N., Liu, J., Fang, S. F., Jiao, F. Y., Pettoello-Mantovani, M., & Somekh, E. (2020). Behavioral and emotional disorders in children during the COVID-19 epidemic. *The Journal of Pediatrics*, 221, 264–266.

Karimi, J., Homayouni, A., & Homayouni, F. (2019). *The prediction of health anxiety based on experiential avoidance and anxiety sensitivity among non-clinical population. Journal of Research in Psychological Health*, 12(4), 66–79.

Kim, S. Y., Lee, N. E., Yoo, D. M., Kim, J. H., Kwon, M. J., Kim, J. H., … & Choi, H. G. (2022). Changes in the mean of medical visits due to psychiatric disease in Korean children and adolescents before and during the COVID-19 pandemic. *Life*, 12(4), 600.

Köteles, F., Freyler, A., Kökönyei, G., & Bárdos, G. (2015). Family background of modern health worries, somatosensory amplification, and health anxiety: a questionnaire study. *Journal of Health Psychology*, 20, 1549–1557. doi:10.1177/1359105313516661.

Lebowitz, E. R., Woolston, J., Bar-Haim, Y., Calvocoressi, L., Dauser, C., Warnick, E., Scahill, L., Chakir, A. R., Shechner, T., Hermes, H., Vitulano, L. A., King, R. A., & Leckman, J. F. (2013). Family accommodation in pediatric anxiety disorders. *Depression and Anxiety*, 30(1), 47–54. doi:10.1002/da.21998.

Lees, A., Mogg, K., & Bradley, B. P. (2005). Health anxiety, anxiety sensitivity, and attentional biases for pictorial and linguistic health-threat cues. *Cognition & Emotion*, 19(3), 453–462.

Leonidou, C. & Panayiotou, G. (2018). How do illness-anxious individuals process health-threatening information? A systematic review of evidence for the cognitive-behavioral model. *Journal of Psychosomatic Research*, 111, 100–115.

Lu, X., Zhang, L., Du, H., Zhang, J., Li, Y. Y., & Qu, J. (2020). SARS-CoV-2 infection in children. *New England Journal of Medicine*, 382, 1663–1665. doi:10.1056/NEJMc2005073.

Marcus, D. K., Gurley, J. R., Marchi, M. M., & Bauer, C. (2007). Cognitive and perceptual variables in hypochondriasis and health anxiety: a systematic review. *Clinical Psychology Review*, 27, 127–139. doi:10.1016/j.cpr.2006.09.003.

Marshall, T., Jones, D. P., Ramchandani, P. G., Stein, A., & Bass, C. (2007). Intergenerational transmission of health beliefs in somatoform disorders: exploratory study. *British Journal of Psychiatry*, 191, 449–450. doi:10.1192/bjp.bp.107.035261.

Martin, A. & Jacobi, F. (2006). Features of hypochondriasis and illness worry in the general population in Germany. *Psychosomatic Medicine*, 68(5), 770–777. doi:10.1097/01.psy.0000238213.04984.b0.

Muris, P., Vlaeyen, J., & Meesters, C. (2001). The relationship between anxiety sensitivity and fear of pain in healthy adolescents. *Behaviour Research and Therapy*, 39(11), 1357–1368.

Muse, K., McManus, F., Leung, C., Meghreblian, B., & Williams, J. M. G. (2012). Cyberchondriasis: fact or fiction? A preliminary examination of the relationship between health anxiety and searching for health information on the Internet. *Journal of Anxiety Disorders*, 26(1), 189–196.

Noyes, R., Jr., Stuart, S., Langbehn, D. R., Happel, R. L., Longley, S. L., & Yagla, S. J. (2002). Childhood antecedents of hypochondriasis. *Psychosomatics: Journal of Consultation and Liaison Psychiatry*, 43(4), 282–289. doi:10.1176/appi.psy.43.4.282.

Offord, D. R., Boyle, M. H., Szatmari, P., Rae-Grant, N. I., Links, P. S., Cadman, D. T., Byles, J. A., Crawford, J. W., Blum, H. M., & Byrne, C. (1987). Ontario Child Health Study. II. Six-month prevalence of disorder and rates of service utilization. *Archives of General Psychiatry*, 44(9), 832–836. https://doi.org/10.1001/archpsyc.1987.01800210084013.

Olatunji, B. O., Etzel, E. N., Tomarken, A. J., Ciesielski, B. G., & Deacon, B. (2011). The effects of safety behaviors on health anxiety: An experimental investigation. *Behaviour Research and Therapy*, 49(11), 719–728.

Parker, H., Carlton, E., Harris, S., & Daniels, J. (2023). Psychological predictors of health anxiety and pain in ambulatory presentations in a hospital emergency department. *Behavioural and Cognitive Psychotherapy*, 51(1), 11–20. doi:10.1017/S1352465822000352.

Rachman, S. (2012). Health anxiety disorders: a cognitive construal. *Behavior and Research Therapy*, 50, 502–512. doi:10.1016/j.brat.2012.05.001.

Rapee R. M. (2012). Family factors in the development and management of anxiety disorders. *Clinical child and family psychology review*, 15(1), 69–80. doi:10.1007/s10567-011-0106-3.

Rask, C. U. (2019). Health anxiety in children and adolescents. In *The Clinician's Guide to Treating Health Anxiety* (pp. 165–176). Academic Press.

Rask, C. U., Elberling, H., Skovgaard, A. M., Thomsen, P. H., & Fink, P. (2012). Parental reported health anxiety symptoms in 5-to 7-year-old children: The Copenhagen Child Cohort CCC 2000. *Psychosomatics*, 53(1), 58–67.

Reiss, S. (1991). Expectancy model of fear, anxiety, and panic. *Clinical Psychology Review*, 11(2), 141–153.

Robbins, J. M. & Kirmayer, L. J. (1996). Transient and persistent hypochondriacal worry in primary care. *Psychological Medicine*, 26(3), 575–589.

Rogers, T. A., Daniel, T. A., & Bardeen, J. R. (2022). Health anxiety and attentional control interact to predict uncertainty-related attentional biases. *Journal of Behavior Therapy and Experimental Psychiatry*, 74. doi:10.1016/j.jbtep.2021.101697.

Salkovskis, P. M. & Warwick, H. M. (1986). Morbid preoccupations, health anxiety and reassurance: A cognitive-behavioural approach to hypochondriasis. *Behaviour Research and Therapy*, 24(5), 597–602. doi:10.1016/0005-7967(86)90041-0.

Shi, C., Taylor, S., Witthöft, M., Du, X., Zhang, T., Lu, S., & Ren, Z. (2022). Attentional bias toward health-threat in health anxiety: A systematic review and three-level meta-analysis. *Psychological Medicine*, 52(4), 604–613. doi:10.1017/S0033291721005432.

Sirri, L., Garotti, M. G. R., Grandi, S., & Tossani, E. (2015). Adolescents' hypochondriacal fears and beliefs: Relationship with demographic features, psychological distress, well-being and health-related behaviors. *Journal of Psychosomatic Research*, 79(4), 259–264.

Starcevic, V. (2013). *Hypochondriasis and health anxiety: conceptual challenges.* The British Journal of Psychiatry, 202(1), 7–8.

Starcevic, V. & Lipsitt, D. R. (Eds). (2001). *Hypochondriasis: Modern perspectives on an ancient malady.* Oxford University Press.

Stokes, E. K., Zambrano, L. D., Anderson, K. N., Marder, E. P., Raz, K. M., Felix, S. E. B., ... & Fullerton, K. E. (2020). Coronavirus disease 2019 case surveillance—United States, January 22–may 30, 2020. *Morbidity and Mortality Weekly Report*, 69(24), 759.

Taylor, S. (1995). Anxiety sensitivity: Theoretical perspectives and recent findings. *Behaviour Research and Therapy*, 33(3), 243–258.

Taylor, S. & Asmundson, G. J. (2004). *Treating Health Anxiety: A Cognitive-Behavioral Approach* (Vol. *494*). New York: Guilford Press.

Thorgaard, M. V., Frostholm, L., & Rask, C. U. (2018). Childhood and family factors in the development of health anxiety: A systematic review. *Children's Health Care*, 47(2), 198–238. doi:10.1080/02739615.2017.1318390.

Tsao, J. C., Allen, L. B., Evans, S., Lu, Q., Myers, C. D., & Zeltzer, L. K. (2009). Anxiety sensitivity and catastrophizing: Associations with pain and somatization in non-clinical children. *Journal of Health Psychology*, 14(8), 1085–1094.

Villadsen, A., Thorgaard, M. V., Hybel, K. A., Jensen, J. S., Thomsen, P. H., & Rask, C. U.(2017). Health anxiety symptoms in children and adolescents diagnosed with OCD. *European child & adolescent psychiatry, 26*(2), 241–251. doi:10.1007/s00787-016-0884-8.

Warwick, H. M. & Salkovskis, P. M. (1990). Hypochondriasis. *Behaviour Research and Therapy*, 28, 105–117.

Watson, D. & Pennebaker, J. W. (1989). Health complaints, stress, and distress: Exploring the central role of negative affectivity. *Psychological Review*, 96(2), 234–254. doi:10.1037/0033–0295X.96.2.234.

Weck, F., Richtberg, S., & MB Neng, J. (2014). Epidemiology of hypochondriasis and health anxiety: Comparison of different diagnostic criteria. *Current Psychiatry Reviews*, 10(1), 14–23.

Wheaton, M. G., Berman, N. C., & Abramowitz, J. S. (2010). The contribution of experiential avoidance and anxiety sensitivity in the prediction of health anxiety. *Journal of Cognitive Psychotherapy*, 24(3), 229–239.

Williams, P. G. (2004). The psychopathology of self-assessed health: A cognitive approach to health anxiety and hypochondriasis. *Cognitive Therapy and Research*, 28(5), 629–644. doi:10.1023/B:COTR.0000045569.25096.44.

World Health Organization (WHO) (2020). *Naming the coronavirus disease (COVID-19) and the virus that causes it.* Retrieved from: www.who.int/emergencies/diseases/novel-coronavirus-2019/technical-guidance/naming-the-coronavirus-disease-(covid-2019)-and-the-virus-that-causes-it.

Wright, K. D. & Asmundson, G. J. (2003). Health anxiety in children: development and psychometric properties of the Childhood Illness Attitude Scales. *Cognitive Behaviour Therapy*, 32, 194–202. doi:10.1080/16506070310014691.

Wright, K. D., Lebell, M. A. A., & Carleton, R. N. (2016). Intolerance of uncertainty, anxiety sensitivity, health anxiety, and anxiety disorder symptoms in youth. *Journal of Anxiety Disorders*, 41, 35–42.

8   Persistent (Chronic) Tic Disorders and Tourette Syndrome

Jordan T. Stiede, Emily Braley, Steven T. Bellows, Joseph Jankovic and Eric A. Storch

Diagnosis

Persistent (chronic) tic disorders (PTDs) are a class of neurodevelopmental disorders marked by motor and/or phonic tics. There are three main diagnostic categories, largely differentiated by the duration and type of tics (i.e., motor and/or phonic) present. In order to receive a diagnosis of Tourette Syndrome (TS), the individual must present with multiple motor tics and at least one phonic tic that have been present at some point, not necessarily simultaneously, for a minimum of one year, and tics must onset before age 18 years and are not due to the physiological effects of a substance or other medical condition. Individuals who receive a provisional tic disorder diagnosis may also present with multiple motor and/or phonic tics or just one tic; however, the tic or tics have not been present for a year. Individuals who have a single or multiple motor or phonic tics, but not both, present for over a year meet criteria for persistent motor or phonic tic disorder. Additionally, the diagnostic categories are hierarchical in the fact that individuals cannot receive a lower-level diagnosis (e.g., provisional tic disorder) after receiving a higher-level diagnosis (e.g., TS; American Psychiatric Association, 2022).

Clinical presentation

Tics, which are the primary symptom of all PTDs, are defined as sudden, rapid, recurrent, non-rhythmic movements and/or sounds (vocalizations). Contrary to conventional understanding, not all phonic tics involve verbalizations. Rather, a tic is categorized as a phonic tic if it involves contraction of the diaphragm or muscles of the throat alongside movement of air through the body. Motor and phonic tics can also be categorized as simple or complex. Simple tics are typically brief, purposeless movements (e.g., head jerking, eye blinking, face scrunching) or vocalizations (e.g., sniffing, throat clearing, animal noises, humming) that involve one area of the body. Complex tics can be a combination of simple tics that involve more than one area of the body, or a longer series of movements

DOI: 10.4324/9781003517429-8

including multiple muscles. Examples of complex motor tics include jumping, spinning, or jerking an arm then head, while complex phonic tics include sentences or phrases, coprolalia (i.e., obscene words), echolalia (i.e., repeating other's words), or palilalia (i.e., repeating own words; American Psychiatric Association, 2022; Bloch & Leckman, 2009). In addition to simple and complex, tics may be classified phenomenologically as clonic, dystonic, tonic (isometric), stereotypic, compulsive and blocking (Baizabal-Carvallo & Jankovic, 2023).

Tics are estimated to affect around 1 percent of the pediatric population, with males impacted more often than females (ratios varying from 2:1 to 4:1; Baizabal-Carvallo & Jankovic, 2022; Robertson, 2012; Scharf et al., 2015). Tics typically fluctuate and change in phenomenology, intensity, frequency, and distribution over time, with simple tics (e.g., sniff, throat clear, rapid blink) typically appearing around age four to six (Bloch & Leckman, 2009). As an individual ages, tics progress in a cephalocaudal trend and may become more complex (Baizabal-Carvallo et al., 2022a; Bloch & Leckman, 2009; Himle et al., 2014).

PTDs remain widely misunderstood by the lay public (Malli et al., 2016). For example, tics like coprolalia (i.e., obscene words) and copropraxia (i.e., obscene gestures), while popular in mainstream media, only affect around 10 percent of the tic population (Robertson, 2012). Initially, tics can also be mistaken as allergies, eye problems, or even other motor behaviors, such as stereotypies, leading to a delay in diagnosis or seeing multiple providers before receiving a diagnosis (Wolicki et al., 2019). Therefore, it is important to highlight how tics differ from other common motor movements, such as stereotypies. Phenomenologically, stereotypies are more rhythmic, coordinated, and longer in duration than tics (Baizabal-Carvallo & Jankovic, 2021). Tics also differ from stereotypies in the fact that stereotypies are often soothing for the individual, whereas tics mitigate unwanted, unpleasant sensations in the body. Furthermore, tics can be temporarily suppressed by an individual, whereas stereotypies are rarely voluntarily suppressed, owing to the pleasurable experience of engaging in them (Nilles et al., 2023).

Premonitory urges

Although not a diagnostic requirement for PTDs, the majority of individuals with tics report experiencing premonitory urges prior to execution of the tic. Premonitory urges are uncomfortable, undesirable physiological sensations that precede tics and are relieved, albeit temporarily, after ticcing. Individuals with tics have described these sensory phenomena as an itch, pressure, energy, tense feeling, or a general sense of not "just right" experiences (Woods et al., 2005). While premonitory urges are common, children typically do not report on or recognize these sensations until around ten years of age (Leckman et al., 1993), and awareness of the premonitory urge appears to increase as individuals age (Woods et al., 2005).

Imaging and neurophysiologic studies of premonitory urges preceding tics have also yielded insights. Multiple functional magnetic resonance imaging (fMRI) and transcranial magnetic stimulation (TMS) studies have noted activation of the anterior cingulate, insular cortex, supplementary motor area, and parietal operculum concurrent with tic urges (Bohlhalter et al., 2006; Neuner et al., 2014; Singer & Augustine, 2019). One fMRI study noted increased activity in the supplementary motor area (SMA) and motor cortices two seconds prior to the onset of tics, increased insular, anterior cingulate, putaminal, and cerebellar activity one second prior, and increased thalamic and primary motor and somatosensory cortical activity at the onset of tics (Neuner et al., 2014). Results were suggestive of preparatory action in the SMA being relayed to monitoring centers in the insula and anterior cingulate before propagating to output pathways from the cortico-basal ganglia-thalamo-cortical (CBGTC) loops. Similarly, SMA overactivation has been noted prior to tics as compared to simulation of tics (Hampson et al., 2009). Urge intensity has correlated with gray matter volume and cortical thickness in left somatosensory and prefrontal cortices (Draganski et al., 2010; Müller-Vahl et al., 2009), and has correlated with connectivity between the right dorsal anterior insula and either SMA (Tinaz et al., 2015). Frequency of urges correlates with the connectivity between the insula and motor cortex as well (He et al., 2022; Johnson et al., 2023; Sigurdsson et al., 2018).

Tic severity and course

Owing to variability in tic presentation, tic severity measures assess multiple dimensions of tics (Chang et al., 2009; Leckman et al., 1989). The Yale Global Tic Severity Scale (YGTSS; Leckman et al., 1989), which is a clinician-rated measure of tic severity and tic-related impairment, is the gold standard assessment instrument for tics and is typically used as the primary outcome measure in treatment trials (Piacentini et al., 2010; Wilhelm et al., 2012). The YGTSS assesses motor and phonic tic number, frequency, intensity, complexity, and interference over the past week, as well as tic-related impairment. The Parent Tic Questionnaire (PTQ; Chang et al., 2009), which is a parent-rated measure of tic severity, is frequently given to parents of patients before treatment sessions to evaluate patient outcomes. The PTQ assesses motor and phonic tic number, frequency, and intensity over the past week, and parents can complete the measure in approximately five minutes.

Tic severity is associated with tic-related impairment (Storch et al., 2007a), with motor tic complexity and phonic tic number, intensity, and interference linked to the most impairment (Stiede et al., 2018). Adults and youth with tics experience impairment in multiple areas of life, including physical, social, familial, academic, and occupational domains (Conelea et al., 2011b; Conelea et al., 2013; Makhoul & Jankovic, 2021). Individuals also report discrimination related to tics, which occasionally leads to social or public avoidance, as well as peer victimization/teasing (Storch et al., 2007b; Zinner et al., 2012). Further, it has been shown that TS impacts quality of life across the lifespan (Evans et al., 2016; Johnson et al., 2023; Wadman et al., 2016).

Several studies have examined the course of tic severity, with results demonstrating that tic severity typically peaks in late childhood at approximately the age of ten (Bloch et al., 2006; Leckman et al., 1998). Bloch and Leckman (2009) found that by early adulthood, 75 percent of youth with TS experienced reduced tic severity, while 33 percent reported no tics. In a review of 100 individuals with TS at ten years post tic-onset, none of the participants were tic free, but 80 percent demonstrated effective tic management (Rizzo et al., 2012), while an 11-year follow up of 80 individuals with TS showed a lower rate of tic reduction, as 40 percent of participants met partial remission criteria (Espil et al., 2022). These findings suggest that tic severity decreases as individuals enter later adolescence and young adulthood. It has also been shown that higher childhood tic severity and female sex predicted increased tic severity in adulthood (Ricketts et al., 2022).

Furthermore, comprehensive behavioral intervention for tics (CBIT), the most well-supported non-pharmacological treatment for tics, can potentially alter the long-term course of tics. Espil et al. (2022) completed a long-term follow up of a randomized controlled trial that examined treatment outcomes of CBIT versus a psychoeducation and supportive therapy (PST) control condition. After controlling for intermediate interventions, they found that tics improved at 11-year follow up for participants in both conditions, but children who initially responded to CBIT improved faster and maintained their gains at follow up. This suggests that the early implementation of effective tic management skills may influence the course of tic severity. Long-term outcomes of pharmacological treatment for tics have not yet been examined.

Comorbidities

Psychiatric comorbidities are common in those with tics, as approximately 78 percent to 90 percent of individuals experience one or more comorbid conditions (Hirschtritt et al., 2015; Johnson et al., 2023; Lebowitz et al., 2012; Robertson, 2015). Attention-deficit hyperactivity disorder (ADHD) is the most common comorbidity, with prevalence rates of approximately 50–60 percent, while approximately 30–50 percent of individuals with tics are diagnosed with obsessive-compulsive disorder (OCD; Freeman et al., 2000; Hirschtritt et al., 2015; Robertson, 2015). Anxiety disorders, which impact approximately 30 percent of individuals with TS, are another common comorbidity (Hirschtritt et al., 2015). Additionally, other comorbid conditions, such as depression, oppositional defiant disorder (ODD), rage attacks (i.e., outbursts of disruptive/explosive behaviors), self-injurious behaviors, and learning disorders, also occur at lower rates (Baizabal-Carvallo et al., 2022b; Hirschtritt et al., 2015; Lebowitz et al., 2012; Sambrani et al., 2016). Studies have shown that individuals with tics plus another comorbid condition are at a greater risk of psychosocial impairment than healthy controls or those with only tics (Eapen et al., 2016).

Biobehavioral Model of Tics

The biobehavioral model incorporates the underlying biological basis of tics with behavioral theory to identify the factors that impact the occurrence and maintenance of tics (Woods et al., 2008). First, the model indicates that TS is a biologically based condition with a strong genetic component, as tics result from structural and functional abnormalities within the CBGTC loop (Deng et al., 2012; Singer & Augustine, 2019). Second, the relationship between tics and premonitory urges is an important factor in tic occurrence and maintenance (Woods et al., 2005). Finally, the model demonstrates that antecedent stimuli and tic-contingent consequences are crucial components in tic expression and suppression (Conelea & Woods, 2008). Although additional research is needed to fully understand each aspect of this model, current supporting evidence is described below.

Biological basis of tics

Genetics

TS has long been recognized to have a genetic component (Deng et al., 2012). Heritability rates have been estimated at 77 percent to 92.4 percent via genome-wide association studies (GWAS), and an 18.69 odds ratio for having a tic disorder in patients with a first-degree relative with a tic disorder has been described (Mataix-Cols et al., 2015; Yu et al., 2019). Diagnostic concordance in monozygotic twins of 0.77 and 0.53 have been shown in twins with tics and formal TS, respectively (Price et al., 1985), with similar rates in later registry studies (Lichtenstein et al., 2010; Polderman et al., 2015). High correlation between TS, OCD, and ADHD have also been noted by GWAS (Domènech et al., 2021), matching the commonly observed clustering of these conditions in clinical practice.

There is no clear single gene that contributes to a significant proportion of TS. Monogenic causes of TS, including *SLITRK 1–6, CELSR3, NRXN1*, and *CNTN6* are found in less than 2 percent of individuals (Yu et al., 2019). A study using whole-exome sequencing (WES) found a 12 percent contribution of risk from de novo variants, but only one high-confidence gene, *WWC1*, was found for TS (S. Wang et al., 2018). Despite frequently comorbid OCD and ADHD, no gene has been determined to be a high-confidence contribution to both TS and OCD (Johnson et al., 2023). Candidate regions in linkage studies, such as *HDC* (Ercan-Sencicek et al., 2010), have not been replicated outside of individual families (Domènech et al., 2021), and similar candidate genes by GWAS, such as *FLT3*, have not been replicated in independent cohorts (Yu et al., 2019).

Copy number variants (CNV) in TS have been studied as well. Rare exonic CNV associated with other neuropsychiatric disorders have been found in TS (Sundaram et al., 2010), and TS patients are more likely to have excessive CNV (OR 2.28; Huang et al., 2017). CNV in *NRXN1* and *CNTN6* in particular have been noted as risk factors for TS (Huang et al., 2017). WES studies of TS cohorts have also identified several probable risk genes, such as *ASH1L* (S. Liu et al., 2020; W. Liu et al., 2022), *NIPBL,* and *FN1* (Willsey et al., 2017). Excessive *de novo* variants have been found in simplex cohorts, with an estimated 10 percent of patients carrying *de novo* variants, with 483 separate genes potentially contributing to TS risk (S. Wang et al., 2018).

Despite the noted heritable nature, TS has complex genetic under-pinnings comprised of rare genetic risk factors and varied polygenic burden (Johnson et al., 2023; Levy et al., 2021), with further interaction of environmental risk factors. Further investigation in the pathophysiology of TS and study of genetic risk factors in larger cohorts is required for better understanding of the genetic architecture of TS.

Cortico-Basal Ganglia-Thalamo-Cortical (CBGTC) Loop

The basal ganglia and their connections have frequently been studied as potential locations in the generation of tics (Singer & Augustine, 2019; Figure 8.1). Early investigations and discussions relied on simpler models of the cortico-basal ganglia pathways, such as the classic indirect and direct pathways. Individual areas in the cortex and basal ganglia have been examined as key sites in tic generation (Johnson et al., 2023; Singer & Augustine, 2019), but localization increasingly appears to lie in aberrant networks rather than singular areas.

Newer models propose that disruption of a number of areas comprising the cortico-basal ganglia-thalamo-cortical (CBGTC) loop could result in dysfunction of the entire circuit, leading to abnormal output to the motor cortex and subsequent generation of tics (Augustine & Singer, 2018). Functional imaging studies have noted aberrant pathway connections in TS. In one study, increased basal ganglia (BG) and cortical connectivity and reduced cortico-cerebellar connectivity, suggestive of predominant excitatory neurotransmission, were noted in 28 TS patients versus 28

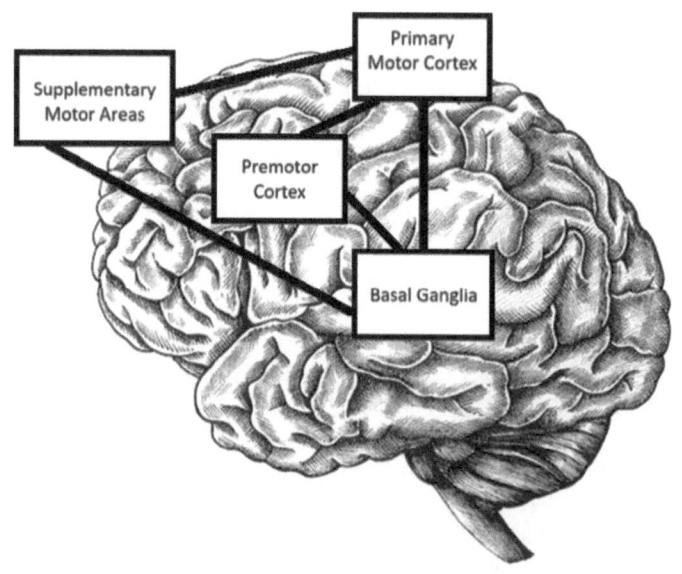

Figure 8.1 Tic Generation Network.

healthy controls (Ramkiran et al., 2019). Another study comparing 13 TS versus 21 healthy control patients noted excessive sensorimotor pathway activity in cortico-BG circuits with actual tics versus simulated tics, and weaker activity in CBGTC circuits implicated in exerting top-down control (such as the caudate and anterior cingulate cortex), also pointing to an excessive excitatory state (Z. Wang et al., 2011). The degree of enhanced cortico-BG connectivity in sensorimotor networks has also correlated with tic severity in some studies of TS patients (Worbe et al., 2015). Tic onset has been associated with activity in the thalamus, central operculum, primary motor and somatosensory cortices, and premotor and lateral prefrontal cortical activation in other fMRI studies (Bohlhalter et al., 2006; Neuner et al., 2014; Polyanska et al., 2017).

Areas comprising the CBGTC circuit have been implicated in tic generation. Involvement of the cortex has often been suggested by the frequent presence of coexisting neuropsychiatric features in TS patients

(Augustine & Singer, 2018). Magnetic resonance imaging (MRI) studies have shown volumetric changes in cortical structures, such as larger dorsal prefrontal and parietal and occipital areas (Peterson et al., 2001), and changes in prefrontal, frontal, sensorimotor, temporal, and cingulate areas (Müller-Vahl et al., 2009). Positron emission tomography (PET) studies have also demonstrated cortical areas of hypermetabolism (Augustine & Singer, 2018). In addition, decreased prefrontal cortical thickness has been described in several studies of patients with TS (Martino et al., 2018). Tic severity correlated with the degree of decreased thickness in some studies, suggesting that tics may result from decreased inhibition of motor programs. TMS studies have noted reduced short-interval intracortical inhibition and short-afferent inhibition in TS patients (Kurvits et al., 2020), and bilateral TMS of the SMA was shown to improve tic severity scores in ten children with TS over 15 sessions (Kahl et al., 2021).

Studies have demonstrated BG involvement in tic generation as well. In animal models, disruption of striatal glutamate/gamma-aminobutyric acid (GABA) balance has generated tic-like behaviors (Singer & Augustine, 2019). Indeed, many studies have suggested that GABAergic deficiency is the primary defect in TS leading to central "disinhibition" (Lerner et al., 2012). Ablation of cholinergic interneurons in mice striatum has also generated tic-like phenomenology (Xu et al., 2015). While variations in the size of striatal structures have been variable in imaging studies, postmortem studies have noted reduced parvalbumin-positive interneurons in the caudate and putamen in TS patients (Kalanithi et al., 2005; Kataoka et al., 2010).

Thalamic involvement has been implicated in several neurophysiologic studies. Bursting activity has been seen in the centromedian-parafascicular (CM-Pf) nucleus prior to tic production (Testini et al., 2016), and reduced alpha and increased gamma band activity has correlated with reduction of tic activity after deep brain stimulation (DBS; Priori et al., 2013). Thalamic synchronization and time locked cross-coherence with cortical structures has been noted to occur before spontaneous motor tics (Bour et al., 2015).

In adults with TS, clinical data have shown improvements in tic severity with DBS targeting the BG and thalamus support the involvement of these structures in tic generation. Common targets for DBS in TS include the CM-Pf thalamic nucleus and both anteromedial and posteroventral globus pallidus internus (GPi; Martinez-Ramirez et al., 2018). In pooled analyses, YGTSS scores in TS patients have been noted to improve by 46.3 percent in patients with CM-Pf, 50.5 percent in anteromedial GPi, and 27.7 percent in posteroventral GPi targeted DBS at 12-month follow-up. Furthermore, positive outcomes of DBS have been correlated with connectivity of targets to CBTGC loops. In a review of TS patients who had undergone DBS, GPi connectivity to limbic and associative networks, caudate, thalamus, and cerebellum correlated with the degree of tic improvement (Johnson et al., 2020). Overlap of the estimated volume of tissue activated with higher regions of stimulation correlated with tic improvement as well. Similarly, in patients with CM thalamic targeting, connectivity of the target with sensorimotor networks, putamen, cerebellum, and other cortical networks predicted improvement in tic scores (Johnson et al., 2020).

Disinhibition in the CBGTC loop has been proposed as the primary abnormality in TS, where tics can be viewed as an "excess of actions" (Beste & Münchau, 2018; Lerner et al., 2012). In this model, BG and fronto-striatal loops serve as selectors of salient action models among competing action programs, modulated by phasic dopaminergic signals (Redgrave & Gurney, 2006). Defective "braking" by the BG results in decreased selection of saliency and unwanted activation of motor programs. Reduced numbers of inhibitory GABA and cholinergic interneurons have been found in the striatum in TS patients in postmortem studies (Kalanithi et al., 2005; Kataoka et al., 2010). Magnetoencephalography studies have shown imbalanced inhibitory and excitatory activity in TS patients (Kurvits et al., 2020), with suggestion of a voluntary component to tics, which may be triggered by impaired motor inhibitory mechanisms (Niccolai et al., 2019). Other inhibitory markers, such as prepulse inhibition of startle responses, are also deficient in patients with tic disorders (Kurvits et al., 2020). Flumazenil PET studies have noted decreased $GABA_A$ receptors in TS patients in the ventral striatum, GP, thalamus, amygdala, and right insula, compatible with disinhibition (Ilyas et al., 2019; Lerner et al., 2012). While many studies support this model of impaired inhibition, there are conflicting results in the literature (Kurvits et al., 2020).

Multiple neurotransmitters have also been implicated in the dysfunction of the CBGTC loop, of which dopamine is most notable (Augustine & Singer, 2018). Involved in movement, processing, reward, learning, and sensorimotor integration pathways, dopamine has been long implicated in TS, as many of the most effective medications for TS involve blocking or reducing dopamine activity (Augustine & Singer, 2018). TS has been associated with increased striatal dopamine release (Testini et al., 2016), which may lead to observed disinhibition (Leckman, 2002). However, results of PET studies examining dopamine receptor levels have been mixed (Augustine & Singer, 2018), and neither increased dopamine nor homovanillic acid have been increased in post-mortem striatal samples (Singer et al., 1991). A lack of receptor regulation may point away from tonic dopamine firing abnormalities, and some have suggested that abnormalities may lie instead in the phasic release of dopamine. Increased extrastriatal phasic dopamine release has been found in TS (Steeves et al., 2010). As phasic dopamine can transition goal-directed behavior to habit formation in animal models (Augustine & Singer, 2018), some have proposed that tics may represent motor habits that are reinforced with excessive phasic dopamine release (Johnson et al., 2023; Maia & Conceição, 2018). Further, dopamine-associated reward-guide learning is increased in TS (Palminteri & Pessiglione, 2013), and successful resolution of urges by completion of tics may generate a positive predictive error with associated phasic dopamine release and reinforcement of tics (Conceição et al., 2017).

In addition to genetic predisposition there are many other pathogenic mechanisms of tics, including neurodevelopmental disorders (e.g. autism, drugs (e.g. antipsychotics, cocaine), structural lesions involving the basal ganglia and it connections), and functional (psychogenic tics). The latter has become particularly prominent since the COVID-19 pandemic (Buts et al., 2022; Hull et al., 2021).

Premonitory urges and tics

The relationship between premonitory urges and tics plays an important role in tic occurrence and maintenance. Some studies have suggested that the functional relationship between premonitory urges and tics develops over time (Leckman et al., 1993; Woods et al., 2005). In contrast, other studies have shown a functional urge-tic relationship within months of tic onset; though, not as strong of a relationship as individuals with tics for a longer period of time (Greene et al., 2015). Premonitory urge strength is hypothesized to temporarily reduce or even be eliminated after ticcing and is referred to as the negative reinforcement, or urge-reduction, model (Evers & van de Wetering, 1994; Woods et al., 2005). This has been corroborated by patient reports (Kwak et al., 2003; Leckman et al., 1993); however, experimental results on the urge-tic relationship are inconsistent, as the relationship varies across age groups and individuals. Furthermore, premonitory urges cannot be objectively rated (Brabson et al., 2016; Himle et al., 2007), as most studies obtain subjective ratings of premonitory urge severity via the Premonitory Urge for Tics Scale (Woods et al., 2005). Studies also use tic suppression/expression to observe changes in premonitory urge severity ratings, with higher urge ratings during tic suppression lending support to the negative reinforcement model (Himle et al., 2007).

Several studies have pointed to the negative reinforcement model as an explanation of how tics are maintained. The first study to investigate the functional relationship between premonitory urges and tics found the majority of participants reported more intense premonitory urges when asked to suppress tics versus when they were allowed to tic freely, providing preliminary support for the negative reinforcement model (Himle et al., 2007). Another study showed a similar pattern of higher urge ratings during reinforced tic suppression periods than free to tic periods, with tics covarying inversely with premonitory urge strength (Capriotti et al., 2014). Other studies on the pathology of tics have indirectly provided support for the negative reinforcement model, as the vast majority of patients report relief from premonitory urges after ticcing (Kwak et al., 2003). Additionally, treatment studies have shown reductions in premonitory urge intensity within and between sessions (Evers & van de Wetering, 1994; Verdellen et al., 2008).

While several studies support this hypothesis, others have failed to replicate findings. In a sample of adolescents with tics, Specht and colleagues (2013) unexpectedly found that premonitory urge intensity did not increase when participants suppressed tics. Additionally, Brabson and colleagues (2016) suggested that there are several different patterns of urges that individuals could present with, rather than one salient model of negative reinforcement. Furthermore, a study with a pooled dataset found that the ability to suppress tics was not significantly correlated with premonitory urger severity, suggesting that not every individual with tics fits within the negative reinforcement model (Conelea et al., 2018). Others pose that poor urge tolerance could likely play a role in tic maintenance (Ramsey et al., 2022; Ramsey et al., 2021). Regardless, while premonitory urges may be a part of tic maintenance, they are most likely not the primary mechanism of tic maintenance.

Influence of contextual variables on tic expression

Although TS has a biological basis, contextual factors interact with biological processes to influence the occurrence of tics. Studies have shown that contextual variables, such as antecedents (e.g., settings, activities, emotions) and consequences (e.g., attention, aversive, or escape-based reactions to tics), play a significant role in tic expression and suppression (Conelea & Woods, 2008). These factors, which can be highly individualized, help explain the situational variability of tics. This section reviews how contextual factors impact tic expression and the possible mechanisms underpinning the relationship between contextual factors and tics.

Antecedent variables

Antecedent variables, which occur immediately before tics, alter the likelihood of tic expression (Conelea & Woods, 2008). Studies have demonstrated that external antecedents, such as specific settings, activities, and people, can both positively and negatively impact tic occurrence. For example, children with tics and their parents reported that activities associated with school (e.g., taking a test, completing homework) were related to tic exacerbation (Himle et al., 2014; Wadman et al., 2016). Further, watching television and playing video games were also associated with increases in tics (Barnea et al., 2016; Caurín et al., 2014; Himle et al., 2014). In contrast, other settings and activities have been linked to tic attenuation. For instance, Doja et al. (2018) demonstrated that physical activity is associated with lower phonic tic severity, while Caurín et al. (2014) reported that sports and outdoor activities were associated with decreases in tics. It has also been shown that musical performances, listening to music, and other creative activities (e.g., dancing, painting) were related to tic attenuation (Bodeck et al., 2015; Caurín et al., 2014), which aligns with studies that suggest there is an improvement in tics during behaviors that require increased attention and fine motor/vocal control (Eapen et al., 2004).

Additionally, internal antecedents, such as premonitory urges and emotions, can influence tic occurrence. Several studies have found that tics alleviate these premonitory sensations and tic suppression is associated with increases in premonitory urge intensity (Brandt et al., 2016; Capriotti et al., 2014). Further, mood states, such as boredom, dissatisfaction, and disinterest, have been related to tic exacerbation (Eapen et al., 2004; O'Connor et al., 2003; Silva et al., 1995), and studies have also found that fatigue and poor sleep were associated with increases in tics (Eapen et al., 2004; Robertson et al., 2002). In addition, there are contrasting findings in the relationship between stress and tics. Descriptive studies have shown that stress is linked to tic exacerbation (Bornstein et al., 1990; Caurín et al., 2014; Eapen et al., 2004), whereas experimental studies have demonstrated that high stress situations do not lead to increases in tics (Conelea et al., 2011a; Conelea et al., 2014). Future studies should continue to examine the stress–tic relationship.

Consequence Variables

Tic-contingent consequences, such as reactions to or accommodations after tics, can also impact tic expression. Capriotti et al. (2015) developed the Tic Accommodation and Reactions Scale (TARS), which assessed immediate consequences of tics in children with TS. They found that tic severity was positively correlated with attention (e.g., parent physically comforts child), aversive (e.g., sibling teases child), and escape-based (e.g., child does not complete homework) consequences of tics. Other studies have also demonstrated that tic-contingent attention and escape are related to tic exacerbation and increases in premonitory urge intensity (Eaton et al., 2017; Himle et al., 2014; Rivera-Navarro et al., 2014; Zinner et al., 2012). Further, Watson and Sterling (1998) showed that the removal of parental attention after tics led to decreases in tic severity. Several studies have also demonstrated that the use of differential reinforcement of zero-rate behavior schedules, in which rewards were delivered for tic-free periods, led to significant reductions in tic expression (Capriotti et al., 2012; Himle & Woods, 2005; Woods & Himle, 2004). In a pooled dataset of 99 children with TS, Conelea et al. (2018) found that 70 percent of children had at least a 50 percent reduction in tic frequency during reward-enhanced tic suppression periods, with 20 percent showing close to complete suppression.

Mechanisms underpinning the relationship between contextual factors and tics

Researchers do not fully understand the mechanisms by which contextual factors impact tic expression. Godar and Bortolato (2017) suggested that antecedent variables that lead to overstimulation (e.g., watching television, playing video games) may be related to tic exacerbation because individuals with tics experience sensory overload, owing to gating deficits. For antecedents that lead to under stimulation (e.g., boredom), tic exacerbation may occur because of increases in interoceptive awareness of premonitory urges (Ganos et al., 2015; Godar & Bortolato, 2017). Further, Conelea et al. (2011a) found that situations that elicit stress impact tic suppressibility, which may explain why individuals with tics report that stress is associated with increases in tics. Fatigue and poor sleep may also be related to tic exacerbation because they decrease an individual's ability to manage other contextual/emotional triggers (Godar & Bortolato, 2017). Finally, in an experimental study, Woods et al. (2009) demonstrated that reinforcing tics in the presence of antecedent stimuli can lead to the antecedent stimuli acquiring some control over tic expression. This may also explain the variability in tic expression based on different environments.

Summary

PTDs are neurological conditions which consist of simple and complex motor and phonic tics. They affect approximately 1 percent of the pediatric population (Scharf et al., 2015) and are associated with impairment in physical, social, familial, and academic/occupational domains (Conelea et al., 2011b). Tics typically peak in severity around age ten, with decreases in tic severity normally occurring as individuals enter late adolescence and young adulthood (Bloch & Leckman, 2009). Most individuals with tics experience comorbidities, with ADHD and OCD being the most common, and those with PTDs and comorbid conditions tend to have increased psychosocial impairment (Eapen et al., 2016; Hirschtritt et al., 2015).

The biobehavioral model of tics helps explain how biological and behavioral factors lead to the occurrence and maintenance of tics (Woods et al., 2008). TS has a strong genetic component, with no clear single gene contributing to a significant proportion of the disorder (Deng et al., 2012). Complex genetic underpinnings interact with environmental variables to explain tic occurrence, and future studies are needed to fully understand the genetic architecture of TS. The CBGTC circuit is also involved in tic generation, with recent findings demonstrating that localization appears to occur in aberrant networks rather than singular areas (Singer & Augustine, 2019). Additionally, the negative reinforcement hypothesis suggests that the relationship between premonitory urges and tics is important in tic maintenance, as urge intensity tends to reduce after the performance of tics (Woods et al., 2005). Finally, contextual variables, which include antecedent stimuli and tic-contingent consequences, play an important role in tic expression and suppression (Conelea & Woods, 2008). Future research should continue to examine the mechanisms underlying the association between contextual factors and tics.

References

American Psychiatric Association. (2022). *Diagnostic and statistical manual of mental disorders* (5th Ed., rev. text). doi:10.1176/appi.books.9780890425787.

Augustine, F. & Singer, H. S. (2018). Merging the Pathophysiology and Pharmacotherapy of Tics. *Tremor and Other Hyperkinetic Movements*, 8, 595. doi:10.7916/D8H14JTX.

Baizabal-Carvallo, J. F., Alonso-Juarez, M., & Jankovic, J. (2022a). Dystonic motor and phonic tics in Tourette syndrome. *Journal of Neurology*, 269, 5312–5318.

Baizabal-Carvallo, J. F., Alonso-Juarez, M., & Jankovic, J. (2022b). Self-injurious behavior in Tourette syndrome. *Journal of Neurology*, 269, 2453–2459.

Baizabal-Carvallo, J. F. & Jankovic, J. (2023). The clinical characterization of blocking tics in patients with Tourette syndrome. *Journal of Movement Disorder*. doi:10.14802/jmd.22122. E-publication ahead of print.

Baizabal-Carvallo, J. F. & Jankovic, J. (2022). Sex differences in patients with Tourette syndrome. *CNS Spectrum*.

Baizabal-Carvallo, J. F. & Jankovic, J. (2021). Beyond tics: Movement disorders in patients with Tourette syndrome. *Journal of Neural Transmission*, 128(8), 1177–1183.

Barnea, M., Benaroya-Milshtein, N., Gilboa-Sechtman, E., Woods, D. W., Piacentini, J., Fennig, S., ... Steinberg, T. (2016). Subjective versus objective measures of tic severity in Tourette syndrome: The influence of environment. *Psychiatry Research*, 242, 204–209. doi:10.1016/j.psychres.2016.05.047.

Beste, C., & Münchau, A. (2018). Tics and Tourette syndrome—Surplus of actions rather than disorder? *Movement Disorders*, 33(2), 238–242. doi:10.1002/mds.27244.

Bloch, M. H. & Leckman, J. F. (2009). Clinical course of Tourette syndrome. *Journal of Psychosomatic Research*, 67, 497–501. doi:10.1016/j.jpsychores.2009.09.002.

Bloch, M. H., Peterson, B. S., Scahill, L., Otka, J., Katsovich, L., Zhang, H., & Leckman, J. F. (2006). Adulthood outcome of tic and obsessive-compulsive symptom severity in children with Tourette syndrome. *Archives of Pediatrics and Adolescent Medicine*, 160, 65–69. doi:10.1001/archpedi.160.1.65.

Bodeck, S., Lappe, C., & Evers, S. (2015). Tic-reducing effects of music in patients with Tourette's syndrome: Self-reported and objective analysis. *Journal of Neurological Sciences*, 352, 41–47. doi:10.1016/j.jns.2015.03.016.

Bohlhalter, S., Goldfine, A., Matteson, S., Garraux, G., Hanakawa, T., Kansaku, K., Wurzman, R., & Hallett, M. (2006). Neural correlates of tic generation in Tourette syndrome: An event-related functional MRI study. *Brain: A Journal of Neurology*, 129(8), 2029–2037. doi:10.1093/brain/awl050.

Bornstein, R. A., Stefl, M. E., & Hammond, L. (1990). A survey of Tourette syndrome patients and their families: The 1987 Ohio Tourette survey. *Journal of Neuropsychiatry*, 2, 275–281. doi:10.1176/jnp.2.3.275.

Bour, L. J., Ackermans, L., Foncke, E. M. J., Cath, D., van der Linden, C., Visser Vandewalle, V., & Tijssen, M. A. (2015). Tic related local field potentials in the thalamus and the effect of deep brain stimulation in Tourette syndrome: Report of three cases. *Clinical Neurophysiology: Official Journal of the International Federation of Clinical Neurophysiology*, 126(8), 1578–1588. doi:10.1016/j.clinph.2014.10.217.

Brabson, L. A., Brown, J. L., Capriotti, M. R., Ramanujam, K., Himle, M. B., Nicotra, C. M., Ostrander, R., Kelly, L. M., Grados, M. A., Walkup, J. T., Perry-Parrish, C., Reynolds, E. K., Hankinson, J. C., & Specht, M. W. (2016). Patterned changes in urge ratings with tic suppression in youth with chronic tic disorders. *Journal of Behavior Therapy and Experimental Psychiatry*, 50, 162–170. doi:10.1016/j.jbtep.2015.07.004.

Brandt, V. C., Beck, C., Sajin, V., Baaske, M. K., Bäumer, T., Beste, C., … Münchau, A. (2016). Temporal relationship between premonitory urges and tics in Gilles de la Tourette syndrome. *Cortex*, 77, 24–37. doi:10.1016/j.cortex.2016.01.008.

Buts, S., Duncan, M., Owen, T., et al. (2022). Paediatric tic-like presentations during the COVID-19 pandemic. *Archives of Disease in Childhood*, 107(3), e17.

Capriotti, M. R., Brandt, B. C., Ricketts, E. J., Espil, F. M., & Woods, D. W. (2012). Comparing the effects of differential reinforcement of other behavior and response-cost contingencies on tics in youth with Tourette syndrome. *Journal of Applied Behavior*, 45(2), 251–263. doi:10.1901/jaba.2012.45-251.

Capriotti, M. R., Brandt, B. C., Turkel, J. E., Lee, H. J., & Woods, D. W. (2014). Negative reinforcement and premonitory urges in youth with Tourette syndrome: An experimental evaluation. *Behavior Modification*, 38, 276–296. doi:10.1177/0145445514531015.

Capriotti, M. R., Piacentini, J. C., Himle, M. B., Ricketts, E. J., Espil, F. M., Lee, H. J., … Woods, D. W. (2015). Assessing environmental consequences of ticcing in youth with chronic tic disorders: The tic accommodation and reactions scale. *Children's Health Care*, 44, 205–220. doi:10.1080/02739615.2014.948164.

Caurín, B., Serrano, M., Fernández-Alvarez, E., Campistol, J., & Pérez-Dueñas, B. (2014). Environmental circumstances influencing tic expression in children. *European Journal of Paediatric Neurology*, 18, 157–162. doi:10.1016/j.ejpn.2013.10.002.

Conceição, V. A., Dias, Â., Farinha, A. C., & Maia, T. V. (2017). Premonitory urges and tics in Tourette syndrome: Computational mechanisms and neural correlates. *Current Opinion in Neurobiology*, 46, 187–199. doi:10.1016/j.conb.2017.08.009.

Chang, S., Himle, M. B., Tucker, B. T. P., Woods, D. W., & Piacentini, J. (2009). Initial psychometric properties of a brief parent-report instrument for assessing tic severity in children with chronic tic disorders. *Child and Family Behavior Therapy*, 31(3), 181–191. doi:10.1080/07317100903099100.

Conelea, C. A., Ramanujam, K., Walther, M. R., Freeman, J. B., & Garcia, A. M. (2014). Is there a relationship between tic frequency and physiological arousal? Examination in a sample of children with co-occurring tic and anxiety disorders. *Behavior Modification*, 38, 217–234. doi:10.1177/0145445514528239.

Conelea, C. A., Wellen, B., Woods, D. W., Greene, D. J., Black, K. J., Specht, M., ... Capriotti, M. (2018). Patterns and predictors of tic suppressibility in youth with tic disorders. *Frontiers in Psychiatry*, 9, 1–10. doi:10.3389/fpsyt.2018.00188.

Conelea, C. A. & Woods, D. W. (2008). The influence of contextual factors on tic expression in Tourette's syndrome: A review. *Journal of Psychosomatic Research*, 65, 487–496. doi:10.1016/j.jpsychores.2008.04.010.

Conelea, C. A., Woods, D. W., & Brandt, B. C. (2011a). The impact of a stress induction task on tic frequencies in youth with Tourette Syndrome. *Behaviour Research and Therapy*, 49, 492–497. doi:10.1016/j.brat.2011.05.006.

Conelea, C. A., Woods, D. W., Zinner, S. H., Budman, C., Murphy, T., Scahill, L. D., Compton, S. N., & Walkup, J. T. (2011b). Exploring the Impact of Tourette Syndrome on Youth: Results from the Tourette Syndrome Impact Survey. *Child Psychiatry and Human Development*, 42 (2), 219–242. doi:10.1007/s10578-010-0211-4.

Conelea, C. A., Woods, D. W., Zinner, S., Budman, C. L., Murphy, T. K., Scahill, L. D., Compton, S., & Walkup, J. T. (2013). The impact of tourette syndrome in adults: Results from the tourette syndrome impact survey. *Community Mental Health Journal, 49(1)*, 110–120. doi:10.1007/s10597-011-9465-y.

Deng, H., Gao, K., & Jankovic, J. (2012). The genetics of Tourette syndrome. *Nature Reviews Neurology*, 8(4), Article 4. doi:10.1038/nrneurol.2012.26.

Doja, A., Bookwala, A., Pohl, D., Rossi-Ricci, A., Barrowman, N., Chan, J., & Longmuir, P. E. (2018). Relationship between physical activity, tic severity and quality of life in children with Tourette syndrome. *Journal of the Canadian Academy of Child and Adolescent Psychiatry*, 27, 222–226.

Domènech, L., Cappi, C., & Halvorsen, M. (2021). Genetic architecture of Tourette syndrome: Our current understanding. *Psychological Medicine*, 51(13), 2201–2209. doi:10.1017/S0033291721000234.

Draganski, B., Martino, D., Cavanna, A. E., Hutton, C., Orth, M., Robertson, M. M., Critchley, H. D., & Frackowiak, R. S. (2010). Multispectral brain morphometry in Tourette syndrome persisting into adulthood. *Brain*, 133(12), 3661–3675. doi:10.1093/brain/awq300.

Eaton, C. K., Jones, A. M., Gutierrez-Colina, A. M., Ivey, E. K., Carlson, O., Melville, L., Kardon, P., & Blount, R. L. (2017). The influence of environmental consequences and internalizing symptoms on children's tic severity. *Child Psychiatry & Human Development, 48(2)*, 327–334. doi:10.1007/s10578-016-0644-5.

Eapen, V., Cavanna, A. E., & Robertson, M. M. (2016). Comorbidities, social impact, and quality of life in Tourette syndrome. *Frontiers in Psychiatry*, 7, 97. doi:10.3389/fpsyt.2016.00097.

Eapen, V., Fox-Hiley, P., Banerjee, S., & Robertson, M. (2004) Clinical features and associated psychopathology in a Tourette syndrome cohort. *Acta Neurolgica Scandinavica*, 109, 255–260.

Ercan-Sencicek, A. G., Stillman, A. A., Ghosh, A. K., Bilguvar, K., O'Roak, B. J., Mason, C. E., Abbott, T., Gupta, A., King, R. A., Pauls, D. L., Tischfield, J.

A., Heiman, G. A., Singer, H. S., Gilbert, D. L., Hoekstra, P. J., Morgan, T. M., Loring, E., Yasuno, K., Fernandez, T., ... State, M. W. (2010). L-Histidine Decarboxylase and Tourette's Syndrome. *New England Journal of Medicine*, 362 (20), 1901–1908. doi:10.1056/NEJMoa0907006.

Espil, F. M., Woods, D W., Specht, M., Bennett, S. M., Walkup, J. T., Ricketts, E. J., McGuire, J. F., Stiede, J. T., Schild, J., Chang, S., Peterson, A., Scahill, L., Wilhelm, S., & Piacentini, J. (2022). Determining the long-term effects of comprehensive behavioral intervention for tics (CBIT). *Journal of the American Academy of Child and Adolescent Psychiatry, 61(6)*, 764–771. doi:10.1016/j. jaac.2021.08.022.

Evans, J., Seri, S., & Cavanna, A. E. (2016). The effects of Gilles de la Tourette syndrome and other chronic tic disorders on quality of life across the lifespan: A systematic review. *European Child & Adolescent Psychiatry, 25(9)*, 939–948. doi:10.1007/s00787-016-0823-8.

Evers, R. A. & van de Wetering, B. J. (1994). A treatment model for motor tics based on a specific tension-reduction technique. *Journal of Behavior Therapy and Experimental Psychiatry*, 25(3), 255–260. doi:10.1016/0005-7916(94)90026–90024.

Freeman, R. D., Fast, D. K., Burd, L., Kerbeshian, J., Robertson, M. M., & Sandor, P. (2000). An international perspective on Tourette syndrome: Selected findings from 3500 individuals in 22 countries. *Developmental Medicine and Child Neurology*, 42, 436–447. doi:10.1017/S0012162200000839.

Ganos, C., Garrido, A., Navalpotro-Gomez, I., Ricciardi, L., Martino, D., Edwards, M. J., Tsakiris, M., Haggard, P., & Bhatia, K. P. (2015). Premonitory urge to tic in Tourette's is associated with interoceptive awareness. *Movement Disorders, 30(9)*, 1198–1202. doi:10.1002/mds.26228.

Godar, S. C. & Bortolato, M. (2017). What make you tic? Transitional approaches to study the role of stress and contextual triggers in Tourette syndrome. *Neuroscience and Biobehavioral Reviews*, 76, 123–133. doi:10.1016/j. neubiorev.2016.10.003.

Greene, D. J., Koller, J. M., Robichaux-Viehoever, A., Bihun, E. C., Schlaggar, B. L., & Black, K. J. (2015). *Reward enhances tic suppression in children within months of tic disorder onset. Developmental Cognitive Neuroscience*, 11, 65–74. doi:10.1016/j.dcn.2014.08.005.

Hampson, M., Tokoglu, F., King, R. A., Constable, R. T., & Leckman, J. F. (2009). Brain Areas Coactivating with Motor Cortex During Chronic Motor Tics and Intentional Movements. *Biological Psychiatry*, 65(7), 594–599. doi:10.1016/j.biopsych.2008.11.012.

He, J. L., Mikkelsen, M., Huddleston, D. A., et al. (2022). Frequency and intensity of premonitory urges-to-tic in Tourette syndrome is associated with supplementary motor area GABA+ Levels. *Movement Disorders*, 37(3), 563–573.

Himle, M. B., Capriotti, M. R., Hayes, L. P., Ramanujam, K., Scahill, L., Sukhodolsky, D. G., ... Piacentini, J. (2014). Variables associated with tic exacerbation in children with chronic tic disorders. *Behavior Modification*, 38, 163–183. doi:10.1177/0145445514531016.

Himle, M. B., & Woods, D. W. (2005). An experimental evaluation of tic suppression and the tic rebound effect. *Science Direct*, 43, 1443–1451. doi:10.1016/j. brat.2004.11.002.

Himle, M. B., Woods, D. W., Conelea, C. A., Bauer, C. C., & Rice, K. A. (2007). Investigating the effects of tic suppression on premonitory urge ratings in children and adolescents with Tourette's syndrome. *Behaviour Research and Therapy*, 45, 2964–2976. doi:10.1016/j.brat.2007.08.007.

Hirschtritt, M.E., Lee, P.C., Pauls, D.L., Dion, Y., Grados, M.A.,…Mathews, C.A. (2015). Lifetime prevalence, age of risk, and genetic relationships of comorbid psychiatric disorders in Tourette syndrome. *JAMA Psychiatry, 72(4)*, 325–333. doi:10.1001/jamapsychiatry.2014.2650.

Huang, A. Y., Yu, D., Davis, L. K., Sul, J. H., Tsetsos, F., Ramensky, V., Zelaya, I., Ramos, E. M., Osiecki, L., Chen, J. A., McGrath, L. M., Illmann, C., Sandor, P., Barr, C. L., Grados, M., Singer, H. S., Nöthen, M. M., Hebebrand, J., King, R. A., … Smit, J. (2017). Rare Copy Number Variants in NRXN1 and CNTN6 Increase Risk for Tourette Syndrome. *Neuron*, 94(6), 1101–1111.e7. doi:10.1016/j.neuron.2017.06.010.

Hull, M., Parnes, M., & Jankovic, J. (2021). Increased incidence of functional (psychogenic) movement disorders in children and adults amid the COVID-19 pandemic: A cross-sectional study. *Neurology Clinical Practice*, 11(5), 686–690.

Ilyas, A., Pizarro, D., Romeo, A. K., Riley, K. O., & Pati, S. (2019). The centromedian nucleus: Anatomy, physiology, and clinical implications. *Journal of Clinical Neuroscience*, 63, 1–7. doi:10.1016/j.jocn.2019.01.050.

Johnson, K. A., Duffley, G., Anderson, D. N., Ostrem, J. L., Welter, M.-L., Baldermann, J. C., Kuhn, J., Huys, D., Visser-Vandewalle, V., Foltynie, T., Zrinzo, L., Hariz, M., Leentjens, A. F. G., Mogilner, A. Y., Pourfar, M. H., Almeida, L., Gunduz, A., Foote, K. D., Okun, M. S., & Butson, C. R. (2020). Structural connectivity predicts clinical outcomes of deep brain stimulation for Tourette syndrome. *Brain*, 143(8), 2607–2623. doi:10.1093/brain/awaa188.

Johnson, K. A., Worbe, Y., Foote, K. D., Butson, C. R., Gunduz, A., & Okun, M. S. (2023). Tourette syndrome: Clinical features, pathophysiology, and treatment. *The Lancet. Neurology*, 22(2), 147–158. doi:10.1016/S1474-4422(22)00303-00309.

Kahl, C. K., Kirton, A., Pringsheim, T., Croarkin, P. E., Zewdie, E., Swansburg, R., Wrightson, J., Langevin, L. M., & Macmaster, F. P. (2021). Bilateral transcranial magnetic stimulation of the supplementary motor area in children with Tourette syndrome. *Developmental Medicine and Child Neurology*, 63(7), 808–815. doi:10.1111/dmcn.14828.

Kalanithi, P. S. A., Zheng, W., Kataoka, Y., DiFiglia, M., Grantz, H., Saper, C. B., Schwartz, M. L., Leckman, J. F., & Vaccarino, F. M. (2005). Altered parvalbumin-positive neuron distribution in basal ganglia of individuals with Tourette syndrome. *Proceedings of the National Academy of Sciences*, 102(37), 13307–13312. doi:10.1073/pnas.0502624102.

Kataoka, Y., Kalanithi, P. S. A., Grantz, H., Schwartz, M. L., Saper, C., Leckman, J. F., & Vaccarino, F. M. (2010). Decreased number of parvalbumin and cholinergic interneurons in the striatum of individuals with Tourette syndrome. *The Journal of Comparative Neurology*, 518(3), 277–291. doi:10.1002/cne.22206.

Kurvits, L., Martino, D., & Ganos, C. (2020). Clinical Features That Evoke the Concept of Disinhibition in Tourette Syndrome. *Frontiers in Psychiatry*, 11, 21. doi:10.3389/fpsyt.2020.00021.

Kwak, C., Vuong, K. D., & Jankovic, J. (2003). Premonitory sensory phenomenon in Tourette's syndrome. *Movement Disorders*, 18, 1530–1533. doi:10.1002/mds.10618.

Lebowitz, E. R., Motlagh, M. G., Katsovich, L., King, R. A., Lombroso, P. J., Grantz, H., ... Leckman, J. F. (2012). Tourette syndrome in youth with and without obsessive compulsive disorder and attention deficit hyperactivity disorder. *European Child and Adolescent Psychiatry*, 21, 451–457. doi:10.1007/s00787-012-0278-5.

Leckman, J. F., Riddle, M. A., Hardin, M. T., Ort, S. I., Swartz, K. L., Stevenson, J., & Cohen, D. J. (1989). The Yale Global Tic Severity Scale: Initial testing of a clinician-rated scale of tic severity. *Journal of the American Academy of Child and Adolescent Psychiatry, 28(4)*, 566–573. doi:10.1097/00004583-198907000-00015.

Leckman, J. F., Walker, D. E., & Cohen, D. J. (1993). Premonitory urges in Tourette's syndrome. *The American Journal of Psychiatry*, 150(1), 98–102. doi:10.1176/ajp.150.1.98.

Leckman, J. F., Zhang, H., Vitale, A., Lahnin, F., Lynch, K., Bondi, C., ... Peterson, B. S. (1998). Course of tic severity in Tourette syndrome: The first two decades. *Pediatrics*, 102, 14–19. doi:10.1542/peds.102.1.14.

Leckman, J. F. (2002). Tourette's syndrome. *The Lancet*, 360(9345), 1577–1586. doi:10.1016/S0140-6736(02)11526–11521.

Lerner, A., Bagic, A., Simmons, J. M., Mari, Z., Bonne, O., Xu, B., Kazuba, D., Herscovitch, P., Carson, R. E., Murphy, D. L., Drevets, W. C., & Hallett, M. (2012). Widespread abnormality of the ⊠-aminobutyric acid-ergic system in Tourette syndrome. *Brain*, 135(6), 1926–1936. doi:10.1093/brain/aws104.

Levy, A. M., Paschou, P., & Tümer, Z. (2021). Candidate Genes and Pathways Associated with Gilles de la Tourette Syndrome – Where Are We? *Genes*, 12(9), 1321. doi:10.3390/genes12091321.

Lichtenstein, P., Carlström, E., Råstam, M., Gillberg, C., & Anckarsäter, H. (2010). The Genetics of Autism Spectrum Disorders and Related Neuropsychiatric Disorders in Childhood. *American Journal of Psychiatry*, 167(11), 1357–1363. doi:10.1176/appi.ajp.2010.10020223.

Liu, S., Tian, M., He, F., Li, J., Xie, H., Liu, W., Zhang, Y., Zhang, R., Yi, M., Che, F., Ma, X., Zheng, Y., Deng, H., Wang, G., Chen, L., Sun, X., Xu, Y., Wang, J., Zang, Y., ... Guan, J.-S. (2020). Mutations in ASH1L confer susceptibility to Tourette syndrome. *Molecular Psychiatry*, 25(2), 476–490. doi:10.1038/s41380-019-0560-8.

Liu, W., Xu, L., Zhang, C., Shen, L., Dong, J., Zhang, H., Liu, S., Che, F., & Zheng, X. (2022). ASH1L may contribute to the risk of Tourette syndrome: Combination of family-based analysis and case-control study. *Brain and Behavior*, 12(4), e2539. doi:10.1002/brb3.2539.

Maia, T. V. & Conceição, V. A. (2018). Dopaminergic Disturbances in Tourette Syndrome: An Integrative Account. *Biological Psychiatry*, 84(5), 332–344. doi:10.1016/j.biopsych.2018.02.1172.

Makhoul, K. & Jankovic, J. (2021). Tourette syndrome and driving. *Movement Disorders Clinical Practice*, 8, 763–768.

Malli, M. A., Forrester-Jones, R., & Murphy, G. (2016). Stigma in youth with Tourette's syndrome: A systematic review and synthesis. *European Child Adolescent Psychiatry*, 25, 127–139.

Martinez-Ramirez, D., Jimenez-Shahed, J., Leckman, J. F., Porta, M., Servello, D., Meng, F.-G., Kuhn, J., Huys, D., Baldermann, J. C., Foltynie, T., Hariz, M. I., Joyce, E. M., Zrinzo, L., Kefalopoulou, Z., Silburn, P., Coyne, T., Mogilner, A. Y., Pourfar, M. H., Khandhar, S. M., ... Okun, M. S. (2018). Efficacy and

Safety of Deep Brain Stimulation in Tourette Syndrome: The International Tourette Syndrome Deep Brain Stimulation Public Database and Registry. *JAMA Neurology*, 75(3), 353–359. doi:10.1001/jamaneurol.2017.4317.

Martino, D., Ganos, C., & Worbe, Y. (2018). Chapter Three: Neuroimaging Applications in Tourette's Syndrome. In M. Politis (Ed.), *International Review of Neurobiology* (Vol. 143, pp. 65–108). Academic Press. doi:10.1016/bs. irn.2018.09.008.

Mataix-Cols, D., Isomura, K., Pérez-Vigil, A., Chang, Z., Rück, C., Larsson, K. J., Leckman, J. F., Serlachius, E., Larsson, H., & Lichtenstein, P. (2015). Familial Risks of Tourette Syndrome and Chronic Tic Disorders: A Population-Based Cohort Study. *JAMA Psychiatry*, 72(8), 787–793. doi:10.1001/jamapsychiatry.2015.0627.

Müller-Vahl, K. R., Kaufmann, J., Grosskreutz, J., Dengler, R., Emrich, H. M., & Peschel, T. (2009). Prefrontal and anterior cingulate cortex abnormalities in Tourette Syndrome: Evidence from voxel-based morphometry and magnetization transfer imaging. *BMC Neuroscience*, 10(1), 47. doi:10.1186/1471-2202-10-47.

Neuner, I., Werner, C. J., Arrubla, J., Stöcker, T., Ehlen, C., Wegener, H. P., Schneider, F., & Shah, N. J. (2014). Imaging the where and when of tic generation and resting state networks in adult Tourette patients. *Frontiers in Human Neuroscience*, 8, 362. doi:10.3389/fnhum.2014.00362.

Niccolai, V., Korczok, S., Finis, J., Jonas, M., Thomalla, G., Siebner, H. R., Müller-Vahl, K., Münchau, A., Schnitzler, A., & Biermann-Ruben, K. (2019). A peek into premonitory urges in Tourette syndrome: Temporal evolution of neurophysiological oscillatory signatures. *Parkinsonism & Related Disorders*, 65, 153–158. https://doi.org/10.1016/j.parkreldis.2019.05.039.

Nilles, C., Amorelli, G., Pringsheim, T. M., & Martino, D. (2023). "Unvoluntary" movement disorders: Distinguishing between tics, akathisia, restless legs, and stereotypies. *Seminars in Neurology*. doi:10.1055/s-0043-1764164.

O'Connor, K., Brisebois, H., Brault, M., Robillard, S., & Loiselle J. (2003). Behavioral activity associated with onset in chronic tic and habit disorder. *Behaviour Research and Therapy*, 41, 241–249.

Palminteri, S. & Pessiglione, M. (2013). Chapter Five: Reinforcement Learning and Tourette Syndrome. In D. Martino & A. E. Cavanna (Eds), *International Review of Neurobiology* (Vol. 112, pp. 131–153). Academic Press. doi:10.1016/ B978-0-12-411546-0.00005-6.

Peterson, B. S., Staib, L., Scahill, L., Zhang, H., Anderson, C., Leckman, J. F., Cohen, D. J., Gore, J. C., Albert, J., & Webster, R. (2001). Regional Brain and Ventricular Volumes in Tourette Syndrome. *Archives of General Psychiatry*, 58 (5), 427–440. doi:10.1001/archpsyc.58.5.427.

Piacentini, J., Woods, D. W., Scahill, L., Wilhelm, S., Peterson, A. L., Chang, S., … Walkup, J. T. (2010). Behavior therapy for children with Tourette disorder: A randomized controlled trial. *JAMA: The Journal of the American Medical Association*, 303, 1929–1937. doi:10.1001/jama.2010.607.

Polderman, T. J. C., Benyamin, B., de Leeuw, C. A., Sullivan, P. F., van Bochoven, A., Visscher, P. M., & Posthuma, D. (2015). Meta-analysis of the heritability of human traits based on fifty years of twin studies. *Nature Genetics*, 47(7), Article 7. doi:10.1038/ng.3285.

Polyanska, L., Critchley, H. D., & Rae, C. L. (2017). Centrality of prefrontal and motor preparation cortices to Tourette Syndrome revealed by meta-analysis of task-based neuroimaging studies. *NeuroImage. Clinical*, 16, 257–267. doi:10.1016/j.nicl.2017.08.004.

Price, R. A., Kidd, K. K., Cohen, D. J., Pauls, D. L., & Leckman, J. F. (1985). A twin study of Tourette syndrome. *Archives of General Psychiatry*, 42(8), 815–820. doi:10.1001/archpsyc.1985.01790310077011.

Priori, A., Giannicola, G., Rosa, M., Marceglia, S., Servello, D., Sassi, M., & Porta, M. (2013). Deep brain electrophysiological recordings provide clues to the pathophysiology of Tourette syndrome. *Neuroscience & Biobehavioral Reviews*, 37(6), 1063–1068. doi:10.1016/j.neubiorev.2013.01.011.

Ramsey, K. A., De Nadai, A. S., Espil, F. M., Ricketts, E., Stiede, J. T., Schild, J., Specht, M. W., Woods, D. W., Bennet, S., Walkup, J. T., Chang, S., Piacentini, J., & McGuire, J. F. (2022). Urge intolerance predicts tic severity and impairment among adults with Tourette syndrome and chronic tic disorders. *Frontiers in Psychiatry*, 13, 929413. doi:10.3389/fpsyt.2022.929413.

Ramkiran, S., Heidemeyer, L., Gaebler, A., Shah, N. J., & Neuner, I. (2019). Alterations in basal ganglia-cerebello-thalamo-cortical connectivity and whole brain functional network topology in Tourette's syndrome. *NeuroImage. Clinical*, 24, 101998. doi:10.1016/j.nicl.2019.101998.

Ramsey, K. A., Essoe, J. K.-Y., Storch, E. A., Lewin, A. B., Murphy, T. K., & McGuire, J. F. (2021). Urge intolerance and impairment among youth with Tourette's and chronic tic disorders. *Child Psychiatry & Human Development*, 52 (5), 761–771. doi:10.1007/s10578-020-01085-3.

Redgrave, P. & Gurney, K. (2006). The short-latency dopamine signal: A role in discovering novel actions? *Nature Reviews Neuroscience*, 7(12), Article 12. doi:10.1038/nrn2022.

Ricketts, E. J., Woods, D. W., Espil, F. M., McGuire, J. F., Stiede, J. T., Schild, J., Yadegar, M., Bennett, S. M., Specht, M. W., Chang, S., Scahill, L., Wilhelm, S., Peterson, A. L., Walkup, J. T., & Piacentini, J. (2022). Childhood Predictors of Long-Term Tic Severity and Tic Impairment in Tourette's Disorder. *Behavior Therapy*, 53(6), 1250–1264. doi:10.1016/j.beth.2022.07.002.

Rivera-Navarro, J., Cubo, E., & Almazán, J. (2014). The impact of Tourette's syndrome in the school and the family: Perspectives from three stakeholder groups. *International Journal for the Advancement of Counselling*, 36, 96–113. doi:10.1007/s10447-013-9193-9.

Rizzo, R., Gulisano, M., Cali, P. V., & Curatolo, P. (2012). Long term clinical course of Tourette syndrome. *Brain & Development*, 34, 667–673. doi:10.1016/j. braindev.2011.11.006.

Robertson, M. M., Banerjee, S., Eapen, V., & Fox-Hiley, P. (2002). Obsessive compulsive behaviour and depressive symptoms in young people with Tourette syndrome: A controlled study. *European Child and Adolescent Psychiatry*, 11, 261–265. doi:10.1007/s00787-002-0301-3.

Robertson, M. M. (2012). The Gilles De La Tourette syndrome: The current status. *Archives of Disease in Childhood – Education & Practice Edition*, 97(5), 166–175. doi:10.1136/archdischild-2011-300585.

Robertson, M. M. (2015). A personal 35 year perspective on Gilles de la Tourette syndrome: Prevalence, phenomenology, comorbidities, and coexistent psychopathologies. *The Lancet Psychiatry*, 2, 68–87. doi:10.1016/S2215-0366(14)00132-00131.

Sambrani, T., Jakubovski, E., & Muller-Vahl, K. R. (2016). New insights into clinical characteristics of Gilles de la Tourette syndrome: Findings in 1032 patients from a single German center. *Frontiers in Neuroscience*, 10, 415. doi:10.3389/fnins.2016.00415.

Scharf, J. M., Miller, L. L., Gauvin, C. A., Alabiso, J., Mathews, C. A., & Ben-Shlomo, Y. (2015). Population prevalence of Tourette Syndrome: A systematic review and meta-analysis. *Movement Disorders*, 30(2), 221–228. doi:10.1002/mds.26089.

Sigurdsson, H. P., Pépés, S. E., Jackson, G. M., Draper, A., Morgan, P. S., & Jackson, S. R. (2018). Alterations in the microstructure of white matter in children and adolescents with Tourette syndrome measured using tract-based spatial statistics and probabilistic tractography. *Cortex*, 104, 75–89. doi:10.1016/j.cortex.2018.04.004.

Silva, R. R., Munoz, D. M., Barickman, J., & Friedhoff, A. J. (1995). Environmental factors and related fluctuation of symptoms in children and adolescents with Tourette's disorder. *Journal of Child Psychology and Psychiatry*, 36, 305–312. doi:10.1111/j.1469-7610.1995.tb01826.x.

Singer, H. S. & Augustine, F. (2019). Controversies Surrounding the Pathophysiology of Tics. *Journal of Child Neurology*, 34(13), 851–862. doi:10.1177/0883073819862121.

Singer, H. S., Hahn, I.-H., & Moran, T. H. (1991). Abnormal dopamine uptake sites in postmortem striatum from patients with tourette's syndrome. *Annals of Neurology*, 30(4), 558–562. doi:10.1002/ana.410300408.

Specht, M. W., Woods, D. W., Nicotra, C. M., Kelly, L. M., Ricketts, E. J., Conelea, C. A., Grados, M. A., Ostrander, R. S., & Walkup, J. T. (2013). Effects of tic suppression: Ability to suppress, rebound, negative reinforcement, and habituation to the premonitory urge. *Behaviour Research and Therapy*, 51(1), 24–30. doi:10.1016/j.brat.2012.09.009.

Steeves, T. D. L., Ko, J. H., Kideckel, D. M., Rusjan, P., Houle, S., Sandor, P., Lang, A. E., & Strafella, A. P. (2010). Extrastriatal dopaminergic dysfunction in tourette syndrome. *Annals of Neurology*, 67(2), 170–181. doi:10.1002/ana.21809.

Stiede, J. T., Alexander, J. R., Wellen, B., Bauer, C. C., Himle, M. B., Mouton-Odum, S., & Woods, D. W. (2018). Differentiating tic-related from non-tic-related impairment in children with persistent tic disorders. *Comprehensive Psychiatry*, 87, 38–45. doi:10.1016/j.comppsych.2018.07.017.

Storch, E. A., Lack, C. W., Simons, L. E., Goodman, W. K., Murphy, T. K., & Geffken, G. R. (2007a). A measure of functional impairment in youth with Tourette's syndrome. *Journal of Pediatric Psychology*, 32, 950–959. doi:10.1093/jpepsy/jsm034.

Storch, E. A., Murphy, T. K., Chase, R. M., Keeley, M., Goodman, W. K., Murray, M., & Geffken, G. R. (2007b). Peer victimization in youth with Tourette's syndrome and chronic tic disorder: Relations with tic severity and internalizing symptoms. *Journal of Psychopathology and Behavioral Assessment*, 29, 211–219.

Sundaram, S. K., Huq, A. M., Wilson, B. J., & Chugani, H. T. (2010). Tourette syndrome is associated with recurrent exonic copy number variants. *Neurology*, 74(20), 1583–1590. doi:10.1212/WNL.0b013e3181e0f147.

Testini, P., Min, H.-K., Bashir, A., & Lee, K. H. (2016). Deep Brain Stimulation for Tourette's Syndrome: The Case for Targeting the Thalamic Centromedian–

Parafascicular Complex. *Frontiers in Neurology*, 7. www.frontiersin.org/articles/ 10.3389/fneur.2016.00193.

Tinaz, S., Malone, P., Hallett, M., & Horovitz, S. G. (2015). Role of the right dorsal anterior insula in the urge to tic in tourette syndrome. *Movement Disorders*, 30(9), 1190–1197. doi:10.1002/mds.26230.

Verdellen, C. W., Hoogduin, C. A., Kato, B. S., Keijsers, G. P., Cath, D. C., & Hoijtink, H. B. (2008). Habituation of premonitory sensations during exposure and response prevention treatment in Tourette's syndrome. *Behavior modification*, 32(2), 215–227. doi:10.1177/0145445507309020.

Wadman, R., Glazebrook, C., Beer, C., & Jackson, G. M. (2016). Difficulties experienced by young people with Tourette syndrome in secondary school: A mixed methods description of self, parent and staff perspectives. *BMC Psychiatry*, 16, 14. doi:10.1186/s12888-016-0717-9.

Wang, S., Mandell, J. D., Kumar, Y., Sun, N., Morris, M. T., Arbelaez, J., Nasello, C., Dong, S., Duhn, C., Zhao, X., Yang, Z., Padmanabhuni, S. S., Yu, D., King, R. A., Dietrich, A., Khalifa, N., Dahl, N., Huang, A. Y., Neale, B. M., ... State, M. W. (2018). De Novo Sequence and Copy Number Variants Are Strongly Associated with Tourette Disorder and Implicate Cell Polarity in Pathogenesis. *Cell Reports*, 24(13), 3441–3454.e12. https://doi.org/ 10.1016/j.celrep.2018.08.082.

Wang, Z., Maia, T. V., Marsh, R., Colibazzi, T., Gerber, A., & Peterson, B. S. (2011). The Neural Circuits That Generate Tics in Tourette's Syndrome. *American Journal of Psychiatry*, 168(12), 1326–1337. doi:10.1176/appi.ajp.2011.09111692.

Watson, T. S., & Sterling, H. E. (1998). Brief functional analysis and treatment of a vocal tic. *Journal of Applied Behavior Analysis*, 31(3), 471–474. doi:10.1901/ jaba.1998.31-471.

Wilhelm, S., Peterson, A. L., Piacentini, J., Woods, D. W., Deckersbach, T., Sukhodolsky, D. G., ... Scahill, L. (2012). Randomized trial of behavior therapy for adults with Tourette syndrome. *Archives of General Psychiatry*, 69, 795–803. doi:10.1001/archgenpsychiatry.2011.1528.

Willsey, A. J., Fernandez, T. V., Yu, D., King, R. A., Dietrich, A., Xing, J., Sanders, S. J., Mandell, J. D., Huang, A. Y., Richer, P., Smith, L., Dong, S., Samocha, K. E., Abdulkadir, M., Bohnenpoll, J., Bromberg, Y., Brown, L. W., Cheon, K.-A., Coffey, B. J., ... Heiman, G. A. (2017). De Novo Coding Variants Are Strongly Associated with Tourette Disorder. *Neuron*, 94(3), 486–499. e9. doi:10.1016/j.neuron.2017.04.024.

Wolicki, S. B., Bitsko, R. H., Danielson, M. L., Holbrook, J. R., Zablotsky, B., Walkup, J. T., Woods, D. W., & Mink, J. W. (2019). Children with Tourette Syndrome in the United States: Parent-reported diagnosis, co-occurring disorders, severity, and influence of activities on tics. *Journal of Developmental and Behavioral Pediatrics*, 40(6), 407–414. doi:10.1097/DBP.0000000000000667.

Woods, D. W., & Himle, M. B. (2004). Creating tic suppression: Comparing the effects of verbal instrument to differential reinforcement. *Journal of Applied Behavior Analysis*, 3(3), 417–420.

Woods, D. W., Piacentini, J. C., Chang, S. W., Deckersbach, T., Ginsburg, G. S., Peterson, A. L., Scahill, L. D., Walkup, J. T., & Wilhelm, S. (2008). *Managing Tourette syndrome: A behavioral intervention for children and adults*. New York: Oxford University Press.

Woods, D. W., Piacentini, J., Himle, M. B., & Chang, S. (2005). Premonitory Urge for Tics Scale (PUTS): Initial psychometric results and examination of the premonitory urge phenomenon in youths with Tic disorders. *Journal of Developmental and Behavioral Pediatrics*, 26(6), 397–403. doi:10.1097/00004703-200512000-00001.

Woods, D. W., Walther, M. R., Bauer, C. C., Kemp, J. J., & Conelea, C. A. (2009). The development of stimulus control over tics: A potential explanation for contextually-based variability in the symptoms of Tourette syndrome. *Behaviour Research & Therapy, 47(1)*, 41–47. doi:10.1016/j.brat.2008.10.013.

Worbe, Y., Marrakchi-Kacem, L., Lecomte, S., Valabregue, R., Poupon, F., Guevara, P., Tucholka, A., Mangin, J.-F., Vidailhet, M., Lehericy, S., Hartmann, A., & Poupon, C. (2015). Altered structural connectivity of cortico-striato-pallido-thalamic networks in Gilles de la Tourette syndrome. *Brain: A Journal of Neurology*, 138(Pt 2), 472–482. doi:10.1093/brain/awu311.

Xu, M., Kobets, A., Du, J.-C., Lennington, J., Li, L., Banasr, M., Duman, R. S., Vaccarino, F. M., DiLeone, R. J., & Pittenger, C. (2015). Targeted ablation of cholinergic interneurons in the dorsolateral striatum produces behavioral manifestations of Tourette syndrome. *Proceedings of the National Academy of Sciences*, 112(3), 893–898. doi:10.1073/pnas.1419533112.

Yu, D., Sul, J. H., Tsetsos, F., Nawaz, M. S., Huang, A. Y., Zelaya, I., Illmann, C., Osiecki, L., Darrow, S. M., Hirschtritt, M. E., Greenberg, E., Muller-Vahl, K. R., Stuhrmann, M., Dion, Y., Rouleau, G., Aschauer, H., Stamenkovic, M., Schlögelhofer, M., Sandor, P., ... on behalf of the Tourette Association of America International Consortium for Genetics, the Gilles de la TouretteGWAS Replication Initiative, the Tourette InternationalCollaborative Genetics Study, and the Psychiatric GenomicsConsortium TouretteSyndrome Working Group. (2019). Interrogating the Genetic Determinants of Tourette's Syndrome and Other Tic Disorders Through Genome-Wide Association Studies. *American Journal of Psychiatry*, 176(3), 217–227. doi:10.1176/appi.ajp.2018.18070857.

Zinner, S. H., Conelea, C. A., Glew, G. M., Woods, D. W., & Budman, C. L. (2012). Peer victimization in youth with Tourette syndrome and other chronic tic disorders. *Child Psychiatry and Human Development*, 43, 124–136. doi:10.1007/s10578-011-024.

9 The Nature, Presentation, and Underlying Theories Behind Body-Focused Repetitive Behaviors (BFRBs) in Youth

Chandni Fredrickson, Theresa Gladstone and Christopher A. Flessner

Pediatric body-focused repetitive behaviors (BFRBs) encompass a broad array of repetitive and ritualistic grooming behaviors including hair pulling, skin picking, nail biting, teeth grinding (bruxism), and cheek/lip biting. These behaviors do not occur exclusively among youths; however, age at onset often occurs during this developmental period. Conversely, the existing body of empirical literature has focused largely upon the experience of adults with BFRBs. The aim of this chapter is to provide an overview of BFRBs among youths. Our aims are to summarize important facets to these conditions including (1) definition and symptoms; (2) incidence/prevalence; (3) age at onset; (4) conceptualizations; (5) clinical course and prognosis; (6) predictors and causes; (7) various types of BFRBs; (8) impairment and disruption, and, finally; (8) evidence-based treatments for BFRBs. To the extent possible, our focus will be upon literature describing these topics pertaining youths with BFRBs; however, the dearth of pediatric literature regarding these topics will be apparent. Much of the discussion that follows will be gleaned from science's understanding regarding the experience of youths with TTM and, in turn, extrapolated, to the experience of those presenting with other BFRBs.

Definition and symptoms

Body-focused repetitive behaviors are a group of behaviors characterized by non-functional and repetitive, self-grooming directed towards one or more body regions (e.g., skin picking, hair pulling, nail biting, etc.; American Psychological Association, 2013; Houazene et al., 2020; McGuire et al., 2012; O'Connor et al., 2005; Snorrason et al., 2012). These difficult-to-resist and sometimes injurious behaviors are thought to be maintained, owing to negative and positive reinforcement (Roberts et al., 2013; Sailly et al., 2020) and can be present across the developmental spectrum. BFRBs can provide instant relief or pleasure to the afflicted individual and have been commonly used to reduce uncomfortable or unpleasant emotions, such as anxiety and frustration. Among youth,

DOI: 10.4324/9781003517429-9

engaging in these habitual behaviors may function as a form of avoidance (Selles et al., 2018). Regardless of the purpose these behaviors serve, BFRBs can lead to functional impairment, physical damage, psychological distress, and a myriad of social problems (Franklin et al., 2008; Houazene et al., 2020; Houghton et al., 2018; Roberts et al., 2013; Sailly et al., 2020; Siddiqui et al., 2012). Despite these negative consequences, both youths and adults with BFRBs report being unsuccessful in controlling or stopping the behaviors (American Psychological Association, 2013; Grant & Chamberlain, 2022; Topal Hangül et al., 2022; Houazene et al., 2020).

The term BFRB encapsulates a myriad of behaviors including trichotillomania (TTM; hair pulling disorder), excoriation disorder (skin-picking disorder [SPD]), onychophagia (nail-biting), lip biting, cheek biting, and other similar behaviors (Grant et al., 2021; Greenberg et al., 2017; La Buissonnière-Ariza et al., 2020; Topal Hangül et al., 2022). Interestingly, these various types of BFRBs often co-occur and share many common features such as comorbidity patterns, etiological models, and a chronic and impulsive nature (Houazene et al., 2020; Houghton et al. 2018; Lochner et al., 2002; Snorrason et al., 2012). Therefore, research supports conceptualizing the group of behaviors as cohesive (Roberts et al., 2013; Teng et al., 2002), rather than entirely distinct presentations or disorders. Of the multiple types of BFRBs noted previously, TTM, SPD, and nail biting have been the most extensively researched (La Buissonnière-Ariza et al., 2020; McGuire et al., 2012). Unlike within the context of adults, limited literature has focused on youth with BFRBs. In turn, limited knowledge exists about the pediatric forms of these behaviors (Grant & Chamberlain., 2021; Ricketts et al., 2022). Most of the evidence discussed in this chapter will be presented within the context of pediatric TTM, since most of the youth literature has focused on this specific BFRB in children and adolescents (Harrison & Franklin, 2012).

Trichotillomania and SPD are the only BFRBs included as independent disorders with distinct criteria in the Obsessive-Compulsive and Related Disorders section of the DSM-5 (American Psychological Association, 2013). A diagnosis of TTM requires the youth or adult to engage in recurrent hair pulling resulting in noticeable hair loss accompanied by repeated attempts to limit or stop the behavior. Alternatively, a diagnosis of SPD necessitates recurrent skin picking resulting in lesions to the skin accompanied by repeated attempts to inhibit the behavior. As is the case with most other psychiatric diagnoses in the DSM-5, neither TTM nor SPD can be due to the effects of a substance or a medical or dermatological condition (e.g., cheek biting, nail biting, etc.). Both TTM and SPD also require hair pulling and skin picking, respectively, to result in clinically significant impairment in functioning. Other BFRBs, such as cheek biting and onychophagia, have not received distinct diagnostic criteria and are typically grouped under the Other Specific Obsessive-Compulsive and Related Disorders nosology in the DSM-5 (American Psychological Association, 2013; Snorrason & Woods, 2014).

Incidence/Prevalence

A dearth of prevalence data exists for youth with BFRBs (Ricketts et al., 2022; Teng et al., 2002). Previous studies in community samples have reported that BFRBs, such as TTM, are more common than previously believed (Houghton et al., 2018; Lewin et al., 2009). Some studies have also suggested that BFRBs are particularly prevalent among youth with Attention-Deficit Hyperactivity Disorder (ADHD), obsessive compulsive disorder (OCD), and some other psychiatric conditions (La Buissonnière-Ariza et al., 2020; Selles et al., 2018). Current estimates suggest that TTM prevalence rates in youth are between.6 percent and 3.5 percent (Grzesiak et al., 2017; Houghton et al., 2018; Moreno-Amador et al., 2022; Topal Hangül et al., 2022), while SPD demonstrates a 1.2 percent to 4.2 percent prevalence rate among youth (Moreno-Amador et al., 2022; Odlaug et al., 2013; Topal Hangül et al., 2022). Nail biting occurs in about 14 to 37 percent of youth, with approximately 7.3 percent experiencing significant distress, owing to the behavior (Ghanizadeh, 2008; Selles et al., 2015; Winebrake et al., 2018). Relative prevalence rates for other forms of BFRBs are not well understood.

Age of onset

The age of onset for BFRBs is typically during childhood and adolescence (Halteh et al., 2017; Ricketts et al., 2022). For example, TTM and SPD typically display an age at onset during adolescence, often coinciding with puberty but can present at any age (Flessner & Woods, 2006; Grant & Chamberlain, 2021; Ricketts et al., 2022; Wright & Holmes, 2003). Very young children can develop TTM. This early onset version of TTM is often referred to as "baby trich" (Snorrason et al., 2022) and is thought to represent a separate developmental subtype of the condition. This form of TTM has been hypothesized to demonstrate greater prevalence in males and present as a more self-limiting course (i.e., not thought to predict continued presence of hair pulling into later childhood and adolescence) compared to later onset presentations. Researchers have also suggested that males presenting with TTM tend to have an earlier age of onset compared to females (Snorrason et al., 2022). Like other psychiatric conditions (e.g., tic disorders and ADHD), this could suggest the involvement of important neurodevelopmental factors in TTM (i.e., problems in brain or central nervous system maturation and growth). A later age of onset in TTM has also been associated with greater risk of a more chronic form of the disorder as well as increased rates of comorbidities (Mancini et al., 2009; Swedo et al., 1993). Although studied less frequently, researchers have hypothesized that SPD may demonstrate a tri-modal age of onset (i.e., childhood, adolescence to young adulthood, and middle adulthood; Grant et al., 2012; Topal Hangül et al., 2022; Torales et al., 2020).

Conceptualization

Multiple theoretical underpinnings have been proposed to aid in the conceptualization of BFRBs (American Psychological Association, 2013). Most prominently, BFRBs have been described as exhibiting facets of both compulsivity and impulsivity. While sometimes viewed as a spectrum, with compulsivity and impulsivity at opposite ends, researchers have more recently theorized that the relationship between compulsivity and impulsivity may be more intricate. For example, a child with TTM may exhibit behaviors with both impulsive and compulsive elements, potentially even simultaneously (Grant & Potenza, 2006; Flessner et al., 2012).

Compulsivity has been described as engaging in a behavior (or failing to suppress a repetitive behavior) to reduce negative affect or an urge (Flessner et al., 2012). For example, individuals with OCD engage in compulsions (e.g., repetitive hand washing) to decrease distress caused by obsessive thoughts (e.g., harm to self or others). Similarly, in BFRBs, a patient may engage in repetitive behavior, such as hair pulling, to regulate a negative emotional state (e.g., frustration or anxiety) or relieve a sensation (i.e., sense of tension at the pulling site). Conversely, previous iterations of the DSM categorized TTM, SPD, and other BFRBs as disorders of impulse control (American Psychological Association, 1994). Impulsivity has been described as difficulty inhibiting behavior motivated by a reward. For example, a child with ADHD may demonstrate difficulty inhibiting oneself (e.g., interrupting others before they are finished speaking). Within the context of BFRBs, this may include difficulty inhibiting hair pulling, nail biting, and so on, especially if the behavior is accompanied by a positive sensation (Flessner et al., 2012; Fineberg et al., 2010). Further highlighting the co-occurring nature of impulsivity and compulsivity, focused pulling, discussed in greater detail below (see Body-Focused Repetitive Behaviors: Various Types below), may show qualities of both impulsivity and compulsivity (e.g., thoughtfully pulling to either decrease a negative emotion or increase a positive one). Although research has pointed to the role of both impulsivity and compulsivity in BFRBs, further investigation is necessary to parse out the intricacies of these respective facets to the conceptualization of BFRBs.

A spectrum of impulsivity-compulsivity is not the only conceptualization of BFRBs. More recently, researchers have posited that an addiction model, providing a more practical application of the impulsivity-compulsivity spectrum notion, may be helpful to understand BFRBs (Grant et al., 2007). Like addiction, BFRBs often occur to eliminate a negative or increase a positive state. For example, increased pleasure seeking, like individuals with substance-related disorders, may be prominent in those with TTM (Grant et al., 2007). Given that BFRBs are reinforced in varying ways and include elements of both impulsivity and compulsivity, targeting the antecedents and consequences surrounding repetitive behaviors has been a major theme in treatments. We discuss that topic later in this chapter (see Evidence-Based Treatments for Pediatric BFRBs below).

Clinical course and prognosis

Although onset often occurs during childhood and adolescence, BFRB symptoms can vary in severity and fluctuate over time (Flessner & Woods, 2006; Grant & Chamberlain, 2021). Research has suggested that relapses are typical among youth with BFRBs treated with current evidence-based treatment approaches; thus, relapse prevention strategies are pertinent in treatment (Ricketts et al., 2022). In lieu of intervention, TTM and SPD exhibit a chronic course with fluctuating symptom severity for many individuals (Grant & Chamberlain, 2021; Snorrason et al., 2012). Further, TTM in youth can worsen and evolve into an episodic presentation with individuals having two to three episodes annually (Henkel et al., 2019; Torales et al., 2021), if left untreated. It is important to note, however, that patients with TTM can have complete remission if the disorder is treated properly (Torales et al., 2021). Owing to the lack of longitudinal studies for the various BFRBs, clinical course information is usually derived from cross-sectional studies or clinical experiences; thus, additional research is needed in this domain (Snorrason et al., 2012; Grant & Chamberlain, 2021).

Predictors/Causes

Limited knowledge exists around the etiology of BFRBs; however, research suggests that the cause of BFRBs is complex and involves the interaction of multiple factors (i.e., genetic, environmental, biological, psychological, and social; Duke et al., 2010; Snorrason et al., 2012). For example, the severity and onset of nail biting has been linked to both genetic and environmental components (Halteh et al., 2017; Ooki, 2005). BFRBs exhibit a familial basis and are heritable with certain individuals having a genetic predisposition for these behaviors (Redden et al., 2016). Specifically, increased rates of BFRBs have been noted among first-degree or immediate relatives of those with BFRBs (e.g., TTM; Torales et al., 2021). Heritability estimates for TTM range from .32 to .78 (Grant & Chamberlain, 2021); however, specific genes that increase the risk of developing BFRBs remain unidentified. The SLITRK1 and SAPAP3 proteins may play a potential role in the development of TTM (Grant,

2019; Okumuş & Akdemir, 2023; Snorrason et al., 2012; Torales et al., 2021; Züchner et al., 2006; Züchner et al., 2009), but evidence is scant and mixed. Further, there is a need to ascertain risk factors for developing BFRBs in youth and how these risk factors relate to genetic variables. Research of this nature has the potential to help identify youth that are at an increased risk for TTM, SPD, and other BFRBs (Grant et al., 2021).

Neuroimaging research has revealed structural changes in various regions of the brain, such as the cerebellum and left putamen, among patients with TTM (Chamberlain et al., 2009; Torales et al., 2021). Several neurotransmitter systems (e.g., glutamate, serotonin, dopamine, nora-drenaline) have also been implicated in the pathophysiology of BFRBs (Grant et al., 2021; Madan et al., 2023; Woods & Houghton, 2014). Fur-thermore, environmental factors (e.g., activity restriction or an under-sti-mulating environment) may have an important role in the development of BFRBs (Grant et al., 2021; Madan et al., 2023; Snorrason et al., 2012).

Inconsistencies exist in the literature regarding sex differences in BFRBs. Multiple studies have found no sex differences among those with BFRBs, while other studies have discovered that BFRBs tend to occur more fre-quently in females compared to males (Chandran et al., 2015; Hayes et al., 2009; Selles et al., 2018). Although there seems to be a female pre-ponderance for TTM, some research has suggested that females and males are equally affected in youth (Lewin et al., 2009). In addition, the female preponderance established in prior research has been attributed to treat-ment-seeking bias and the greater social acceptance of hair loss among male patients (Greenberg et al., 2018; Roberts et al., 2013; Snorrason et al., 2012).

Body-focused repetitive behaviors: various types

As noted above, multiple manifestations of BFRBs exist (e.g., TTM, SPD, nail biting, teeth grinding, etc.). All are directed towards one's own body; however, only two BFRBs – TTM and SPD – have received most of the attention from the research community. In turn, we focus upon these spe-cific BFRBs below.

Trichotillomania

Trichotillomania, or hair pulling disorder, in youth is characterized by self-induced and repetitive pulling out of one's hair resulting in hair loss (alo-pecia) and non-scarring bald spots (Houazene et al., 2020; Woods et al., 2006). Like other BFRBs, TTM is thought to develop as the result of a complex interaction of psychological, biological, and social variables (Duke et al., 2010). This chronic and heterogeneous disorder can become severe, extremely challenging to manage, and can exhibit a fluctuating course (Flessner et al., 2008; Harrison & Franklin, 2012; Roberts et al.,

2013; Tolin et al., 2007). While individuals may pull from any site of their body with hair, most youth with trichotillomania commonly pull hair from the scalp, eyebrows, eyelashes, legs, arms, or the pubic area (in peri puberty; Franklin et al., 2008; Grant et al., 2021; Harrison & Franklin, 2012; Henkel et al., 2019; McGuire et al., 2012). Hair pulling can last anywhere from a couple of minutes to several hours and is usually symmetrical (Grant & Chamberlain, 2021). Pulling may occur using an instrument (i.e., tweezers) or hands (nondominant and/or dominant; Grant et al., 2021; Torales et al., 2021). Limited evidence suggests that symptoms tend to fluctuate in frequency and intensity and changes in pulling sites co-occur with these fluctuations (McGuire et al., 2012). Youth with TTM are less likely to pull from multiple sites compared to adults (Franklin et al., 2008). It has been postulated that an increase in the number of pulling sites during adulthood may be due to a developmental progression of the disorder (Franklin et al., 2008; Henkel et al., 2019; Tolin et al., 2007).

Triggers for pulling are present in a variety of realms, including sensory (e.g., how the hair or scalp feels), emotional (e.g., anxious, bored, angry), and cognitive (e.g., rigid thinking/hair and appearance thoughts; Grant et al., 2021). Additionally, researchers have identified two distinct pulling styles among youth with TTM (Flessner et al., 2008). For example, youths may pull their hair unconsciously (automatic pulling) and/or in response to an emotional state (focused pulling; e.g., anxiety, depression, stress, uncomfortable urge, etc.; Grant et al., 2021; Harrison & Franklin, 2012). Automatic pulling frequently occurs while reading, watching tv, or engaging in any other stationary activity (Flessner et al., 2008; Lee et al., 2020). Focused pulling tends to be more goal-oriented, intentional, and may occur when a hair feels coarse, kinky, out of place, or feels different compared to others (Flessner et al., 2008; Grant & Chamberlain, 2021). Most youth and adults with TTM engage in both types of pulling to varying extents (Grant et al., 2021; Lee et al., 2020; Murphy et al., 2017). Youths reporting high levels of both pulling styles are three times more likely to report that their behavior impedes their ability to study, for example, compared to those with low levels of both types of pulling (Flessner et al., 2008).

TTM demonstrates a high rate of comorbidity, with approximately 33 percent to 70 percent of youth with the condition meeting criteria for one or more disorders (Lewin et al., 2009; Tolin et al., 2007). For example, youth with TTM have reported increased prevalence rates of comorbid internalizing and externalizing disorders (La Buissonnière-Ariza et al., 2020; Singal & Daulatabad, 2017; Tolin et al., 2007), The most common comorbidities in youth with TTM are mood and anxiety disorders, eating disorders, substance use disorders, and disruptive behavior disorders (particularly ADHD; Franklin et al., 2008; Harrison & Franklin, 2012;

Henkel et al., 2019; Lewin et al., 2009; Ricketts et al., 2022; Tolin et al., 2007; Woods & Houghton, 2014).

Trichotillomania can lead to significant distress or functional impairment, especially in younger individuals, as hair-pulling and concealing bald spots can be time-consuming (Franklin et al., 2008; Grant et al., 2021; Harrison & Franklin, 2012; Henkel et al., 2019; Woods et al., 2006). There are many physical consequences of TTM, which include scalp irritation, damage to follicles, enamel erosion, gingivitis if hair mouthing is present, and carpal tunnel syndrome (Roberts et al., 2013, Woods et al., 2006). The minority of patients with TTM who consume their hair are more likely to develop trichobezoars (i.e., hair masses accumulating within the GI tract; Snorrason et al., 2022; Woods et al., 2006). These trichobezoars can require surgical interventions and cause vomiting, loss of weight, obstruction, ulceration, and perforation (Snorrason et al., 2022; Torales et al., 2021). In addition, it is common for youth with TTM to engage in associated behaviors, such as nose-pinching, lip biting, and nail biting (Torales et al., 2021). Despite these negative sequelae, it is rare for individuals with TTM to seek treatment (Torales et al., 2021).

Excoriation disorder

Excoriation Disorder, or SPD, refers to recurrent and intentional picking of skin resulting in noticeable skin lesions or tissue damage that can lead to significant distress or functional impairment (Flessner & Woods, 2006; Grant et al., 2021; Hayes et al., 2009; Roberts et al., 2015). Skin-picking usually involves multiple body sites and can occur on any area of the body with the face being the most common site (Gallinat et al., 2021; Nemeh & Hogeling, 2022). Fingers, teeth, or instruments (e.g., tweezers, pins, or needles) can be used to pick the skin, and time spent engaging in skin picking varies from a couple of minutes to several hours a day (Flessner & Woods, 2006; Gallinat et al., 2021; Hayes et al., 2009). Skin picking can result in infections, skin erosions, ulcerations, and scars (Ekore & Ekore, 2021; Hayes et al., 2009; Yeo & Lee, 2017). In addition, skin picking appears to demonstrate the same clinical presentation across age groups and cultures (Grant et al., 2021). Repeated unsuccessful attempts to stop the behavior are common and can cause shame, anxiety, or depression within the individual (Flessner & Woods, 2006; Lochner et al., 2017; Roberts et al., 2015).

Multiple triggers for skin picking are common and can vary across multiple domains and those afflicted with SPD (Grant & Chamberlain, 2021; Lochner et al., 2017). For example, common dermatological triggers for the onset of skin picking include acne, eczema, psoriasis, and other skin conditions (Lochner et al., 2017; Odlaug & Grant, 2008). Emotions, such as stress, anxiety, and anger, can also serve as triggers. Additional catalysts for skin picking include boredom, sedentary activities (e.g., reading and watching television), visual stimuli (i.e., scabs or scars), somatosensory triggers (i.e., itchiness), and fatigue (Grant & Chamberlain, 2021; Lochner et al., 2017; Mehrmann et al., 2020; Odlaug & Grant, 2008). As is the case amongst those afflicted with TTM, at least two disparate yet related skin picking styles exist – focused and automatic picking (Ricketts et al., 2022). Unlike the TTM literature, however, the validity of these picking styles has yet to be examined among youths.

Like TTM, skin picking in youth is linked to an increased prevalence of comorbid externalizing and internalizing disorders (La Buissonnière-Ariza et al., 2020). The most common comorbidities include other BFRBs (predominantly TTM), mood and anxiety disorders, OCD, body dysmorphic disorder, as well as substance use disorders (Lochner et al., 2017; McGuire et al., 2012; Odlaug & Grant, 2008; Ricketts et al., 2018; Snorrason et al., 2012).

Impairment and disruption

BFRBs can result in substantial distress and impairments, owing to the wounds associated with the behaviors and efforts to hide them (Hayes et al., 2009; Tucker et al., 2011). BFRBs may also impose a significant personal and societal burden. Affected youth may experience impairment in multiple areas including emotional (e.g., guilt, embarrassment, shame, anxiety, depression), social, academic, as well as family functioning domains (Harrison & Franklin, 2012; Ricketts et al., 2022). Individuals with BFRBs report avoiding social activities because of the shame and embarrassment caused by the behaviors (Flessner & Woods, 2006; Houghton et al., 2018; Tucker et al., 2011). Furthermore, youth with BFRBs exhibit increased impulsivity as well as poorer quality of life, enjoyment, satisfaction, and distress tolerance compared to youth without BFRBs (Ricketts et al., 2022). Youth who engage in hair-pulling and skin picking show lower adaptive functioning and greater distress compared to peers (Moreno-Amador et al., 2022; Selles et al., 2015). Adolescents with TTM may also demonstrate anxiety about their peers potentially noticing their bald spots (Harrison & Franklin, 2012). Furthermore, hair-pulling may cause negative evaluations or reduced social acceptance by peers, which can result in bullying and isolation (Boudjouk et al., 2000; Harrison & Franklin, 2012; Henkel et al., 2019; Ricketts et al., 2022). Among youth with TTM, the effects of childhood bullying or teasing can be long-term and cause psychological sequelae (e.g., low self-esteem; Henkel et al., 2019). Additionally, avoidance behaviors, body dissatisfaction, and negative affective states (e.g., irritability or feeling unattractive) have been reported among those with TTM (Duke et al., 2010). Youth with SPD also show an increased likelihood of facing stigmatization and bullying, which can also lead to negative psychological sequelae (e.g., depression or anxiety; Ekore & Ekore, 2021).

Evidence-based treatments for pediatric BFRBs

Behavioral treatments are the most researched interventions to target BFRBs. It is important to understand, however, that the research literature examining *any* treatment for youths with BFRBs is scant; thus, limited empirical research is an important caveat to consider when evaluating interventions for BFRBs in youth. Habit reversal treatment (HRT) is one treatment, grounded in learning principles, that has received the greatest degree of empirical support, thus far, among youth (Azrin & Nunn, 1973; Woods & Houghton, 2016; Franklin et al., 2011). From a learning theory perspective, BFRBs can be understood from an antecedent, behavior, and consequence model (ABC model). For example, when pulling decreases a negative emotional state, one might view the antecedent as the stressor (e. g., individual with TTM stressed about an upcoming exam), the behavior as the pulling, and the consequence as immediate relief and decreased stress in that moment. Therefore, with this conceptualization, hair pulling is negatively reinforced as it provides relief from the negative affective state. The main components of HRT include awareness training, stimulus control, and competing response training. Awareness training helps the child and their family increase their awareness of when the BFRB occurs. This element may be particularly important with automatic pulling, as it is often out of the individual's conscious awareness. Awareness training brings attention to the BFRB and allows for manipulation of it. Stimulus control targets the antecedent to reduce the chances that the individual will start to engage in the BFRB in the first place. For example, if the youth's hair pulling or skin picking often occurs in a specific environment (e.g., while watching television after school), then changing that environment (e.g., engaging in a different activity after school and watching television at a different time) can help to decrease the BFRB. Competing response training involves learning an action that one cannot do at the same time as the BFRB (e.g., making a fist instead of nail biting). This method is designed to inhibit the behavior from occurring. Competing response training is conceptualized as response prevention as it teaches the individual that the urge to engage in the BFRB will subside over time without engagement in the BFRB. Social reinforcement (e.g., parents praising individual for practicing not engaging in the BFRBs) and relapse prevention (e.g., managing flare-ups of BFRBs following treatment) are additional strategies utilized to treat BFRBs within these behavioral treatments (Sarah et al., 2013; Woods & Houghton, 2016).

Summary and conclusions

Body-focused repetitive behaviors occur across the developmental spectrum, although they most frequently begin during late childhood and adolescence. While BFRBs can take a variety of forms (i.e., TTM, SPD, nail biting, teeth grinding, lip/cheek biting), TTM and SPD are among the most often studied of this class of behavior and are more prevalent than expected by some. Despite the impairment and disruption that results from BFRBs in youths, a disturbingly small body of empirical literature has examined the experience of youths with TTM and even less so with respect to SPD or other forms of BFRBs. Continued research is needed across a variety of domains including the development, course, and treatment of BFRBs. We acknowledge that the areas in need of further study are broad. At the same time and as the overview above suggests, remarkably little is known regarding BFRBs in youths; thus, the need for research within this population is all encompassing and important.

References

American Psychiatric Association. (1994). *Diagnostic and statistical manual of mental disorders: DSM-IV* (Fourth Ed.).

American Psychiatric Association. (2013). *Diagnostic and statistical manual of mental disorders: DSM-5* (Vol. 5, No. 5). Washington, DC: American Psychiatric Association.

Azrin, N. H. & Nunn, R. G. (1973). Habit-reversal: a method of eliminating nervous habits and tics. *Behaviour research and therapy*, 11(4), 619–628.

Boudjouk, P. J., Woods, D. W., Miltenberger, R. G., & Long, E. S. (2000). Negative Peer Evaluation in Adolescents: Effects of Tic Disorders and Trichotillomania. *Child & Family Behavior Therapy*, 22(1), 17–28. doi:10.1300/j019v22n01_02.

Chamberlain, S. R., Odlaug, B. L., Boulougouris, V., Fineberg, N. A., & Grant, J. E. (2009). Trichotillomania: neurobiology and treatment. *Neuroscience and biobehavioral reviews*, 33(6), 831–842. doi:10.1016/j.neubiorev.2009.02.002.

Chandran, N. S., Novak, J., Iorizzo, M., Grimalt, R., & Oranje, A. P. (2015). Trichotillomania in Children. *Skin appendage disorders*, 1(1), 18–24. doi:10.1159/000371809.

Duke, D. C., Keeley, M. L., Geffken, G. R., & Storch, E. A. (2010). Trichotillomania: A current review. *Clin Psychol Rev*, 30(2), 181–193. doi:10.1016/j.cpr.2009.10.008.

Ekore, R. I. & Ekore, J. O. (2021). Excoriation (skin-picking) disorder among adolescents and young adults with acne-induced postinflammatory hyperpigmentation and scars. *Int J Dermatol*, 60(12), 1488–1493. doi:10.1111/ijd.15587.

Fineberg, N. A., Potenza, M. N., Chamberlain, S. R., Berlin, H. A., Menzies, L., Bechara, A., & Hollander, E. (2010). Probing compulsive and impulsive behaviors, from animal models to endophenotypes: a narrative review. *Neuropsychopharmacology*, 35(3), 591–604.

Flessner, C. A., Knopik, V. S., & McGeary, J. (2012). Hair pulling disorder (trichotillomania): genes, neurobiology, and a model for understanding impulsivity and compulsivity. *Psychiatry research*, 199(3), 151–158.

Flessner, C. A. & Woods, D. W. (2006). Phenomenological characteristics, social problems, and the economic impact associated with chronic skin picking. *Behav Modif*, 30(6), 944–963. doi:10.1177/0145445506294083.

Flessner, C. A., Woods, D. W., Franklin, M. E., Keuthen, N. J., Piacentini, J., & Trichotillomania Learning Center-Scientific Advisory Board. (2008). Styles of pulling in youths with trichotillomania: exploring differences in symptom severity, phenomenology, and comorbid psychiatric symptoms. *Behav Res Ther*, 46 (9), 1055–1061. doi:10.1016/j.brat.2008.06.006.

Franklin, M. E., Edson, A. L., Ledley, D. A., & Cahill, S. P. (2011). Behavior therapy for pediatric trichotillomania: a randomized controlled trial. *Journal of the American. Academy of Child & Adolescent Psychiatry*, 50(8), 763–771.

Franklin, M. E., Flessner, C. A., Woods, D. W., Keuthen, N. J., Piacentini, J. C., Moore, P., Stein, D. J., Cohen, S. B., Wilson, M. A., & Trichotillomania LearningCenter-Scientific Advisory Board (2008). The child and adolescent trichotillomania impact project: descriptive psychopathology, comorbidity, functional impairment, and treatment utilization. *Journal of developmental and behavioral pediatrics: JDBP*, 29(6), 493–500. doi:10.1097/DBP.0b013e31818d4328.

Gallinat, C., Stürmlinger, L. L., Schaber, S., & Bauer, S. (2021). Pathological Skin Picking: Phenomenology and Associations With Emotions, Self-Esteem, Body Image, and Subjective Physical Well-Being. *Frontiers in psychiatry*, 12, 732717. doi:10.3389/fpsyt.2021.732717.

Ghanizadeh, A. (2008). Association of nail biting and psychiatric disorders in children and their parents in a psychiatrically referred sample of children. *Child and adolescent psychiatry and mental health*, 2(1), 13. doi:10.1186/1753-2000-2-13.

Grant J. E. (2019). Trichotillomania (hair pulling disorder). *Indian journal of psychiatry*, 61 (Suppl 1), S136–S139. doi:10.4103/psychiatry. IndianJPsychiatry_529_18.

Grant, J. E. & Chamberlain, S. R. (2021). *Trichotillomania and Skin-Picking Disorder: An Update. Focus (Am Psychiatr Publ)*, 19(4), 405–412. doi:10.1176/ appi.focus.20210013.

Grant, J. E. & Chamberlain, S. R. (2022). The role of compulsivity in body-focused repetitive behaviors. *J Psychiatr Res*, 151, 365–367. doi:10.1016/j. jpsychires.2022.05.001.

Grant, J. E., Odlaug, B. L., Chamberlain, S. R., Keuthen, N. J., Lochner, C., & Stein, D. J. (2012). Skin picking disorder. *The American journal of psychiatry*, 169(11), 1143–1149. doi:10.1176/appi.ajp.2012.12040508.

Grant, J. E., Odlaug, B. L., & Potenza, M. N. (2007). Addicted to hair pulling? How an alternate model of trichotillomania may improve treatment outcome. *Harvard review of psychiatry*, 15(2), 80–85.

Grant, J. E., Peris, T. S., Ricketts, E. J., Lochner, C., Stein, D. J., Stochl, J., Chamberlain, S. R., Scharf, J. M., Dougherty, D. D., Woods, D. W., Piacentini, J., & Keuthen, N. J. (2021). Identifying subtypes of trichotillomania (hair pulling disorder) and excoriation (skin picking) disorder using mixture modeling in a multicenter sample. *J Psychiatr Res*, 137, 603–612. doi:10.1016/j. jpsychires.2020.11.001.

Grant, J. E. & Potenza, M. N. (2006). Compulsive aspects of impulse-control disorders. *Psychiatric Clinics*, 29(2), 539–551.

Greenberg, E., Grant, J. E., Curley, E. E., Lochner, C., Woods, D. W., Tung, E. S., Stein, D. J., Redden, S. A., Scharf, J. M., & Keuthen, N. J. (2017). Predictors of comorbid eating disorders and association with other obsessive-compulsive spectrum disorders in trichotillomania. *Comprehensive psychiatry*, 78, 1–8. doi:10.1016/j.comppsych.2017.06.008.

Greenberg, E., Tung, E. S., Gauvin, C., Osiecki, L., Yang, K. G., Curley, E., Essa, A., Illmann, C., Sandor, P., Dion, Y., Lyon, G. J., King, R. A., Darrow, S., Hirschtritt, M. E., Budman, C. L., Grados, M., Pauls, D. L., Keuthen, N. J., Mathews, C. A., Scharf, J. M., … Tourette Association of America International Consortium for Genetics. (2018). Prevalence and predictors of hair pulling disorder and excoriation disorder in Tourette syndrome. *European child & adolescent psychiatry*, 27(5), 569–579. doi:10.1007/s00787-017-1074-z.

Grzesiak, M., Reich, A., Szepietowski, J. C., Hadryś, T., & Pacan, P. (2017). Trichotillomania Among Young Adults: Prevalence and Comorbidity. *Acta dermato-venereologica*, 97(4), 509–512. doi:10.2340/00015555-2565.

Halteh, P., Scher, R. K., & Lipner, S. R. (2017). Onychophagia: A nail-biting conundrum for physicians. *J Dermatolog Treat*, 28(2), 166–172. doi:10.1080/09546634.2016.1200711.

Harrison, J. P. & Franklin, M. E. (2012). Pediatric trichotillomania. *Curr Psychiatry Rep*, 14(3), 188–196. doi:10.1007/s11920-012-0269-8.

Hayes, S. L., Storch, E. A., & Berlanga, L. (2009). Skin picking behaviors: An examination of the prevalence and severity in a community sample. *J Anxiety Disord*, 23(3), 314–319. doi:10.1016/j.janxdis.2009.01.008.

Henkel, E. D., Jaquez, S. D., & Diaz, L. Z. (2019). Pediatric trichotillomania: Review of management. *Pediatr Dermatol*, 36(6), 803–807. doi:10.1111/pde.13954.

Houazene, S., Aardema, F., Leclerc, J. B., & O'Connor, K. (2020). The Role of Self-Criticism and Shame in Body-Focused Repetitive Behaviour Symptoms. *Behaviour Change*, 38(1), 10–24. doi:10.1017/bec.2020.16.

Houghton, D. C., Alexander, J. R., Bauer, C. C., & Woods, D. W. (2018). Body-focused repetitive behaviors: More prevalent than once thought?. *Psychiatry Res*, 270, 389–393. doi:10.1016/j.psychres.2018.10.002.

La Buissonnière-Ariza, V., Alvaro, J., Cavitt, M., Rudy, B. M., Cepeda, S. L., Schneider, S. C., McIngvale, E., Goodman, W. K., & Storch, E. A. (2020). Body-focused repetitive behaviors in youth with mental health conditions: A preliminary study on their prevalence and clinical correlates. *International Journal of Mental Health*, 50(1), 33–52. doi:10.1080/00207411.2020.1824111.

Lee, E. B., Homan, K. J., Morrison, K. L., Ong, C. W., Levin, M. E., & Twohig, M. P. (2020). Acceptance and Commitment Therapy for Trichotillomania: A Randomized Controlled Trial of Adults and Adolescents. *Behavior modification*, 44(1), 70–91. doi:10.1177/0145445518794366.

Lewin, A. B., Piacentini, J., Flessner, C. A., Woods, D. W., Franklin, M. E., Keuthen, N. J., Moore, P., Khanna, M., March, J. S., Stein, D. J., & TLC Scientific Advisory Board. (2009). Depression, anxiety, and functional impairment in children with trichotillomania. *Depress Anxiety*, 26(6), 521–527. doi:10.1002/da.20537.

Lochner, C., Roos, A., & Stein, D. J. (2017). Excoriation (skin-picking) disorder: a systematic review of treatment options. *Neuropsychiatr Dis Treat*, 13, 1867–1872. doi:10.2147/NDT.S121138.

Lochner, C., Simeon, D., Niehaus, D. J. H., & Stein, D. (2002). Trichotillomania and skin-picking: A phenomenological comparison. *Depression and anxiety*, 15, 83–86. doi:10.1002/da.10034.

Madan, S. K., Davidson, J., & Gong, H. (2023). Addressing body-focused repetitive behaviors in the dermatology practice. *Clinics in dermatology*, 41(1), 49–55. doi:10.1016/j.clindermatol.2023.03.004.

Mancini, C., Van Ameringen, M., Patterson, B., Simpson, W., & Truong, C. (2009). Trichotillomania in youth: a retrospective case series. *Depress Anxiety*, 26(7), 661–665. doi:10.1002/da.20579.

McGuire, J. F., Kugler, B. B., Park, J. M., Horng, B., Lewin, A. B., Murphy, T. K., & Storch, E. A. (2012). Evidence-Based Assessment of Compulsive Skin Picking, Chronic Tic Disorders and Trichotillomania in Children. *Child Psychiatry & Human Development*, 43(6), 855–883. doi:10.1007/s10578-012-0300-7.

Mehrmann, L. M., Urban, A., & Gerlach, A. L. (2020). Visual Triggers of Skin Picking Episodes: An Experimental Study in Self-Reported Skin Picking Disorder and Atopic Dermatitis. *Clinical psychology in Europe*, 2(4), e2931. doi:10.32872/cpe.v2i4.2931.

Moreno-Amador, B., Falcó, R., Marzo, J. C., & Piqueras, J. A. (2022). Body-dysmorphic, hoarding, hair-pulling, and skin-picking symptoms in a large sample of adolescents. *Current Psychology*. doi:10.1007/s12144-022-03477-1.

Murphy, Y. E., Flessner, C. A., Altenburger, E. M., Pauls, D. L., & Keuthen, N. J. (2017). The impact of family functioning on pulling styles among adolescents with trichotillomania (hair pulling disorder). *Journal of Obsessive-Compulsive and Related Disorders*, 14, 27–35. doi:10.1016/j.jocrd.2017.05.002.

Nemeh, M. N. & Hogeling, M. (2022). Pediatric skin picking disorder: A review of management. *Pediatr Dermatol*, 39(3), 363–368. doi:10.1111/pde.14953.

O'Connor, K. P., Lavoie, M. E., Robert, M., Stip, E., & Borgeat, F. (2005). Brain-behavior relations during motor processing in chronic tic and habit disorder. *Cognitive and behavioral neurology: official journal of the Society for Behavioral and Cognitive Neurology*, 18(2), 79–88. doi:10.1097/01.wnq.0000151131.06699.af.

Odlaug, B. L. & Grant, J. E. (2008). Trichotillomania and Pathologic Skin Picking: clinical comparison with an examination of comorbidity. *Ann Clin Psychiatry*, 20(2), 57–63. doi:10.1080/10401230802017027.

Odlaug, B. L., Lust, K., Schreiber, L. R., Christenson, G., Derbyshire, K., & Grant, J. E. (2013). Skin picking disorder in university students: health correlates and gender differences. *General hospital psychiatry*, 35(2), 168–173. doi:10.1016/j.genhosppsych.2012.08.006.

Okumuş, H. G. & Akdemir, D. (2023). Body Focused Repetitive Behavior Disorders: Behavioral Models and Neurobiological Mechanisms. Beden Odaklı Tekrarlayıcı Davranış Bozuklukları: Davranış Modelleri ve Nörobiyolojik Mekanizmalar. *Turk psikiyatri dergisi = Turkish journal of psychiatry*, 34(1), 50–59. doi:10.5080/u26213.

Ooki S. (2005). Genetic and environmental influences on finger-sucking and nail-biting in Japanese twin children. *Twin research and human genetics: the official journal of the International Society for Twin Studies*, 8(4), 320–327. doi:10.1375/1832427054936637.

Redden, S. A., Leppink, E. W., & Grant, J. E. (2016). Body focused repetitive behavior disorders: Significance of family history. *Compr Psychiatry*, 66, 187–192. doi:10.1016/j.comppsych.2016.02.003.

Ricketts, E. J., Peris, T. S., Grant, J. E., Valle, S., Cavic, E., Lerner, J. E., Lochner, C., Stein, D. J., Dougherty, D. D., O'Neill, J., Woods, D. W., Keuthen, N. J., & Piacentini, J. (2022). Clinical Characteristics of Youth with Trichotillomania (Hair-Pulling Disorder) and Excoriation (Skin-Picking) Disorder. *Child Psychiatry Hum Dev*. doi:10.1007/s10578-022-01458-w.

Ricketts, E. J., Snorrason, Í., Kircanski, K., Alexander, J. R., Thamrin, H., Flessner, C. A., Franklin, M. E., Piacentini, J., & Woods, D. W. (2018). A latent profile analysis of age of onset in pathological skin picking. *Comprehensive psychiatry*, 87, 46–52. doi:10.1016/j.comppsych.2018.08.011.

Roberts, S., O'Connor, K., Aardema, F., & Belanger, C. (2015). The impact of emotions on body-Focused repetitive behaviors: evidence from a non-treatment-seeking sample. *J Behav Ther Exp Psychiatry*, 46, 189–197. doi:10.1016/j.jbtep.2014.10.007.

Roberts, S., O'Connor, K., & Belanger, C. (2013). Emotion regulation and other psychological models for body-focused repetitive behaviors. *Clin Psychol Rev*, 33(6), 745–762. doi:10.1016/j.cpr.2013.05.004.

Sailly, S., Khanande, R. V., Munda, S. K., & Mehta, V. S. (2020). Body-focused repetitive behaviors in school-going children and adolescents and its relationship with state-trait anxiety and life events. *Indian journal of psychiatry*, 62(6), 703–706. doi:10.4103/psychiatry.IndianJPsychiatry_607_19.

Sarah H. M., Hana, F. Z., Hilary E. D., & Martin, E. F. (2013). Habit reversal training in trichotillomania: guide for the clinician. *Expert review of neurotherapeutics*, 13(9), 1069–1077.

Selles, R. R., La Buissonniere Ariza, V., McBride, N. M., Dammann, J., Whiteside, S., & Storch, E. A. (2018). Initial psychometrics, outcomes, and correlates of the Repetitive Body Focused Behavior Scale: Examination in a sample of youth with anxiety and/or obsessive-compulsive disorder. *Compr Psychiatry*, 81, 10–17. doi:10.1016/j.comppsych.2017.11.001.

Selles, R. R., Nelson, R., Zepeda, R., Dane, B. F., Wu, M. S., Novoa, J. C., Guttfreund, D., & Storch, E. A. (2015). Body focused repetitive behaviors among Salvadorian youth: Incidence and clinical correlates. *Journal of Obsessive-Compulsive and Related Disorders*, 5, 49–54. doi:10.1016/j.jocrd.2015.01.008.

Siddiqui, E. U., Naeem, S. S., Naqvi, H., & Ahmed, B. (2012). Prevalence of body-focused repetitive behaviors in three large medical colleges of Karachi: a cross-sectional study. *BMC research notes*, 5, 614. doi:10.1186/1756-0500-5-614.

Singal, A. & Daulatabad, D. (2017). Nail tic disorders: Manifestations, pathogenesis and management. *Indian journal of dermatology, venereology and leprology*, 83(1), 19–26. doi:10.4103/0378-6323.184202.

Snorrason, I., Belleau, E. L., & Woods, D. W. (2012). How related are hair pulling disorder (trichotillomania) and skin picking disorder? A review of evidence for comorbidity, similarities and shared etiology. *Clin Psychol Rev*, 32(7), 618–629. doi:10.1016/j.cpr.2012.05.008.

Snorrason, I., Ricketts, E. J., Stein, A. T., Thamrin, H., Lee, S. J., Goldberg, H., Hu, Y., & Bjorgvinsson, T. (2022). Sex Differences in Age at Onset and Presentation of Trichotillomania and Trichobezoar: A 120-Year Systematic Review of Cases. *Child Psychiatry Hum Dev*, 53(1), 165–171. doi:10.1007/s10578-020-01117-y.

Snorrason, I. & Woods, D. W. (2014). Hair pulling, skin picking, and other body-focused repetitive behaviors. In E. A. Storch & D. McKay (Eds), *Obsessive-compulsive disorder and its spectrum: A life-span approach* (pp. 163–184). American Psychological Association. doi:10.1037/14323-009.

Swedo, S. E., Lenane, M. C., & Leonard, H. L. (1993). Long-term treatment of trichotillomania (hair pulling). *The New England journal of medicine*, 329(2), 141–142. doi:10.1056/NEJM199307083290220.

Teng, E. J., Woods, D. W., Twohig, M. P., & Marcks, B. A. (2002). Body-focused repetitive behavior problems. Prevalence in a nonreferred population and differences in perceived somatic activity. *Behavior modification*, 26(3), 340–360. doi:10.1177/0145445502026003003.

Tolin, D. F., Franklin, M. E., Diefenbach, G. J., Anderson, E., & Meunier, S. A. (2007). Pediatric trichotillomania: descriptive psychopathology and an open trial of cognitive behavioral therapy. *Cogn Behav Ther*, 36(3), 129–144. doi:10.1080/16506070701223230.

Topal Hangül, Z., Tuman, T. C., Altunay-Tuman, B., Saygılı, G. Y., & Tufan, A. E. (2022). Body-focused repetitive behaviors in children and adolescents, clinical characteristics, and the effects of treatment choices on symptoms: a single-center retrospective cohort study. *Acta Dermatovenerologica Alpina Pannonica et Adriatica*, 31(4). doi:10.15570/actaapa.2022.24.

Torales, J., Díaz, N. R., Barrios, I., Navarro, R., García, O., O'Higgins, M., Castaldelli-Maia, J. M., Ventriglio, A., & Jafferany, M. (2020). Psychodermatology of skin picking (excoriation disorder): A comprehensive review. *Dermatologic therapy*, 33(4), e13661. doi:10.1111/dth.13661.

Torales, J., Ruiz Diaz, N., Ventriglio, A., Castaldelli-Maia, J. M., Barrios, I., Garcia, O., Navarro, R., Gonzalez-Urbieta, I., O'Higgins, M., & Jafferany, M. (2021). Hair-pulling disorder (Trichotillomania): Etiopathogenesis, diagnosis and treatment in a nutshell. *Dermatol Ther*, 34(1), e13466. doi:10.1111/dth.14366.

Tucker, B. T., Woods, D. W., Flessner, C. A., Franklin, S. A., & Franklin, M. E. (2011). The Skin Picking Impact Project: phenomenology, interference, and treatment utilization of pathological skin picking in a population-based sample. *J Anxiety Disord*, 25(1), 88–95. doi:10.1016/j.janxdis.2010.08.007.

Winebrake, J. P., Grover, K., Halteh, P., & Lipner, S. R. (2018). Pediatric Onychophagia: A Survey-Based Study of Prevalence, Etiologies, and Co-Morbidities. *American journal of clinical dermatology*, 19(6), 887–891. doi:10.1007/s40257-018-0386-1.

Woods, D. W., Flessner, C. A., Franklin, M. E., Keuthen, N. J., Goodwin, R. D., Stein, D. J., Walther, M. R., & Trichotillomania Learning Center-Scientific Advisory Board. (2006). The Trichotillomania Impact Project (TIP): exploring phenomenology, functional impairment, and treatment utilization. *The Journal of clinical psychiatry*, 67(12), 1877–1888. doi:10.4088/jcp.v67n1207.

Woods, D. W. & Houghton, D. C. (2014). Diagnosis, evaluation, and management of trichotillomania. *The Psychiatric clinics of North America*, 37(3), 301–317. doi:10.1016/j.psc.2014.05.005.

Woods, D. W. & Houghton, D. C. (2016). Evidence-based psychosocial treatments for pediatric body-focused repetitive behavior disorders. *Journal of Clinical Child & Adolescent. Psychology*, 45(3), 227–240.

Wright, H. H. & Holmes, G. R. (2003). Trichotillomania (hair pulling) in toddlers. *Psychological reports*, 92(1), 228–230. doi:10.2466/pr0.2003.92.1.228.

Yeo, S. K. & Lee, W. K. (2017). The relationship between adolescents' academic stress, impulsivity, anxiety, and skin picking behavior. *Asian J Psychiatr*, 28, 111–114. doi:10.1016/j.ajp.2017.03.039.

Züchner, S., Cuccaro, M. L., Tran-Viet, K. N., Cope, H., Krishnan, R. R., Pericak-Vance, M. A., Wright, H. H., & Ashley-Koch, A. (2006). SLITRK1 mutations in trichotillomania. *Molecular psychiatry*, 11(10), 887–889. doi:10.1038/sj.mp.4001898.

Züchner, S., Wendland, J. R., Ashley-Koch, A. E., Collins, A. L., Tran-Viet, K. N., Quinn, K., Timpano, K. C., Cuccaro, M. L., Pericak-Vance, M. A., Steffens, D. C., Krishnan, K. R., Feng, G., & Murphy, D. L. (2009). Multiple rare SAPAP3 missense variants in trichotillomania and OCD. *Molecular psychiatry*, 14(1), 6–9. doi:10.1038/mp.2008.83.

10 Body Dysmorphic Disorder in Youth

A. D. Jassi and G. Krebs

Nature of BDD

Body Dysmorphic Disorder (BDD) is characterized by a preoccupation with perceived flaw(s) in one's appearance which appear minimal or non-existent to others. This leads sufferers to engage in repetitive behaviors as attempts to hide or fix the perceived flaw(s) e.g. camouflaging, grooming etc., and avoidance. The accumulation of this preoccupation and behavioral consequences leads to distress and impairment in functioning for the sufferer (American Psychiatric Association, 2013; World Health Organization, 2018). BDD is a common condition with prevalence in approximately 2 percent in community samples of youth (Schneider et al., 2017) and adults (Veale et al., 2016; Enander et al., 2018). Higher rates of BDD are found in certain settings such as psychiatric adolescent inpatient settings, with a weighted prevalence of 7.4 percent (Veale et al., 2016).

BDD typically develops in adolescence, with two thirds of adults retrospectively reporting onset during this period, with the most common age of onset being 12 years old (Bjornsson et al., 2013). In a group of 172 adolescents diagnosed with BDD in two specialist clinics, the largest sample exploring clinical characteristics to date, the mean age of onset was 12.6 years (Rautio et al., 2020). In this sample the range of age of onset was 4 to 17 years (Rautio et al., 2020), which is similar to the range of 5–17 years reported in a smaller sample of 33 adolescents (Albertini & Phillips, 1999). This suggests that pre-pubertal onset is possible, although relatively rare. The mean age of presentation to specialist BDD clinics was 15.6 years, which suggests a delay of around three years from onset to accessing specialist clinics, although a proportion will access other services first (Rautio et al., 2020). BDD is an under-recognized and under-diagnosed condition, with a survey of adults in Germany indicating only 15–23 percent of adults with BDD received an accurate diagnosis (Schulte et al., 2020; Marques et al., 2011), which contribute to delays in accessing appropriate services.

One of many challenges in identifying BDD in adolescents is that appearance worries, and associated behaviors, may be disregarded as 'normal' for that developmental stage given how prevalent they are in

DOI: 10.4324/9781003517429-10

adolescence (Voelkar et al., 2015). BDD worries and behaviors are likely to be an extreme manifestation of normal appearance worries and behaviors (Bala et al., 2021). In fact, adolescents with subthreshold BDD symptoms have been found to have poorer quality of life and elevated rates of psychiatric comorbidity (Schneider et al., 2017). The main way to differentiate normal appearance concerns from BDD is to consider the impact and distress of appearance worries and associated repetitive behaviors; that is, in order to meet threshold for a diagnosis the appearance concerns and/or repetitive and avoidant behaviors must be causing significant distress to the individual, and/or functional impairment (American Psychiatric Association, 2013; World Health Organization, 2018).

Presentation of BDD

Typically, sufferers report multiple areas of appearance preoccupations (Rautio et al., 2020). While specific areas are often highlighted, some sufferers report an overall sense of being ugly, hideous or report that the features do not fit well together. In adolescents, the top reported areas of concern were skin, nose, hair, face and stomach (Rautio et al., 2020). Adults report similar areas of concern, with skin and hair being the top two reported by both adults and adolescents (Phillips et al., 2006). In terms of repetitive behaviors, mirror checking, comparing oneself to others, camouflaging, applying make-up, grooming and reassurance seeking are the most frequently reported by adolescents (Rautio et al., 2020). Figure 10.1 below illustrates the top reported areas of concern and repetitive behaviors in a sub-sample (n=99) of adolescents from this study. In a smaller sample comparing adolescents (n=36) with adults (n=164), there were no differences in reported repetitive behaviors (Phillips et al., 2006).

In terms of gender distribution of BDD, in a large sample of 15 (n=6968), 18 (n=3738) and 20–28-year-olds (n= 4671), there was a significantly higher prevalence of clinically significant BDD symptoms among females (1.3–3.3 percent) compared to males (0.2–0.6 percent) (Enander et al., 2018). The female preponderance has also been found in smaller studies with adolescents (n=464) with 2.8 percent of females and 1.7 percent of males (ratio 1.64) scoring over threshold on a self-report measure of BDD (Mayville et al., 1999). In clinical samples of BDD, the sex differences are stark among adolescence, with approximately 80 percent being female (Phillips et al., 2006; Rautio et al., 2020) but there less pronounced in adults (66 percent females) (Phillips et al., 2006). While the reasons for these sex differences are not well understood, the latter results raise the possibility that males tend to have a later age at onset of BDD. In terms of clinical presentation, overall, this is similar across the sexes in adolescents (Rautio et al., 2020) with the exception of muscle dysmorphia, a subtype of BDD which is characterized by sufferers feeling they are insufficiently muscular or too slight, which is typically seen more in boys and men (Rautio et al., 2020).

Risk is high in BDD and can present in a range of ways including suicidal ideation and attempts, self-harm and undertaking cosmetic procedures. BDD has been found to be associated with an increased risk for both suicidal ideation (OR = 3.63, 95 percent CI 1.44 to 3.69) and suicide attempts (OR 3.30, 95 percent CI 2.18 to 4.43) (Angelakis, Gooding & Panagioti, 2016). Rates of reported suicidal ideation in adolescents varies from 57 percent (Rautio et al., 2020) to 81 percent (Phillips et al., 2006), with 11 percent (Rautio et al., 2020), to 44 percent (Phillips et al., 2006) having made a suicidal attempt. Of note, reported suicide attempts has been found to be higher in adolescents compared to adults (Phillips et al., 2006). In terms of self-harm, 52.1 percent report current or past self-harming behavior, most often cutting (Rautio et al., 2020). Rates of self-harm have been found not to differ between adolescents and adults (Phillips et al., 2006).

Between 46.7 percent and 53.7 percent of adolescents reported a desire to have cosmetic procedures (Mataix-Cols et al., 2015; Rautio et al., 2020) and 9.8 percent reported they had conducted a cosmetic procedure (Rautio et al., 2020). This poses a significant risk for BDD sufferers as the outcomes following such procedures are poor in terms of continued distress about the perceived flaw or a shift in foci of appearance concern (Bowyer et al., 2016). Veale and colleagues (2000) found that nine out of 25 (36 percent) of adults with BDD attempted self or 'DIY' surgery, however the rates in adolescents are unknown. It is possible that rates of DIY surgery may be higher in this group, owing to limited to access to some procedures.

The impact of BDD can affect youth in multiple ways; social activities and school attendance have been reported by parents and youth to be the most impaired (Phillips et al., 2006; Albertini & Phillips, 1999; Rautio et al., 2020), with up to a third reporting not attending school at all, owing to BDD (Phillips et al., 2006; Albertini & Phillips, 1999; Rautio et al., 2020; Mataix-Cols et al., 2015). Social functioning, such as peer relationships, have also been reported to be significantly impaired (Phillips et al., 2006; Albertini & Phillips, 1999; Rautio et al., 2020; Mataix-Cols et al., 2015). Adolescence is a critical period of development, the impact of BDD on these aspects of functioning could lead to missed developmental opportunities and impact, i.e., missed education.

Adolescents have significantly poorer insight into their BDD compared to adults as measured by the Brown Assessment of Beliefs Scale (BABS) (Eisen et al., 1998), indicating limited awareness of the excessiveness or irrationality of their appearance-related beliefs, with a significantly higher proportion of adolescents falling in the "delusional" insight category compared to adults (59 percent vs. 33 percent respectively) (Phillips et al., 2006). This finding was echoed in study of 30 adolescents with BDD, with 51.7 percent reporting delusional insight on the BABS (Mataix-Cols et al., 2015). In a larger sample of 172 adolescents using a single item measure of insight on the BDD Yale-Brown Obsessive-Compulsive Scale for Adolescents (Philllips et al., 1997), 51.9 percent were rated as having delusional or poor insight into their BDD (Rautio et al., 2020). This level of insight could potentially hinder access to appropriate support and services.

There are high rates of comorbid psychiatric conditions with BDD, with reported rates of up to 71.5 percent of adolescents having at least one comorbid condition (Rautio et al., 2020; Mataix-Cols et al., 2015). Among the most common comorbid conditions in adolescents are mood disorders (33.3–81 percent) and social anxiety disorder (30–39 percent) (Rautio et al., 2020; Albertini & Phillips, 1999; Phillips et al., 2006; Mataix-Cols et al., 2015). Some of these comorbidities have overlapping and similar symptoms to BDD, which will be considered next.

Differential diagnosis

BDD can be misdiagnosed in mental health settings, owing to the similarities and overlap with other conditions. Obsessive compulsive disorder (OCD) and related conditions such as excoriation disorder and trichotillomania described in other chapters have overlapping features with BDD, given it is a related condition, which can make it difficult to differentiate. However, there are distinguishing features of each condition which can help to disentangle them. For example, excoriation disorder and trichotillomania involve skin picking and hair pulling, respectively, which are behaviors considered to be habitual with the aim of tension relief. These behaviors can also be seen in BDD, however the driver for these differs in that are used as attempts to 'fix' a perceived flaw or improve appearance (Jassi & Krebs, 2022).

There are conditions that are not part of the OCD and related disorders family that can often cause confusion in clinical assessments. Social anxiety disorder, while a common co-occurring condition with 10.5 percent of youth with BDD having this diagnosis, (Rautio et al., 2020), can often be misdiagnosed as BDD. The commonality is around fear and distress of social situations, but in BDD this is driven by fear of negative judgement, owing to a perceived flaw in appearance rather doing or saying something embarrassing, which is characteristic of social anxiety disorder.

Body image disturbance is common in both eating disorders and BDD, which can often lead to diagnostic confusion and misdiagnosis. While 10 percent of youth with BDD were reported to have a comorbid eating disorder (Rautio et al., 2020), sometimes BDD can be missed in eating disorder populations. For example, in a study of 41 patients with anorexia nervosa, 16 (39 percent) were diagnosed with BDD once they had been assessed for it, despite this initially not being diagnosed (Grant et al., 2002). This illustrates potential misdiagnosis or missed diagnosis of BDD in this group. In eating disorders, the focus of appearance concerns is about shape and weight, which leads sufferers to engage in unhealthy eating behaviors, compensatory behaviors, and exercise in an attempt to lose weight. In BDD, the appearance concern can be focused on any part of the body, most commonly facial features, but concerns can focus on weight and shape. In a clinical sample of adolescents with BDD, about 40 percent of girls reported concerns about their weight (Rautio et al., 2020), highlighting that this is a common presentation. Importantly, an exclusion criterion for a diagnosis of BDD is appearance concerns that are *exclusively* focused on weight and shape in an individual whose symptoms meet diagnostic criteria for an eating disorder (American Psychiatric Association, 2013). That is, if an individual fulfils diagnostic criteria for an eating disorder and does not report any significant appearance concerns beyond weight and shape, then they would not be diagnosed with BDD. Conversely, if an individual reports a distressing and impairing preoccupation with their body weight and shape but no dysfunctional eating behaviors, they could be diagnosed with BDD if all other criteria are fulfilled (e.g. presence of appearance-related repetitive behaviors).

There has been a sharp increase in young people presenting to services with gender incongruence in recent years (Zucker, 2017). Appearance concerns are common in gender incongruence and are central to BDD, however the drivers for these are different. In gender incongruence, appearance worries may be focused on sex signifiers e.g. penis, breasts, as they represent the gender the person does not identify with. In gender incongruence there would not only be appearance concerns, there would also be distress of possessing other sex signifiers unrelated to appearance, such as tone of voice. In BDD, sex signifiers can be an area of concern but not because of what they represent, but primarily to do with their appearance. It is common for young people with gender incongruence to be concerned about their prospective body (i.e. how their body will be in the future), and also aspects of their internal body (e.g. possessing ovaries). However, in BDD the focus typically is on the current body and its external appearance. For young people with BDD, their central concern is that there is something wrong with their appearance (e.g. they look deformed or ugly) and they typically want to change or improve certain features, whereas young people with gender incongruence do not see their body parts as defective or flawed, but rather *not belonging* to them, and often want to remove them.

In depression, people can communicate feelings of ugliness and low self-esteem, which is seen in BDD. However, BDD differs in that appearance worries are the primary preoccupation and there are associated repetitive behaviors e.g. camouflaging, grooming etc. In depression, there may be other aspects that people communicate they feel low about in addition to their appearance and they may not engage in behaviors to try to hide or fix a perceived flaw.

Underlying theories

The underlying causes and maintaining mechanisms of BDD are poorly understood. However, over the last decade there has been increasing interest and research into this question, which has started to shed light on possible mechanisms. Figure 10.1 indicates a number of *putative* biological, psychological and social/environmental factors that underly BDD, which are discussed below. This is not an exhaustive list, but instead provides example of some of the mostly well-researched factors to date. It is also important to note that the categories of biological, psychological and social/environmental are independent of one another, and in fact it is well-established that there is considerable overlap between them. For example, many 'psychological' traits, such as perfectionism, are partly genetic in origin (Iranzo-Tatay et al., 2015). Similarly, many so called 'environmental' factors, such as bullying, are influenced by an individual's genetic make-up (Knafo & Jaffee, 2013). Lastly, it is important to recognise that many of the studies examining 'risk factors' for BDD to date have used cross-sectional designs. Therefore, while they have highlighted some potentially important associations, they do not reveal the direction of effects. Prospective studies are needed to determine whether these factors contribute the development and/or maintenance of BDD.

Biological risk factors

The diathesis-stress model of BDD (Fang et al., 2014) suggests that the disorder arises as a result of an interplay between biological predisposing factors, such as a genetic liability, and environmental stressors. Consistent with this, twin studies have indicated that variance in BDD symptoms is indeed accounted for by both genetic and environmental factors (Enander et al., 2018; Lopez-Sola et al., 2016; Monzani et al., 2014). In the first twin study of BDD symptoms, conducted with 3,544 adult female twins in the United Kingdom, genetic factors were found to account for approximately 44 percent of the variance in symptoms, with the remaining 56 percent accounted for by non-shared environmental factors (Monzani et al., 2012). This finding has since been broadly replicated using twin cohort data in Sweden (Enander et al., 2018) and Australia (López-Solà et al., 2014), encompassing adolescents and adults, and natal males and females. Twin studies have also shown that there is overlap in the genetic factors that influence BDD and other obsessive-compulsive related disorders (obsessive-compulsive disorder, hoarding disorder, trichotillomania and skin-picking disorder) (Monzani et al., 2014). It is important to note that all of these twin studies used the Dysmorphic Concerns Questionnaire, and while this measure has been shown to be a valid and reliable measure of BDD symptoms (Oosthuizen et al., 1998), it may capture broader body dissatisfaction and concerns relating to bodily dysfunction (e.g. body odour). Furthermore, while there is good evidence for a genetic influence on BDD symptoms from twin studies, there have not been any genomic studies (e.g. genome-wide association studies) to date, and therefore no specific risk genes have been identified.

Several other biological factors have been highlighted as being relevant to BDD. Natal sex may be a risk factor, given that population-based studies show that BDD is more common in females than males, especially in adolescent populations, as outlined above (Enander et al., 2018; Veale et al., 2016). The reason for this imbalance is unclear, and while it could reflect sex differences in sociocultural pressures and/or exposure to environmental stressors, it may also result from sex-related biological processes. For example, it has been suggested that sex-specific hormonal activation (e.g. estrogen and testosterone) during puberty may partly explain sex differences in BDD young people (Enander et al., 2018). There is also tentative evidence that different genetic influences may underlie BDD in males versus females (López-Solà et al., 2014), and while this finding has yet to be replicated, it could suggest that different biological risk factors underlie the BDD symptoms.

Second, considerable attention has been given to neural circuitry in BDD. A systematic review, which included 19 studies, found evidence of differences in neural activation, structure, and connectivity in frontostriatal, limbic, and visual system regions among individuals with BDD compared to healthy control and other clinical groups (Grace et al., 2017). However, it is unclear whether these are *trait* differences that *precede* BDD onset and play a causal role in the development of the disorder. For example, it is possible that brain differences lie on the causal pathway between genetic vulnerability and BDD. That is, genetic liability for BDD, may give rise to brain differences, which in turn influence the development of the disorder. On the other hand, neurobiological differences may arise as a *consequence* of having BDD and be a *state* effect. Longitudinal research is needed to tease these two possibilities apart. For example, neuroimaging studies could examine brain differences in at-risk groups who have not yet developed BDD, or in treatment cohorts to determine if differences persist after successful treatment of BDD.

Psychological risk factors

Cognitive behavioral models propose that dysfunctional appearance-related beliefs (e.g. 'My appearance is the most important thing about me', 'People will reject me if my appearance is not acceptable') drive certain cognitive proposes that are central to BDD (Veale, 2004; Wilhelm, Phillips & Steketee, 2012). These include selective attention to appearance and catastrophic appraisals of perceived appearance flaws (e.g "My nose is too broad so everybody will think I am a disgusting and won't want to be friends with me"). This in turn gives rise to negative emotions, such as anxiety, shame, disgust and sadness. In response to the negative cognitive appraisals and distress, BDD sufferers engage in repetitive behaviors often aimed at checking, concealing, and/or correcting their perceived flaws, and also avoidant behaviors (e.g. avoiding social situations). These repetitive and avoidant behaviors often provide some temporary distress-relief and are therefore negatively reinforced, and it is proposed that they fuel a negative cycle of appearance anxiety.

In addition to the maintenance cycle described above, cognitive behavioral models also propose that certain psychological traits are risk factors for BDD (Veale, 2004). Several studies have found empirical support for a relationship between perfectionism and BDD (Bartsch, 2007; Hartmann et al., 2014; Krebs et al., 2019; Schieber et al., 2013). Perfectionism encompasses self-oriented perfectionism, which is defined as having excessively high personal standards, and socially prescribed perfectionism, which is defined as a belief that others hold excessively high standard for oneself. High levels of self-oriented perfectionism may contribute to a tendency to notice minor flaws in appearance and to be self-critical of them. High levels of socially prescribed perfectionism could lead individuals to believe that others are judging them against excessively high appearance standards. Therefore, both aspects of perfectionism could theoretically fuel appearance preoccupation and distress in relation to perceived flaws. In support of this, both self-oriented and socially prescribed perfectionism have been shown to be associated with BDD symptoms (Bartsch, 2007; Hanstock & O'Mahony, 2002) including in young people (Krebs et al., 2019). Although most research has been cross-sectional, there is preliminary evidence found that self-oriented perfectionism, but not socially prescribed perfectionism, prospectively predicts BDD symptoms in youth, even when controlling for coexisting psychopathology (Krebs et al., 2019).

Another psychological trait highlighted in cognitive behavioral models of BDD is aesthetic sensitivity (Veale, 2004). Aesthetic sensitivity refers to the ability to recognize and value beauty and compositional excellence (e.g. symmetry, proportionality). It has been proposed that aesthetic sensitivity may be a specific risk for BDD (Feusner et al., 2010), by predisposing individuals to notice slight flaws in their appearance and to have a negative emotional response to such perceptions (Lambrou et al., 2011). In support of this, some studies in adult samples have found support for an association between aesthetic sensitivity and BDD (Lambrou et al., 2011). Indirect evidence also comes from the observation that adults with BDD frequently have an occupation in art or design (Veale et al., 2002). However, not all studies have found a relationship between aesthetic sensitivity and BDD symptoms (Schieber et al., 2013), and therefore further research is needed to clarify the potential association, and to determine if aesthetic sensitivity is a trait that predisposes individuals to BDD or a consequence of having BDD symptoms.

Beyond aesthetic sensitivity, other aspects of visual perception have been proposed to be related to BDD. A considerable number of studies have used neuropsychological paradigms to examine detail-focused versus global processing. Detail-focused processing refers to a tendency to process a visual image in a piecemeal style and to focus on specific features. In contrast, global processing refers to a tendency to integrate individuals features and focus on the "bigger picture." It has been suggested that individuals with BDD may have an increased tendency towards detail-focused processing, which may mean that they are more prone to: a) notice slight differences or blemishes in their appearance; and b) fixate on features that concern them rather than seeing 'the bigger picture'. In support of this, a meta-analysis of 16 studies found evidence for greater detail-focussed processing in adults with BDD relative to controls (pooled effect size of $g = -0.44$) (Lang et al., 2021). Interestingly, a recent study of adults with BDD found that detailed-focused improvement with treatment (CBT or supportive psychotherapy), suggesting that it is a modifiable process and potentially a consequence of BDD symptomatology (Greenberg, Phillips, et al., 2023). In this study, detailed-focused processing did not mediate BDD symptom improvement, suggesting that it is not a mechanism of change in psychological treatment.

Another psychological trait that has received considerable empirical attention in relation to BDD is rejection sensitivity. Rejection sensitivity can be defined as a tendency to anxiously expect, readily perceive, and overreact (emotionally and/or behaviorally) to social rejection. One specific form of rejection sensitivity is appearance-based rejection sensitivity, defined as anxiety-provoking expectations of social rejection based on physical appearance. Appearance-based rejection sensitivity appears to be a key feature of BDD and has been shown to be associated with self-reported BDD symptoms, above and beyond general rejection sensitivity (Calogero et al., 2010; Park et al., 2010). A recent prospective study found that rejection sensitivity and BDD symptoms mutually influenced each other over a four-year period during adolescence (Zimmer-Gembeck et al., 2022); that is, higher rejection sensitivity lead to subsequent increases in BDD symptoms, but elevated BDD symptoms also gave rise to increases in rejection sensitivity.

Social and environmental risk factors

The twin studies described above demonstrate that the risk for developing BDD is not only due to our genes, but also factors that we experience in our environment. In fact, the results of the twin studies suggest that these environmental factors might play an even bigger role than genetics in the development of BDD. Identifying and understanding these environmental factors is crucial, since they may be modifiable and therefore indicate potential targets for preventions.

Bullying is perhaps the most widely studied environmental risk factor for BDD to date. The role of peer victimization in the development of BDD has been highlighted in clinical models (Fang & Wilhelm, 2015), as well as patients' own accounts (Weingarden et al., 2017). In a survey study of adults who screened positive for BDD, bullying was identified as the most commonly reported triggering event for BDD (Weingarden et al., 2017). Furthermore, a recent meta-analysis examined the association between peer victimisation and BDD and found a pooled effect size of $r = 0.28$ for bullying and $r = 0.42$ for appearance-based teasing (Longobardi et al., 2022). However, the vast majority of studies identified were cross-sectional and related to retrospective reporting of previous bullying/teasing, which may be heavily influenced by memory and other biases. Only two studies identified in this review were longitudinal. The first found evidence for peer victimisation predicting change in BDD symptoms over a 12-month period during adolescence (Webb et al., 2016). The second found that appearance-based peer victimisation predicted BDD over a 12-month period and this association was moderated by certain mindfulness-related traits (Lavell et al., 2018).

In addition to bullying, several other Adverse Childhood Experiences (ACEs) have been proposed as risk factors for the development of BDD, including emotional, sexual and physical abuse, and emotional and physical neglect. Theoretical models propose that emotional abuse and neglect could lead to internalised criticism, undermine self-concept, and heighten rejection sensitivity (Gao et al., 2017; Longobardi et al., 2022) Similarly, sexual abuse may lead to body shame, which in turn may increase vulnerability to developing BDD (Malcolm et al., 2021). A recent meta-analysis showed significant, albeit modest, association of abuse and neglect with BDD symptoms ($r = 0.22$ and $r = .17$, respectively; Longobardi et al., 2022). However, all studies were cross-sectional and relied on retrospective recall.

There is much speculation about the role of sociocultural influences on BDD. It has been suggested that living in an appearance-focused society with narrowly defined beauty standards may predispose individuals to developing body image problems and appearance anxiety. There has been strikingly little research of sociocultural factors in relation to BDD, but emerging evidence supports the hypothesis for a link between sociocultural attitudes towards appearance and BDD symptoms (Ahmadpanah et al., 2019). There is also preliminary evidence for a cross-sectional relationship between use of appearance-focused social media platforms and BDD symptoms (Alsaidan et al., 2020; Ryding & Kuss, 2020), although the direction of this association remains unclear. It may be that exposure to highly curated and enhanced images of physical appearance on social media leads to appearance dissatisfaction and thereby increases risk for BDD. Conversely, BDD symptoms may lead to increased use of appearance-based social media, for example to compare appearance, which is one of the most common BDD-related repetitive behaviors (Rautio et al., 2020). Prospective and experimental studies are needed to determine causal relationships, particular in youth samples given the high levels of social media use in this age group.

Aspects of the family environment may also be important for understanding the origins and/or maintenance of BDD, although this has also received little empirical attention. For example, parents may provide appearance-related reassurance to their child with BDD, accommodate BDD-related routines (e.g., by providing cosmetic products), and/or facilitate avoidance (Jassi et al., 2020). Although such behaviors are generally intended to minimise the child's distress or risk, they may have the unintended consequence of fuelling BDD (Jassi et al., 2020). In addition, parental beliefs about appearance might play a role in the development of BDD in young. It is well-recognised that individuals with BDD typically place a high-level of important on appearance, endorsing statements such as "If my appearance is defective, I am worthless" (Veale et al., 1996).

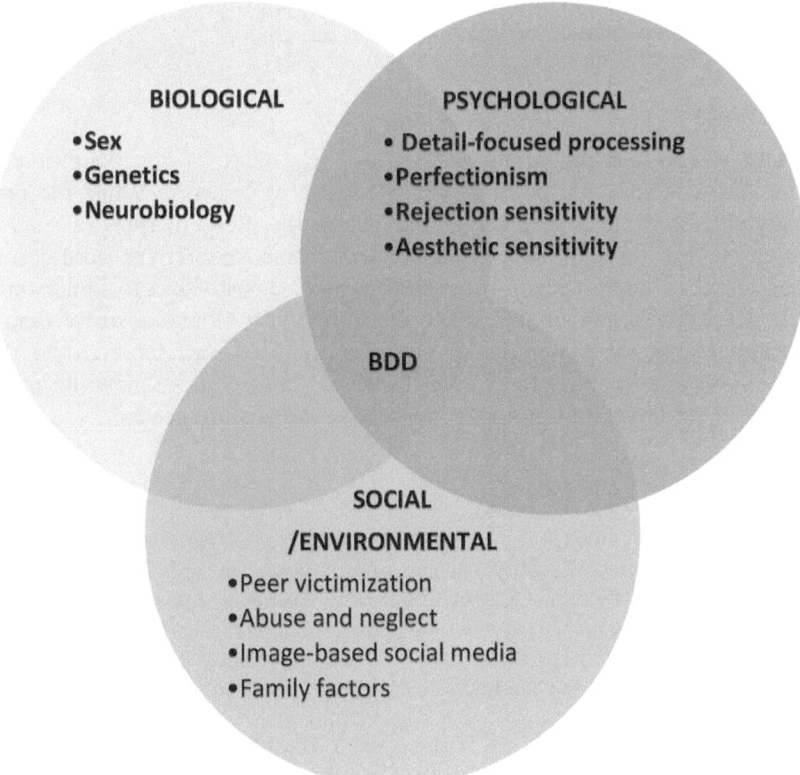

Figure 10.1 Putative risk factors for body dysmorphic disorder.

These beliefs may be partly explained by broader sociocultural influences and interpersonal experiences such as bullying, as mentioned above, but they may also be shaped by experiences within the family (Neziroglu et al., 2004). For example, growing up with a parent who is highly appearance-focused (e.g. who is highly self-critical of their own appearance, or spends a lot of time on their own grooming routines) may inadvertently lead a child to develop the belief that appearance is of central importance and that one must look a certain way in order to be accepted or to be happy. Tentative support for this notion comes from a cross-sectional study of undergraduate students, which found that the relationship between parenting style (maternal rejection) and body dysmorphic symptoms was partially mediated by idealized values of appearance (Farrell et al., 2016). Further longitudinal studies are needed to test whether family factors truly influence idealized values of appearance, which in turn contributes to the development of BDD symptoms.

Note: These are candidate risk factors, and empirical support is currently limited by the small number of studies and methodological limitations (e.g. over-reliance on cross-sectional designs).

Summary

BDD is common in young people and the onset of the condition is thought to commonly occur in early- to mid-adolescence. While the presentation of BDD is broadly similar across the lifespan, rates of suicide attempts are thought to be higher, and insight poorer, in adolescents compared to adults. Several theories have been postulated to understand the development and maintenance of BDD and a biopsychosocial model captures some of the potential contributors. However, research on the nature and underlining theories of BDD in youth is in infancy and more studies with larger samples and prospective designs are needed.

References

Ahmadpanah, M., Arji, M., Arji, J., Haghighi, M., Jahangard, L., Sadeghi Bahmani, D., & Brand, S. (2019). Sociocultural attitudes towards appearance, self-esteem and symptoms of body-dysmorphic disorders among young adults. *International journal of environmental research and public health*, 16(21), 4236.

Albertini, R. S. & Phillips, K. A. (1999). Thirty-three cases of body dysmorphic disorder in children and adolescents. *J Am Acad Child Adolesc Psychiatry*, 38(4), 453–459.

Alsaidan, M. S., Altayar, N. S., Alshmmari, S. H., Alshammari, M. M., Alqahtani, F. T., & Mohajer, K. A. (2020). The prevalence and determinants of body dysmorphic disorder among young social media users: a cross-sectional study. *Dermatology Reports*, 12(3).

American Psychiatric Association. (2013) *The diagnostic and statistical manual of mental disorders*, 5th Edition. Washington, DC: American Psychiatric Association.

Angelakis, I., Gooding, P. A., & Panagioti, M. (2016). Suicidality in body dysmorphic disorder (BDD): a systematic review with meta-analysis. *Clinical psychology review*, 49, 55–66.

Bala, M., Quinn, R., Jassi, A., Monzani, B., & Krebs, G. (2021). Are body dysmorphic symptoms dimensional or categorical in nature? A taxometric investigation in adolescents. *Psychiatry Research*, 305, 114201.

Bartsch, D. (2007). Prevalence of body dysmorphic disorder symptoms and associated clinical features among Australian university students. *Clinical Psychologist*, 11(1), 16–23.

Bjornsson, A. S., Didie, E. R., Grant, J. E., Menard, W., Stalker, E., & Phillips, K. A. (2013). Age at onset and clinical correlates in body dysmorphic disorder. *Compr Psychiatry*, 54(7), 893–903.

Bowyer, L., Krebs, G., Mataix-Cols, D., Veale, D., & Monzani, B. (2016). A critical review of cosmetic treatment outcomes in body dysmorphic disorder. *Body Image*, 19, 1–8.

Calogero, R. M., Park, L. E., Rahemtulla, Z. K., & Williams, K. C. (2010). Predicting excessive body image concerns among British university students: The unique role of appearance-based rejection sensitivity. *Body Image*, 7(1), 78–81.

Eisen, J. L., Phillips, K. A., Baer, L., Beer, D. A., Atala, K. D., & Rasmussen, S. A. (1998). The brown assessment of beliefs scale: reliability and validity. *American Journal of Psychiatry*, 155(1), 102–108.

Enander, J., Ivanov, V. Z., Mataix-Cols, D., Kuja-Halkola, R., Ljótsson, B., Lundström, S., Pérez-Vigil, A., Monzani, B., Lichtenstein, P., & Rück, C. (2018). Prevalence and heritability of body dysmorphic symptoms in adolescents and young adults: a population-based nationwide twin study. *Psychological Medicine*, 48(16), 2740–2747. doi:10.1017/S0033291718000375.

Fang, A., Matheny, N. L., & Wilhelm, S. (2014). Body Dysmorphic Disorder. *Psychiatric Clinics of North America*, 37(3), 287–300. doi:10.1016/j.psc.2014.05.003.

Fang, A. & Wilhelm, S. (2015). Clinical features, cognitive biases, and treatment of body dysmorphic disorder. *Annual Review of Clinical Psychology*, 11, 187–212.

Farrell, L. J., Gregertsen, E. C., Donovan, C. L., Pammenter, A., & Zimmer-Gembeck, M. (2016). Maternal rejection and idealized value of appearance: Exploring the origins of body dysmorphic concerns among young adults. *Journal of Cognitive Psychotherapy*, 30(3), 154–167.

Feusner, J. D., Neziroglu, F., Wilhelm, S., Mancusi, L., & Bohon, C. (2010). What causes BDD: Research findings and a proposed model. *Psychiatric annals*, 40(7), 349–355.

Gao, S., Assink, M., Cipriani, A., & Lin, K. (2017). Associations between rejection sensitivity and mental health outcomes: A meta-analytic review. *Clinical psychology review*, 57, 59–74.

Grace, S. A., Labuschagne, I., Kaplan, R. A., & Rossell, S. L. (2017). The neurobiology of body dysmorphic disorder: A systematic review and theoretical model. *Neuroscience & Biobehavioral Reviews*, 83, 83–96.

Grant, J. E., Kim, S. W., & Eckert, E. D. (2002). Body dysmorphic disorder in patients with anorexia nervosa: prevalence, clinical features, and delusionality of body image. *International Journal of Eating Disorders*, 32(3), 291–300.

Greenberg, J. L., Phillips, K. A., Hoeppner, S. S., Jacobson, N. C., Fang, A., & Wilhelm, S. (2023). Mechanisms of cognitive behavioral therapy vs. supportive psychotherapy in body dysmorphic disorder: An exploratory mediation analysis. *Behaviour Research and Therapy*, 104251.

Hanstock, T. L. & O'Mahony, J. F. (2002). Perfectionism, acne and appearance concerns. *Personality and Individual Differences*, 32(8), 1317–1325.

Hartmann, A. S., Thomas, J. J., Greenberg, J. L., Matheny, N. L., & Wilhelm, S. (2014). A comparison of self-esteem and perfectionism in anorexia nervosa and body dysmorphic disorder. *The Journal of Nervous and Mental Disease*, 202(12), 883–888.

Iranzo-Tatay, C., Gimeno-Clemente, N., Barberá-Fons, M., Rodriguez-Campayo, M. Á., Rojo-Bofill, L., Livianos-Aldana, L., Beato-Fernandez, L., Vaz-Leal, F., & Rojo-Moreno, L. (2015). Genetic and environmental contributions to perfectionism and its common factors. *Psychiatry Research*, 230(3), 932–939.

Jassi, A. & Krebs, G. (2022). Body Dysmorphic Disorder. *Psychiatric Clinics.*

Jassi, A. D., Baloch, A., Thomas-Smith, K., & Lewis, A. (2020). Family accommodation in pediatric body dysmorphic disorder: A qualitative study. *Bulletin of the Menninger Clinic*, 84(4), 319–336.

Knafo, A. & Jaffee, S. R. (2013). Gene–environment correlation in developmental psychopathology. *Development and Psychopathology*, 25(1), 1–6.

Krebs, G., Quinn, R., & Jassi, A. (2019). Is perfectionism a risk factor for adolescent body dysmorphic symptoms? Evidence for a prospective association. *Journal of Obsessive-Compulsive and Related Disorders*, 22, 100445.

Lambrou, C., Veale, D., & Wilson, G. (2011). The role of aesthetic sensitivity in body dysmorphic disorder. *Journal of Abnormal Psychology*, 120(2), 443.

Lang, K., Kerr-Gaffney, J., Hodsoll, J., Jassi, A., Tchanturia, K., & Krebs, G. (2021). Is poor global processing a transdiagnostic feature of Body Dysmorphic Disorder and Anorexia Nervosa? A meta-analysis. *Body Image*, 37, 94–105.

Lavell, C. H., Webb, H. J., Zimmer-Gembeck, M. J., & Farrell, L. J. (2018). A prospective study of adolescents' body dysmorphic symptoms: Peer victimization and the direct and protective roles of emotion regulation and mindfulness. *Body image*, 24, 17–25.

Longobardi, C., Badenes-Ribera, L., & Fabris, M. A. (2022). Adverse childhood experiences and body dysmorphic symptoms: A meta-analysis. *Body Image*, 40, 267–284. doi:10.1016/j.bodyim.2022.01.003.

Lopez-Sola, C., Fontenelle, L. F., Bui, M., Hopper, J. L., Pantelis, C., Yücel, M., Menchon, J. M., Alonso, P., & Harrison, B. J. (2016). Aetiological overlap between obsessive–compulsive related and anxiety disorder symptoms: multivariate twin study. *The British Journal of Psychiatry*, 208(1), 26–33.

López-Solà, C., Fontenelle, L. F., Alonso, P., Cuadras, D., Foley, D. L., Pantelis, C., Pujol, J., Yücel, M., Cardoner, N., & Soriano-Mas, C. (2014). Prevalence and heritability of obsessive-compulsive spectrum and anxiety disorder symptoms: A survey of the Australian Twin Registry. *American Journal of Medical Genetics Part B: Neuropsychiatric Genetics*, 165(4), 314–325.

Malcolm, A., Pikoos, T. D., Grace, S. A., Castle, D. J., & Rossell, S. L. (2021). Childhood maltreatment and trauma is common and severe in body dysmorphic disorder. *Comprehensive Psychiatry*, 109, 152256.

Marques, L., Weingarden, H. M., LeBlanc, N. J., & Wilhelm, S. (2011). Treatment utilization and barriers to treatment engagement among people with body dysmorphic symptoms. *Journal of psychosomatic research*, 70(3), 286–293.

Mataix-Cols, D., de la Cruz, L. F., Isomura, K., Anson, M., Turner, C., Monzani, B., ... & Krebs, G. (2015). A pilot randomized controlled trial of cognitive-behavioral therapy for adolescents with body dysmorphic disorder. *Journal of the American Academy of Child & Adolescent Psychiatry*, 54(11), 895–904.

Mayville, S., Katz, R. C., Gipson, M. T., & Cabral, K. (1999). Assessing the prevalence of body dysmorphic disorder in an ethnically diverse group of adolescents. *Journal of child and family studies*, 8, 357–362.

Monzani, B., Rijsdijk, F., Anson, M., Iervolino, A. C., Cherkas, L., Spector, T., & Mataix-Cols, D. (2012). A twin study of body dysmorphic concerns. *Psychological Medicine*, 42(9), 1949–1955. doi:10.1017/s0033291711002741.

Monzani, B., Rijsdijk, F., Harris, J., & Mataix-Cols, D. (2014). The structure of genetic and environmental risk factors for dimensional representations of DSM-5 obsessive-compulsive spectrum disorders. *JAMA Psychiatry*, 71(2), 182–189. doi:10.1001/jamapsychiatry.2013.3524.

Neziroglu, F., Roberts, M., & Yaryura-Tobias, J. A. (2004). A behavioral model for body dysmorphic disorder. *Psychiatric Annals*, 34(12), 915–920. doi:10.3928/0048-5713-20041201-13.

Oosthuizen, P., Lambert, T., & Castle, D. J. (1998). Dysmorphic concern: prevalence and associations with clinical variables. *Australian & New Zealand Journal of Psychiatry*, 32(1), 129–132. doi:10.3109/00048679809062719.

Park, L. E., Calogero, R. M., Young, A. F., & Diraddo, A. M. (2010). Appearance-based rejection sensitivity predicts body dysmorphic disorder symptoms and cosmetic surgery acceptance. *Journal of Social and Clinical Psychology*, 29 (5), 489–509.

Phillips K, Didie ER, Menard W, Pagano ME, Fay C, Weisberg R. B. (2006). Clinical features of body dysmorphic disorder in adolescents and adults. *Psychiatry Res*, 141(3), 305–314.

Phillips, K. A., Hollander, E., Rasmussen, S. A., & Aronowitz, B. R. (1997). A severity rating scale for body dysmorphic disorder: development, reliability, and validity of a modified version of the Yale-Brown Obsessive Compulsive Scale. *Psychopharmacology bulletin*, 33(1), 17.

Rautio, D., Jassi, A., Krebs, G., Andrén, P., Monzani, B., Gumpert, M., Lewis, A., Peile, L., Sevilla-Cermeño, L., & Jansson-Fröjmark, M. (2020). Clinical characteristics of 172 children and adolescents with body dysmorphic disorder. *European child & adolescent psychiatry*, 1–12.

Ryding, F. C. & Kuss, D. J. (2020). The use of social networking sites, body image dissatisfaction, and body dysmorphic disorder: A systematic review of psychological research. *Psychology of Popular Media*, 9(4), 412.

Schieber, K., Kollei, I., de Zwaan, M., Müller, A., & Martin, A. (2013). Personality traits as vulnerability factors in body dysmorphic disorder. *Psychiatry Research*, 210(1), 242–246.

Schneider, S. C., Turner, C. M., Mond, J., & Hudson, J. L. (2017). Prevalence and correlates of body dysmorphic disorder in a community sample of adolescents. *Aust N Z J Psychiatry*, 51(6), 595–603.

Schulte, J., Schulz, C., Wilhelm, S., & Buhlmann, U. (2020). Treatment utilization and treatment barriers in individuals with body dysmorphic disorder. *BMC psychiatry*, 20(1), 1–11.

Veale, D., Gournay, K., Dryden, W., Boocock, A., Shah, F., Willson, R., & Walburn, J. (1996). Body dysmorphic disorder: A cognitive behavioural model and pilot randomised controlled trial. *Behaviour Research and Therapy*, 34(9), 717–729. doi:10.1016/0005-7967(96)00025-00023.

Veale, D. (2000). Outcome of cosmetic surgery and 'DIY'surgery in patients with body dysmorphic disorder. *Psychiatric Bulletin*, 24(6), 218–221.

Veale, D. (2004). Advances in a cognitive behavioural model of body dysmorphic disorder. *Body Image*, 1(1), 113–125.

Veale, D., Ennis, M., & Lambrou, C. (2002). Possible association of body dysmorphic disorder with an occupation or education in art and design. *American Journal of Psychiatry*, 159(10), 1788–1790.

Veale, D., Gledhill, L. J., Christodoulou, P., & Hodsoll, J. (2016). Body dysmorphic disorder in different settings: A systematic review and estimated weighted prevalence. *Body Image*, 18, 168–186. doi:10.1016/j.bodyim.2016.07.003.

Voelker, D. K., Reel, J. J., & Greenleaf, C. (2015). Weight status and body image perceptions in adolescents: current perspectives. *Adolescent health, medicine and therapeutics*, 149–158.

Webb, H. J., Zimmer-Gembeck, M. J., & Mastro, S. (2016). Stress exposure and generation: A conjoint longitudinal model of body dysmorphic symptoms, peer acceptance, popularity, and victimization. *Body Image*, 18, 14–18.

Weingarden, H., Curley, E. E., Renshaw, K. D., & Wilhelm, S. (2017). Patient-identified events implicated in the development of body dysmorphic disorder. *Body Image*, 21, 19–25.

Wilhelm, S., Phillips, K. A., & Steketee, G. (2012). *Cognitive-behavioral therapy for body dysmorphic disorder: A treatment manual*. Guilford Press.

World Health Organization. (2018). The ICD-11 classification of mental and behavioral disorders: clinical descriptions and diagnostic guidelines. World Health Organization.

Zimmer-Gembeck, M. J., Rudolph, J., & Pariz, J. (2022). A cascade of rejection and appearance preoccupation: Adolescents' body dysmorphic symptoms and appearance rejection sensitivity over 4 years. *British Journal of Developmental Psychology*, 40(1), 17–34.

Zucker, K. J. (2017). Epidemiology of gender dysphoria and transgender identity. *Sexual health*, 14(5), 404–411.

11 Hoarding in Youth

Molly J. Church, Katie H. Mangen and Samuel D. Spencer

Hoarding disorder (HD) is a serious mental health condition that affects an estimated 2–6 percent of the population (Hojgaard & Skarphedinsson, 2020). Although most common in older adults, HD can also impact children and adolescents; the onset of HD symptoms frequently occurs in childhood or adolescence (Cath et al., 2017; Park et al., 2014). To date, the majority of research and clinical efforts related to HD have primarily focused on adults, and literature focused on children and adolescents with HD has been largely limited to clinical case studies (e.g., McKay, 2016) and theoretical or review papers (e.g., Morris et al., 2016). As a result, an increased understanding of hoarding in youth offers potential for increasing early intervention efforts and furthering a developmental/lifespan approach for conceptualizing HD (Chabaud, 2014; Guzick et al., 2020; Ivanov et al., 2021). In this chapter we: (a) provide an overview of the symptomology and nature of HD; (b) discuss key differences between adult and youth clinical presentations, including the differentiation between hoarding symptoms and developmentally appropriate behaviors and other psychological disorders, respectively; (c) explicate evidence-based cognitive-behavioral frameworks for assessment and treatment; and (d) articulate future directions for assessment, intervention, and research endeavors. Through these efforts, we hope to spur further research and understanding of HD in youth.

Introduction to Hoarding Disorder

Clinical Characteristics. HD is characterized by 1) a perceived need to save items; and 2) distress and difficulty discarding items, regardless of the value of these items, resulting in the accumulation of possessions that leads to significant clutter in an individual's living areas and limitations in the usability of these areas for their intended purposes (American Psychiatric Association, 2022). In as many as 80–90 percent cases, these symptoms are accompanied by excessive acquisition, or an urge to collect additional unneeded items. Additionally, HD results in clinically significant distress and/or impairment across major areas of life functioning

DOI: 10.4324/9781003517429-11

(Ong et al., 2015). Individuals with HD may have insight into their symptoms ranging from good (i.e., recognizing that the behaviors are problematic) to absent (i.e., delusional beliefs that behaviors are not problematic despite objective evidence to the contrary). In previous editions of the *Diagnostic and Statistical Manual* (DSM), HD was classified as a subtype of OCD. Since then, however, a long line of research has identified differences between OCD and HD in phenomenology, neurobiological factors (e.g., genetic predispositions), and treatment response, allowing for more nuanced differentiation of these distinct, yet related disorders. As a result, HD is now classified as a separate psychiatric disorder under the category of OCRDs (American Psychiatric Association, 2022; Mataix-Cols et al., 2010).

Differences in presentations of Hoarding Disorder between children and adults

HD commonly presents differently in children than in adults. Differences stem from children's decreased levels of control over their physical environments, and in turn, are not able to accumulate positions to the extent characteristic of HD. This difference in control impacts the assessment process and applicability of the diagnostic criteria for HD to children in several ways. First, parents often control children's finances and, therefore, their purchasing power. This may preclude children from obtaining the items that they would otherwise hoard if given the opportunity (Ivanov et al., 2021). Second, other individuals in the home, such as parents and siblings, may be more likely to discard the hoarded items of children rather than adults. For these reasons, children and adolescents may appear not to meet criteria related to excessive clutter, even though they might meet these criteria without parental intervention – and, in fact, often do later in life (Ivanov et al., 2013). These logistical barriers to accumulation of clutter in children with a predisposition to hoarding may serve to mask early identification efforts, which may allow hoarding psychopathology to manifest over time undetected. Children also may hoard seemingly useless objects, such as trash, rocks, or other objects given lack of financial resources and access to readily available money (Bratiotis et al., 2021). Similar to adults, children with HD experience a perceived need to save possessions and experience distress with discarding them (Tolin, 2023). Most frequent reasons for saving behaviors in children are that the items might be useful in the future and the sentimental value of the item (Ivanov et al.).

Distinguishing clinically significant hoarding behaviors from typical, developmentally appropriate collecting is another important factor to consider particular to hoarding behaviors in children. For example, children commonly have collections of objects, but typically not to an excessive degree, and do not have intense emotional attachments to the objects or exhibit distress upon parting with the objects. As discussed in more detail later in this chapter, such a distinction becomes even more challenging in the context of comorbid mental health concerns that may impact a child's relationship with their possessions or organizational abilities/executive functioning, including ADHD and autism (Guzick et al., 2020; Hacker et al., 2016; La Buissonnière-Ariza et al., 2018; Storch et al., 2016). In sum, the inherent lack of control of children over many aspects of their environment, coupled with the lack of means and time necessary to accumulate excessive volume of possessions, means that unique considerations and more nuanced assessment is needed to conceptualize HD in youth.

Gaps in the literature and areas for further investigation

Research on the phenomenology and treatment of HD in children is limited in several areas that suggest important avenues for future research (see Guzick et al. 2020 for an extended discussion of this). More specifically, much of the current literature for conceptualizing and treating HD in youth is primarily limited to case studies (e.g., McKay, 2016) and retrospective surveys examining the developmental trajectory of symptoms in adult populations (e.g., Ivanov et al., 2021). Given these limitations, more conceptual and empirical work is needed to bolster our understanding of the phenomenology, assessment, treatment, and prevention of childhood HD.

As described elsewhere (e.g., Guzick et al., 2020; Park et al., 2014), and highlighted throughout this chapter, most of the work on HD has been done with adults, further perpetuating the significant disparity in research concerning child and adolescent presentations of HD. In order to bridge this gap and better understand the developmental trajectory of HD, several retrospective studies have been conducted in adults with HD to identify typical age of symptom onset. Findings indicate that hoarding symptoms typically onset between 11 and 15 years of age, i.e., around middle adolescence (Grisham et al., 2006; Tolin et al., 2010). Establishing such a timeline is important from a developmental perspective, as HD symptoms most commonly are chronic for individuals, continuing into adulthood (Tolin et al., 2010; Tolin, 2023). Additionally, individuals with HD have difficulty with recognizing the impact of HD on their functioning, lack insight into the impairment caused by their symptoms, and may not consciously identify their hoarding symptoms oftentimes until a decade after symptoms began (Grisham et al., 2006). Perhaps owing to a lack of awareness concerning early identification of HD, parents also rarely seek out behavioral health services for HD in isolation (Guzick et al., 2020). Earlier identification and intervention for this condition are needed to prevent the worsening of HD symptoms over time. Furthermore, greater understanding of childhood hoarding will help understand the etiology of this disorder and tailor assessment strategies. Most importantly, early clinical intervention can occur before HD symptoms increase in severity.

While HD symptoms may be less frequently identified in and of themselves, children may present for other mental health concerns that are often comorbid with HD (see 'Comorbidity' section below for more details). Hoarding in children has most frequently been studied in relation to its presence with other disorders. For example, one study researching hoarding within a sample of children with ADHD found that 29 percent of the sample reported clinical levels of HD symptoms (Hacker et al., 2016). ADHD has been identified as a common comorbid presentation with similar cognitive contributing factors. Prader Willi syndrome (genetically based developmental condition), autism and OCD are additional disorders in which hoarding has been investigated. Hoarding (and possibly a clinical diagnosis of HD) impacts a substantial number of children and adolescents, including those with other mental health conditions, suggesting the possibility of underlying shared cognitive/attentional and neurobiological etiological factors (Tolin, 2023). Further understanding of such shared etiological pathways could also facilitate early identification efforts for childhood hoarding and accurate differential diagnosis.

A limited number of studies have researched the longitudinal progression of HD in children. For example, Ivanov et al. (2021) followed twins with and without hoarding for a three-year duration. Of the individuals who initially screened positive for HD, 40 percent met criteria for difficulty parting with possessions out of perceived need and distress upon parting with them. Notably, none of the adolescents screened positive for clutter symptomology, illustrating how this criterion may not apply as well to childhood presentations of HD. However, the paucity of work in this area suggests that further research is needed to fully understand the developmental trajectory of childhood HD, as such psychopathology seems likely to continue into adulthood in a deteriorating course (Tolin et al., 2010).

HD across the lifespan also contributes to substantial individual and societal costs (Ong et al., 2015). Moreover, comorbid HD contributes to poorer prognosis for other psychiatric conditions (Frost, Steketee, & Tolin, 2015). Additionally, it may increase the risk of other psychiatric diagnoses occurring (Burton et al., 2016; Hacker et al., 2016). HD also has an impact on a societal level. That is, HD in adults has been associated with health risks, loss of homes, and strained relationships (Burton et al.; Landau et al., 2011). From a community perspective, a large proportion of public health complaints received are related to HD symptoms, further contributing to the societal costs of the disorder (Frost et al., 2000). However, little has been done or studied regarding childhood HD individual and societal costs. As a result, more research is needed to identify the costs of HD in youth and understand the developmental trajectory of HD symptoms starting in youth in order to curb the aforementioned individual and societal costs associated with chronic HD in adults.

Presentations of Hoarding Disorder in children and adolescents

Prevalence

Despite some overlap with HD, collecting and saving items is a typical, developmentally appropriate behavior in children. For example, in one study of six-year-old children, 70 percent reported having a collection of some type of item (Evans et al., 1997). Elevated HD symptoms have been observed in nearly 9 percent of a community sample of children ages 6–17 (Burton et al., 2016). The pervasiveness of these behaviors in children complicates epidemiological research on hoarding in youths, as parents and clinicians may experience difficulties differentiating problematic hoarding symptoms from typical, developmentally appropriate collecting and saving behaviors (Morris et al., 2016). While research in this area remains limited, existing studies have placed prevalence estimates of clinically significant hoarding in adolescents at 2–3 percent (Hojgaard & Skarphedinsson, 2020), which is comparable to estimated prevalence rates of hoarding in adults, which range from 2–5 percent (American Psychiatric Association, 2022).

A recent meta-analysis of studies of HD in adults has indicated a mean age of onset for these symptoms of 16.7 years (Zaboski et al., 2019). The authors of this meta-analysis observed patterns of clustering consistent with previous studies that have suggested a bimodal distribution of hoarding onset. That is, research has indicated an average age of onset of 37 years, with more than a third of one particular sample reporting onset of symptoms prior to age 20 and nearly 40 percent reporting onset after age 50 (Steketee et al., 2012). While some individuals with clinically significant hoarding report links between the onset of their symptoms and stressful life events (e.g., trauma), this association is significantly less common when hoarding onsets in childhood (Landau et al., 2011).

Diagnostically, HD was once considered to be a category of OCD. However, as of the publication of the DSM-5, it has been reclassified as a separate disorder (American Psychiatric Association, 2022). The primary reason for this separation was the identification of significant phenomenological differences between hoarding and other presentations of OCD; for example, obsessions related to hoarding are rarely experienced as intrusive or unpleasant as are the obsessions of other OCD symptom dimensions, but rather tend to be associated with positive emotions (Frost et al., 2012). Furthermore, research indicated that many people with significant hoarding problems did not endorse other symptoms of OCD

(Mataix-Cols et al., 2010). Because of the recency of the separation of HD from OCD, much of the existing epidemiological literature related to hoarding was conducted prior to its official classification as its own disorder and may not reflect the most updated criteria for identifying hoarding.

Comorbidity

In youth, hoarding-related psychopathology has historically been studied in the context of other psychiatric conditions with known onset in childhood. More specifically, significant instances of hoarding behaviors have been noted in ADHD (Hacker et al., 2016), autism (La Buissonnière-Ariza et al., 2018; Storch et al., 2016), and OCD (Frank et al., 2014; Hojgaard et al., 2020; Storch et al., 2007), with levels of comorbid psychopathological hoarding ranging from 7–30 percent, depending on the condition under investigation and sample. Additionally, hoarding behaviors have also been observed in youth with Prader-Willi syndrome, a genetic condition defined by intellectual disability, abnormalities in endocrine functioning, obesity, and disrupted eating behavior (Cassidy et al., 2012). However, conceptually differentiating food-specific hoarding driven by disrupted eating behavior in Prader Willi Syndrome, and perseverative collecting of items related to a special interest in autism, respectively, from clinically independent hoarding psychopathology will be important to guide differential diagnosis and prevalence research efforts in this area (see Guzick et al., 2020).

Of these psychiatric conditions in which hoarding behaviors frequently co-occur, ADHD likely shares the most overlap with hoarding, and demonstrates significant promise for furthering our understanding of shared etiological factors and early identification efforts of hoarding concerns in children (Guzick et al., 2020). As described in more detail in the section below on cognitive-behavioral models of HD, *executive dysfunction, cognitive biases*, and *information processing deficits* play a central role in the maintenance of HD in adults (Frost & Hartl, 1996; Tolin, 2023). Difficulties in fluent categorization of items, visuospatial processing, and problem-solving skills have also been observed in adults with HD (Woody et al., 2014).

These executive functioning deficits are also hallmarks of ADHD, particularly within the inattentive and sluggish cognitive tempo domains (Barkley et al., 2010). Based on this symptom overlap (Lynch et al., 2015), as well as notable comorbidity of ADHD symptoms and hoarding behaviors in youth (Burton et al., 2016; Hacker et al., 2016), it seems likely that ADHD and HD possess shared neurobiological etiological underpinnings. Additional research in this area may uncover whether shared etiological factors account for comorbid ADHD and HD in youth, or if one symptom constellation has temporal precedence over another (e.g., ADHD manifesting in childhood predicts development of HD in adulthood). Further investigation of similarities and differences in ADHD and HD in youth holds promise, especially in light of existing infrastructure in behavioral healthcare systems for early identification of ADHD in childhood– an area that is relatively lacking in HD (Guzick et al., 2020).

Assessment of Hoarding Disorder in youth

Thorough assessment of HD symptoms in children and adolescents is necessary for: (a) comprehensive understanding of the phenomenology of the condition; (b) early identification/detection of symptoms in healthcare and school settings; and (c) optimal case conceptualization and treatment planning where appropriate. Moving beyond sole reliance on the topographical level of clutter in a child's room (which could be attributed to compliance/conduct concerns or organizational deficits in ADHD), assessing children's acquisition motives (i.e., function), compulsive saving behaviors, and difficulty with discarding items (i.e., beliefs about possessions) are all important factors to thoroughly elucidate for assessing HD in youth. However, few measures have been developed specifically for this purpose, and thus more work is needed in this area.

The *Children's Saving Inventory* (CSI; Storch et al., 2011) is currently the only validated assessment of hoarding behaviors in children (Morris et al., 2016). The measure was based on *Saving Inventory- Revised* (SI-R; Frost et al., 2004), which was originally designed for adults. The parent-rated CSI scale contains 23 questions, and ratings are along ordinal response choices (none, a little/minimal, some/moderate, most/much, almost all/completely). Higher scores suggest more hoarding behavior; however, no clinical cutoff scores have been identified to date. Four factors comprise the measure: difficulty discarding, clutter, excessive acquisition, and distress and impairment. Psychometric research from the original measure development study provided evidence of construct validity and reliability in terms of good internal consistency for both the total score and scores of each subscale (⊠=.84-.96; Storch et al.).

The *Children's Yale-Brown Obsessive Compulsive Scale* (CY-BOCS; Scahill et al., 1997) peripherally assesses hoarding behaviors in children. This clinician administered measure was developed to assess OCD and has two questions assessing hoarding behavior symptom clusters (based on the original conceptualization of hoarding as a sub-type of OCD). Fear of losing items and difficulty discarding items are assessed. While the CY-BOCS consistently demonstrates strong evidence of reliability and validity, its utility in assessing hoarding symptoms is limited as it does not yield a hoarding severity score separate from OCD severity. While the inclusion of some items assessing hoarding behavior on the CY-BOCS allows for assessment of this relatively underexamined phenomenon in a widely used clinical measure, the proliferation of an outdated grouping of hoarding within OCD may contribute to further incoherence and misinformation among providers and researchers.

Additional measures designed to assess OCD in children identify hoarding behaviors, due in part to the long history of HD as a sub-type of OCD. For example, the *Obsessive-Compulsive Inventory: Child Version* (OCI-CV; Foa et al., 2010) is a child self-report measure assessing OCD symptoms and has a hoarding behavior factor assessed via three questions on hoarding behaviors rated along a 0–2 scale. However, this measure is limited in the range of hoarding symptoms assessed (Hojgaard & Skarphedinsson, 2020). The *Children's Obsessional Compulsive Inventory* (CHOCI; Shafran et al., 2003) and the *Children's Florida Obsessive Compulsive Inventory* (C-FOCI; Storch et al., 2009) are used to assess OCD symptoms and severity in children and contain hoarding behavior items. However, as discussed above in relation to the CY-BOCS, the range of hoarding symptoms is limited in these measures and the severity, and hoarding symptom severity is not indicated separately but rather combined with OCD symptom severity (Hojgaard & Skarphedinsson, 2020).

Cognitive-behavioral model of Hoarding Disorder in youth

Current gaps in the literature surrounding youth HD have precluded the formation of a full intervention model of pediatric hoarding. Therefore, pediatric HD remains best understood through the cognitive behavioral therapy (CBT) model for adult HD (Steketee & Frost, 2013; Tolin, 2023), with some emphasis on specific aspects of the model that are more relevant to children and adolescents than to adults (i.e., downward extension of the adult CBT model of HD to children; Guzick et al., 2020). The seminal CBT model of HD proposed by Frost and Hartl (1996) describes several cognitive and behavioral maintaining factors thought to underpin hoarding-related psychopathology, including *information processing deficits, emotional attachment patterns, behavioral avoidance*, and *beliefs about one's possessions*. Together, these factors result in excessive acquisition of items and difficulty discarding them– ultimately resulting in significant functional impairment. Fortunately, a developmentally sensitive adaptation of this model for childhood HD has been proposed by Park and colleagues (2014). This adaptation accounts for the factors described in Frost and Hartl's model as well as special considerations relevant to children, including differences between adult and child presentations of hoarding in cognitive functioning, emotional attachment, and the role of family members in maintaining distress and avoidance.

Frost and Hartl (1996) proposed three major information processing deficits that contribute to compulsive hoarding: *difficulties with decision-making, difficulties with organization and categorization*, and *memory problems*. Problems with decision-making tend to arise when an individual with hoarding symptoms must decide what to discard or how to organize items that are saved (Steketee et al., 2012). In children with HD, information processing deficits may be observed in terms of impulsiveness related to acquisition of items, excessive distractibility, difficulty following through with and completing tasks, and problems with disorganization (Park et al., 2014). Information processing deficits may also be relevant to the strong association between HD and ADHD in children. As described in the previous section on comorbidity, these deficits suggest the possibility of a shared neurological underpinning between HD and ADHD and may present as barriers to treatment for either disorder in the presence of the other (Hacker et al., 2016).

Additionally, Frost and Hartl (1996) proposed that three types of cognitive distortions are particularly significant in understanding hoarding. These include an *inflated sense of responsibility for possessions, a need to maintain control over possessions,* and *erroneous beliefs about the attainability of perfection.* Subsequent research has identified specific belief domains that seem to play an important role in the development and maintenance of HD symptoms. For example, Steketee and colleagues (2012) identified beliefs related to memory (e.g., needing to remember, fear of forgetting information), control (e.g., others having no right to touch one's possessions), and responsibility (e.g., needing to preserve an item for its potential usefulness or value) as major factors predicting hoarding symptoms. Children with hoarding issues may report similar cognitions, such as beliefs about the significance of their control or ownership over items (Park et al., 2014). Such beliefs, while less complex than the beliefs that may present in adults, are often developmentally analogous; for example, both adults and children may derive a sense of comfort and safety in stressful or chaotic situations by asserting control over their possessions.

Another important factor in Frost and Hartl's (1996) model includes dysfunction resulting from *exaggerated emotional attachment to possessions.* More specifically, beliefs related to emotional attachment to possessions have been shown to distinguish individuals with HD from individuals with OCD and from community controls (Steketee et al., 2012). Among these attachment-related beliefs are 1) beliefs that one's possessions are more valuable and/or important than they actually are; 2) beliefs that one's possessions afford them a special level of emotional comfort; and 3) beliefs that the loss of one's possessions would result in adverse consequences (Steketee et al., 2012). This excessive attachment has been thought to reflect a personification of or attribution of human-like attachment qualities to possessions (Frost & Steketee, 2013) and may reflect maladaptive attachment patterns resulting in the perception that relationships with objects are safer than those with humans (Grisham et al., 2018). Emotional attachment is thought to play a central role in HD symptoms among children, who may use control over treasured possessions as a means of coping with lack of control over their general environment (Park et al., 2014), which may be especially relevant for youth exposed to trauma or other adverse childhood experiences (Tolin, 2023). These emotional attachments may be formed with different items and/or with exaggerated intensity than what is observed in developmentally appropriate attachment to comforting items (e.g., teddy bears, blankets; Park et al., 2014).

The final factor in Frost and Hartl's (1996) model is *behavioral avoidance*. Here, maladaptive avoidance of discarding items often results from difficulties with decision-making, fear of making mistakes, and intense distress associated with the loss of an item to which one is deeply attached. Owing to the particular relevance of emotional attachment to objects in children with HD, avoidance of discarding may be particularly severe and attempts to do so may be experienced as extremely distressing (Bratiotis et al., 2021). Therefore, children with HD tendencies may demonstrate avoidance of discarding by maintaining careful organization of items, reacting strongly when a family member touches their possessions, and attempting to prevent their parents from entering their bedrooms (Bratiotis & Steketee, 2015). These responses frequently result in family accommodation of HD symptoms (i.e., maladaptive behaviors on the part of parents or loved ones to facilitate symptomatic behaviors), which in turn reinforces behavioral avoidance (Park et al., 2014). However, as described in more detail elsewhere (e.g., Guzick et al., 2020), it is important to note that careful examination of the motivators for hoarding behavior is paramount for differentiating bona fide clinical HD from related reasons for youth difficulty in organizing or decluttering their room (e.g., aversion to unpleasant cleaning tasks, oppositional behavior).

Since the development of Frost and Hartl's (1996) model, several novel findings have emerged detailing the psychological and biological underpinnings of HD. More specifically, Tolin (2023) has synthesized these findings and proposed a *biopsychosocial expansion* to the original CBT model of HD. According to this biopsychosocial model of HD, a variety of vulnerability factors in combination with one another form a baseline predisposition for the development of hoarding psychopathology. These include genetic and heritability factors, structural abnormalities in the brain, stressful and traumatic life events, personality traits and disorders, and impairments in cognitive functioning. Together, these vulnerability factors contribute to 1) blunted resting-state activity in the nervous system; and 2) heightened brain activity and physiological arousal when one is making decisions about one's possessions. This combination of responses results in the individual experiencing dampened subjective distress at baseline but exaggerated distress when making decisions about possessions, leading to distorted beliefs and impaired decision-making around this process. Subsequently, individuals excessively acquire but avoid organizing and discarding items. These behavioral patterns are reinforced through operant conditioning (i.e., positive and negative reinforcement of acquiring possessions, negative reinforcement of avoiding discarding). However, it is important to note that this updated model of HD has been predominantly developed with research on adults with HD, and more research is needed to extend this model to youth with hoarding-related concerns.

Developmental considerations for Hoarding Disorder in youth

Although much of our current understanding about HD in children derives from, and overlaps with, research on hoarding in adults, there are several special considerations that must be taken into account when working with youth who present with hoarding-related concerns. For instance, the clutter component of hoarding likely manifests differently in children and adolescents than in adults (Guzick et al., 2020). That is, the degree of clutter present in the child's environment and associated parental concern may be an imprecise indicator of HD symptoms in youth, as parents commonly report concerns about their children's bedrooms being messy, which, as discussed above, may reflect children's dislike of cleaning as opposed to clinically significant hoarding (Guzick et al.). Furthermore, avoidance of cleaning may reflect executive dysfunction unrelated to hoarding, such as the difficulty initiating and completing tasks that is characteristic of children with ADHD (Hacker et al., 2016). Children who would otherwise meet criteria for HD may not exhibit any problematic clutter which can impact proper identification and diagnosis. As described throughout this chapter, the lack of clutter may be due to their typically limited financial resources and parental intervention, such as discarding items or enforcing limitations that keep clutter confined to the child's bedroom (Guzick et al.; Park et al., 2014). Therefore, assessment of hoarding in children requires consideration of the DSM-5-TR specification that clutter may be absent in individuals as long as the absence is due solely to intervention by others, such as family members (American Psychiatric Association, 2022).

Another important consideration in hoarding in children and adolescents is the significance of accompanying family difficulties. Park and colleagues' (2014) adapted model of childhood HD places a special emphasis on familial dysfunction and parenting difficulties related to the distress associated with youth HD symptoms. Because children often do not understand the irrationality of hoarding-related beliefs, they are likely to react with intense emotional outbursts (e.g., screaming, crying) when confronted with worry about or the actual loss of a possession. Parents frequently report accommodating their children's hoarding symptoms to minimize distress and conflict, both for the child and for other members of the family, often with the paradoxical effect of maintaining and worsening these symptoms (i.e., negative reinforcement; Tolin, 2023). This results in further conflict and distress, which can damage familial relationships (Storch et al., 2011).

In examining the impact of HD on children, it is also important to consider children of parents who hoard. These children experience disruptions in their life and development as a result of their parent's HD, including unsanitary living conditions, a loss of physical space, familial tension, possible financial hardships, and social isolation (Guzick et al., 2020; Neziroglu et al. 2020). Additionally, research has indicated that as many as one in 25 individuals diagnosed with HD have had a child, elder, or animal in their care removed from their home (Tolin et al., 2008). Removal from the home can create a deep sense of uncertainty and confusion for affected youth, which can lead to lasting trauma for both the children and their families (Sankaran et al., 2018). The psychological impact that results from disruptions in children's lives, owing to their parents' hoarding may also last well into adulthood. These adult children frequently report feelings of grief around the loss of their relationships with their parents as well as feelings of shame and embarrassment that negatively impact their self-esteem (Neziroglu et al.).

Finally, an important but understudied consideration in youth HD relates to presentations of hoarding symptoms among children in foster care. In one study of caretakers of foster children, 59 percent reported that the children in their care had engaged in hoarding of food (i.e., often by storing it in hidden places in private spaces such as their bedrooms or school lockers; Norrish et al., 2019). Curewitz and colleagues (2011) presented an unpublished series of case studies of eight children in foster care who demonstrated behaviors consistent with hoarding. Seven of the children exhibited hoarding of food, which was often hidden in their bedrooms, sometimes with other hoarded objects. Each of these children had experienced a history of adverse life events (e.g., neglect, abuse) and displayed concurrent behavioral problems, sometimes overlapping with disordered eating behaviors. Curewitz et al. linked these symptoms to deficits in attachment resulting from lacking or negative interactions with parents in early childhood. Such findings suggest that special consideration is needed when assessing HD in children of parents with hoarding issues or those in foster care.

Future directions for Hoarding Disorder in youth

Assessment

As described earlier in the chapter, current measures assessing HD in youth remain limited. Future psychometric research is needed to develop clinical cut off scores on measures of youth HD with discriminant validity for differentiating developmentally typical behaviors of saving/difficulty discarding, common comorbid conditions, and clinically significant HD in children. One promising measure in this area is the CSI, which was developed to address the aforementioned gap in assessment tools for children with HD. Nevertheless, differentiation of developmentally appropriate collecting/relating to one's possessions in youth from pathological hoarding behavior remains a significant psychometric challenge. Additionally, without empirically validated clinical cut scores indicative of genuine HD psychopathology, diagnosis of HD in youth will be challenging for clinicians.

Furthermore, practices that can aid ready identification of symptoms and presentations of children and adolescents that are at risk for developing HD can facilitate early clinical intervention to mitigate the developmental progression of HD. Moreover, information regarding the motivators for hoarding in youth (i.e., function) may be a beneficial addition for assessment measures and further identify individuals at risk for HD. For example, several studies have found that *sentimental attachment* may differentiate youth HD psychopathology from ADHD, where the latter may involve children saving items because cleaning is viewed as uninteresting (Guzick et al., 2020). In sum, individuals at risk for HD may be identified more easily if assessments are adjusted to include motivation for saving/collecting behaviors.

Treatment

Treatment for HD in youth is commonly adapted from evidence-based treatment for adults (i.e., Steketee & Frost, 2013). However, research is limited regarding what specific aspects of such treatments are most effective for children. Taking into consideration the differences between youth and adult HD presentations (e.g., youth presentations have clutter limited to a specific area and parental involvement), future research into the effectiveness of treatment and standardized adaptations for hoarding in youth is needed (Akınici et al., 2022).

Including parent-focused interventions that have demonstrated efficacy for treating other childhood mental health disorders, such as parent management training for ADHD, may be a beneficial addition to treatment for youth with HD, especially in light of possible familial maintaining factors (e.g., family accommodation). Additionally, since comorbid disorders frequently occur with childhood hoarding, including concurrent interventions for comorbidities may be prudent. Assessing the effectiveness and potential moderators of such multimodal treatment packages will also be important (Guzick et al., 2020). Finally, since hoarding in youth may be likely to continue into adulthood and progress into chronic HD if left unchecked, preventative interventions for youth with HD tendencies and their families may be one way to disrupt this maladaptive developmental progression.

Research

The substantial discrepancy in the literature on hoarding between youth and adult populations suggests that further research is needed to increase our understanding of this condition in youth. Several fruitful topics for such research are briefly reviewed here. First, in light of the common onset of HD relatively during teenage and young adult years and gradual progression of the disorder throughout the lifespan (Zaboski et al., 2019), more prospective studies that longitudinally follow youth identified as being at risk for developing HD are needed. Echoing Guzick et al. (2020), one way to identify such samples could involve specifically recruiting children of adult patients with HD or utilizing samples of youth with common childhood psychiatric conditions known to overlap with hoarding, such as ADHD (Hacker et al., 2016).

Second, in order to facilitate such longitudinal research examining the developmental trajectory of HD, more psychometrically sound measures of hoarding psychopathology are sorely needed. Such measures should prioritize specificity and discriminant validity in terms of differentiating clinically significant hoarding from related conditions and normative childhood collecting/resistance to tidying. Ideally, these instruments should also have identifiable clinical cut-points (sensitivity) in full consideration of differences in the presentation of HD between youth and adults (e.g., deemphasis on the 'clutter' criterion in youth). Development of such measures may catalyze further research that investigates longitudinal developmental pathways of HD, as well as the interactions of such pathways with common psychopathological processes, including executive functioning deficits implicated in adult HD (Woody et al., 2014).

Finally, more research is needed within the area of early intervention, prevention, and outreach concerning youth HD. Given the low prevalence of HD in younger children, future work in this area focused on teenagers and young adults may be most useful. At present, there is a lack of clarity on the differentiation of pathological hoarding from normative collecting/ saving in youth within both the clinical science literature and layperson vernacular. To that end, further outreach, and prevention-based efforts in the domain of development related to fostering healthy relationships between youth and their possessions, along with elucidation of warning signs for when such relationships tend toward dysfunction, would be helpful. The inclusion of these prevention and outreach efforts in mental health awareness programs for high school and college students may be one way to target youth at highest risk for developing HD. Advances in assessment practices and interventions specific to youth with HD, and the dissemination and implementation of such practices, may also help to destigmatize and demystify pathological hoarding (Chasson et al., 2018). Increasing awareness of, and accessibility to interventions for, hoarding in youth could facilitate more opportunities to address this impairing psychiatric condition, for which barriers to treatment have been historically salient (Robertson et al., 2020).

Conclusion

HD is a debilitating psychological condition predicated on excessive accumulation of possessions with concomitant difficulty in discarding and organizing one's possessions, ultimately resulting in significant impairment in numerous life domains, with particular concern related to potentially hazardous living conditions (Steketee & Frost, 2013). While relatively less studied in youth, the notable trajectory of HD across the lifespan, coupled with research suggesting the onset of HD in childhood, suggests that more work is needed to understand hoarding in youth (Guzick et al., 2020; Park et al., 2014). In the present chapter, we sought to address this gap by reviewing relevant literature on the phenomenology, assessment, and treatment of HD in youth, as well as highlighting areas ripe for future research. Some promising avenues include developing measures with greater sensitivity for differentiating pathological HD from typical collecting behavior and related psychological conditions that commonly manifest in youth (e.g., ADHD, autism), as well as further intervention development, testing, and dissemination efforts. Further research and clinical efforts directed to youth HD have potential to not only alleviate suffering in afflicted youth and their families, but also may lead to preventative efforts to disrupt psychopathological developmental pathways related to HD.

References

Achenbach, T. M. (1999). The Child Behavior Checklist and related instruments. In M. E. Maruish (Ed.), *The use of psychological testing for treatment planning and outcomes assessment* (pp. 429–466). Lawrence Erlbaum Associates Publishers.

Akıncı, M. A., Turan, B., Esin, İ. S., & Dursun, O. B. (2022). Prevalence and correlates of hoarding behavior and hoarding disorder in children and adolescents. *European Child and Adolescent Psychiatry*, 31(10), 1623–1634. doi:10.1007/s0078702101847-x.

American Psychiatric Association. (2022). *Diagnostic and statistical manual of mental disorders* (5th Ed., rev. text). doi:10.1176/appi.books.9780890425787.

Barkley, R. A., Murphy, K. R., & Fischer, M. (2010). *ADHD in adults: What the science says*. Guilford Press.

Bratiotis, C., Muroff, J., & Lin, N. X. (2021). Hoarding disorder: development in conceptualization, intervention, and evaluation. *Focus*, 19(4), 392–404. doi:10.1176/appi.focus.20210016.

Bratiotis, C. & Steketee, G. (2015). Hoarding disorder: models, interventions, and efficacy. *Focus*, 13(2), 175–183. doi:10.1176/appi.focus.130202.

Burton, C. L., Crosbie, J., Dupuis, A., Mathews, C. A., Soreni, N., Schachar, R., & Arnold, P. D. (2016). Clinical correlates of hoarding with and without comorbid obsessive-compulsive symptoms in a community pediatric sample. *Journal of the American Academy of Child and Adolescent Psychiatry*, 55(2), 114–121. doi:10.1016/j.jaac.2015.11.014.

Cassidy, S. B., Schwartz, S., Miller, J. L., & Driscoll, D. J. (2012). Prader-Willi syndrome. *Genetics in Medicine*, 14(1), 10–26. doi:10.1038/gim.0b013e31822bead0.

Cath, D. C., Nizar, K., Boomsma, D., & Mathews, C. A. (2017). Age-specific prevalence of hoarding and obsessive compulsive disorder: A population-based study. *American Journal of Geriatric Psychiatry*, 25(3), 245–255. doi:10.1016/j.jagp.2016.11.006.

Chabaud, S. (2014). *Benefits of early identification and intervention for hoarding*. In P. F. Knerr (Ed.), *The ICD guide to collaborating with professional organizers: Forrelated professionals* (pp. 314–317). Institute for Challenging Disorganization.

Curewitz, A., Plimpton, E., & Frost, R. (2011). Hoarding behaviors in foster care: A series of case studies [PowerPoint Presentation]. Retrieved from: https://scholarworks.umass.edu/cgi/viewcontent.cgi?article=1059&context=rudd_conf.

Chasson, G. S., Guy, A. A., Bates, S., & Corrigan, P. W. (2018). They aren't like me, they are bad, and they are to blame: A theoretically-informed study of stigma of hoarding disorder and obsessive-compulsive disorder. *Journal of Obsessive-Compulsive and Related Disorders*, 16, 56–65. doi:10.1016/j.jocrd.2017.12.006.

Evans, D. W., Leckman, J. F., Carter, A., Reznick, J. S., Henshaw, D., King, R. A., & Pauls, D. (1997). Ritual, habit, and perfectionism: The prevalence and development of compulsive-like behavior in normal young children. *Child Development*, 68(1), 58–68. doi:10.2307/1131925.

Foa, E. B., Coles, M., Huppert, J. D., Pasupuleti, R., Franklin, M. E., & March, J. (2010). Development and validation of a child version of the obsessive compulsive inventory. *Behavior Therapy*, 41(1), 121–132. doi:10.1016/j.beth.2009.02.001.

Frank, H., Stewart, E., Walther, M., Benito, K., Freeman, J., Conelea, C., & Garcia, A. (2014). Hoarding behavior among young children with obsessive–compulsive disorder. *Journal of obsessive-compulsive and related disorders*, 3(1), 6–11.

Frost, R. O. & Hartl, T. L. (1996). A cognitive-behavioral model of compulsive hoarding. *Behaviour research and therapy*, 34(4), 341–350.

Frost, R. O., Steketee, G., & Tolin, D. F. (2015). Comorbidity in Hoarding Disorder. *FOCUS*, 13(2), 244–251. doi:10.1176/appi.focus.130218.

Frost, R. O., Steketee, G., & Tolin, D. F. (2012). Diagnosis and assessment of hoarding disorder. *Annual Review of Clinical Psychology*, 8, 219–242. doi:10.1146/annurev-clinpsy-032511-143116.

Frost, R. O., Steketee, G., & Williams, L. (2000). Hoarding: A community health problem. *Health and Social Care in the Community*, 8(4), 229–234. doi:10.1046/j.1365-2524.2000.00245.x.

Frost, R. O., Steketee, G., & Grisham, J. (2004). Measurement of compulsive hoarding: Saving inventory-revised. *Behaviour Research and Therapy*, 42(10), 1163–1182. doi:10.1016/j.brat.2003.07.006.

Frost, R. O., Steketee, G., & Tolin, D. F. (2015). Comorbidity in hoarding disorder. *Depression and Anxiety*, 28(10), 876–884. doi:10.1002/da.20861.

Grisham, J. R., Frost, R. O., Steketee, G., Kim, H. J., & Hood, S. (2006). Age of onset of compulsive hoarding. *Journal of Anxiety Disorders*, 20(5), 675–686. doi:10.1016/j.janxdis.2005.07.004.

Grisham, J. R., Martyn, C., Kerin, F., Baldwin, P. A., & Norberg, M. M. (2018). Interpersonal functioning in hoarding disorder: An examination of attachment styles and emotion regulation in response to interpersonal stress. *Journal of Obsessive-Compulsive and Related Disorders*, 16, 43–49. https://doi.org/10.1016/j.jocrd.2017.12.001.

Guzick, A. G., Schneider, S. C., & Storch, E. A. (2020). Future research directions in children and hoarding. *Children Australia, 45(3)*, 175–181. https://doi.org/10.1017/cha.2020.13.

Hacker, L. E., Park, J. M., Timpano, K. R., Cavitt, M. A., Alvaro, J. L., Lewin, A. B., Murphy, T. K., & Storch, E. A. (2016). Hoarding in Children With ADHD. *Journal of Attention Disorders*, 20(7), 617–626. doi:10.1177/1087054712455845.

Hojgaard, D. R. M. A., & Skarphedinsson, G. (2020). Assessment, treatment and the importance of early intervention of childhood hoarding. In *Children Australia*, 45(3), 145–152. https://doi.org/10.1017/cha.2020.17.

Ivanov, V. Z., Mataix-Cols, D., Serlachius, E., Lichtenstein, P., Anckarsäter, H., Chang, Z., … & Rück, C. (2013). Prevalence, comorbidity and heritability of hoarding symptoms in adolescence: a population based twin study in 15-year olds. *PloS One*, 8(7). doi:10.1371/journal.pone.0069140.

Ivanov, V. Z., Mataix-Cols, D., Serlachius, E., Brander, G., Elmquist, A., Enander, J., & Rück, C. (2021). The developmental origins of hoarding disorder in adolescence: A longitudinal clinical interview study following an epidemiological survey. *European Child and Adolescent Psychiatry*, 30(3), 415–425. doi:10.1007/s00787-020-01527-2.

La Buissonnière-Ariza, V., Wood, J. J., Kendall, P. C., McBride, N. M., Cepeda, S. L., Small, B. J., Lewin, A. B., Kerns, C., & Storch, E. A. (2018). Presentation and correlates of hoarding behaviors in children with autism spectrum disorders and comorbid anxiety or obsessive-compulsive symptoms. *Journal of Autism and Developmental Disorders*, 48(12), 4167–4178. doi:10.1007/s10803-018-3645-3.

Landau, D., Iervolino, A. C., Pertusa, A., Santo, S., Singh, S., & Mataix-Cols, D. (2011). Stressful life events and material deprivation in hoarding disorder. *Journal of Anxiety Disorders*, 25(2), 192–202.

Lynch, F. A., McGillivray, J. A., Moulding, R., & Byrne, L. K. (2015). Hoarding in attention deficit hyperactivity disorder: Understanding the comorbidity. *Journal of Obsessive-Compulsive and Related Disorders*, 4, 37–46. doi:10.1016/j.jocrd.2014.12.001.

Mataix-Cols, D., Frost, R. O., Pertusa, A., Clark, L. A., Saxena, S., Leckman, J. F., Stein, D. J., Matsunaga, H., & Wilhelm, S. (2010). Hoarding disorder: A new diagnosis for DSM-V? *Depression and Anxiety*, 27(6), 556–572. doi:10.1002/da.20693.

McKay, D. (2016). Cognitive-behavioral treatment of hoarding in youth: A case illustration. *Journal of Clinical Psychology*, 72(11), 1209–1218.

Morris, S. H., Jaffee, S. R., Goodwin, G. P., & Franklin, M. E. (2016). Hoarding in children and adolescents: A review. *Child Psychiatry and Human Development*, 47(5), 740–750. doi:10.1007/s10578-015-0607-2.

Neziroglu, F., Upston, M., & Khemlani-Patel, S. (2020). The psychological, relational and social impact in adult offspring of parents with hoarding disorder. *Children Australia*, 45(3), 153–158. doi:10.1017/cha.2020.42.

Norrish, A., Cox, R., Simpson, A., Bergmeier, H., Bruce, L., Savaglio, M., ... & Skouteris, H. (2019). Understanding problematic eating in out-of-home care: The role of attachment and emotion regulation. *Appetite*, 135, 33–42. doi:10.1016/j.appet.2018.12.027.

Ong, C., Pang, S., Sagayadevan, V., Chong, S. A., & Subramaniam, M. (2015). Functioning and quality of life in hoarding: A systematic review. *Journal of Anxiety Disorders*, 32, 17–30. doi:10.1016/j.janxdis.2014.12.003.

Park J. M., McGuire J. F., Storch E. A. (2014) *Compulsive hoarding in children. In R. O. Frost and G. Steketee (Eds) The Oxford Handbook of Hoarding and Acquiring* (pp. 331–340). Oxford University Press.

Robertson, L., Paparo, J., & Wootton, B. M. (2020). Understanding barriers to treatment and treatment delivery preferences for individuals with symptoms of hoarding disorder: A preliminary study. *Journal of Obsessive-Compulsive and Related Disorders*, 26, 100560. doi:10.1016/j.jocrd.2020.100560.

Sankaran, V., Church, C., & Mitchell, M. (2018). A cure worse than the disease: The impact of removal on children and their families. *Marquette Law Review*, 102(4), 1163–1194. https://repository.law.umich.edu/articles/2055.

Scahill, L., Riddle, M. A., McSwiggin-Hardin, M., Ort, S. I., King, R. A., Goodman, W. K., Cicchetti, D., & Leckman, J. F. (1997). Children's Yale-Brown Obsessive Compulsive Scale: Reliability and validity. *Journal of the American Academy of Child and Adolescent Psychiatry*, 36(6), 844–852. doi:10.1097/00004583-199706000-00023.

Shafran, R., Frampton, I., Heymann, I., Reynolds, M., Teachman, B., & Rachman, S. (2003). The preliminary development of a new self-report measure for OCD in young people. *Journal of Adolescence*, 26(1), 137–142. doi:10.1016/S0140-1971(02)000830.

Steketee, G. & Frost, R. O. (2013). *Treatment for hoarding disorder: Therapist guide* (2nd Ed.). Oxford University Press. doi:10.1093/med:psych/9780199334964.001.0001.

Steketee, G., Schmalisch, C. S., Dierberger, A., DeNobel, D., & Frost, R. O. (2012). Symptoms and history of hoarding in older adults. *Journal of Obsessive-Compulsive and Related Disorders*, 1(1), 1–7. doi:10.1016/j.jocrd.2011.10.001.

Storch, E. A., Khanna, M., Merlo, L. J., Loew, B. A., Franklin, M., Reid, J. M., Goodman, W. K., & Murphy, T. K. (2009). Children's Florida obsessive compulsive inventory: Psychometric properties and feasibility of a self-report measure of obsessive-compulsive symptoms in youth. *Child Psychiatry and Human Development*, 40(3), 467–483. doi:10.1007/s10578-009-0138-9.

Storch, E. A., Lack, C. W., Merlo, L. J., Geffken, G. R., Jacob, M. L., Murphy, T. K., & Goodman, W. K. (2007). Clinical features of children and adolescents with obsessive-compulsive disorder and hoarding symptoms. *Comprehensive psychiatry*, 48(4), 313–318.

Storch, E. A., Muroff, J., Lewin, A. B., Geller, D., Ross, A., McCarthy, K., Morgan, J., Murphy, T. K., Frost, R., & Steketee, G. (2011). Development and preliminary psychometric evaluation of the Children's saving inventory. *Child Psychiatry and Human Development*, 42(2), 166–182. doi:10.1007/s10578-010-0207-0.

Storch, E. A., Nadeau, J. M., Johnco, C., Timpano, K., McBride, N., Jane Mutch, P., ... & Murphy, T. K. (2016). Hoarding in youth with autism spectrum disorders and anxiety: incidence, clinical correlates, and behavioral treatment response. *Journal of autism and developmental disorders*, 46, 1602–1612.

Storch, E. A., Rahman, O., Park, J. M., Reid, J., Murphy, T. K., & Lewin, A. B. (2011). Compulsive hoarding in children. *Journal of Clinical Psychology*, 67(5), 507–516. doi:10.1002/jclp.20794.

Tolin, D. F. (2023). Toward a biopsychosocial model of hoarding disorder. *Journal of Obsessive-Compulsive and Related Disorders*, 36. doi:10.1016/j.jocrd.2022.100775.

Tolin, D. F., Frost, R. O., Steketee, G., Gray, K. D., & Fitch, K. E. (2008). The economic and social burden of compulsive hoarding. *Psychiatry Research*, 160 (2), 200–211. doi:10.1016/j.psychres.2007.08.008.

Tolin, D. F., Meunier, S. A., Frost, R. O., & Steketee, G. (2010). Course of compulsive hoarding its relationship to life events. *Depression and Anxiety*, 27(9), 829–838. doi:10.1002/da.20684.

Woody, S. R., Kellman-McFarlane, K., & Welsted, A. (2014). Review of cognitive performance in hoarding disorder. *Clinical Psychology Review*, 34(4), 324–336. doi:10.1016/j.cpr.2014.04.002.

Zaboski, B. A., Merritt, O. A., Schrack, A. P., Gayle, C., Gonzalez, M., Guerrero, L. A., Dueñas, J. A., Soreni, N., & Mathews, C. A. (2019). Hoarding: A meta-analysis of age of onset. *Depression and Anxiety*, 36(6), 552–564. doi:10.1002/da.22896.

12 Misophonia as a New Obsessive-compulsive Related Disorder?

The evidence suggests otherwise

Samuel D. Spencer, Ogechi "Cynthia" Onyeka and Dean McKay

Misophonia is characterized by decreased tolerance to particular ordinary and repetitive human-generated sounds and associated visual stimuli (e.g., chewing, sniffing, lip smacking), coupled with adverse affective and physiological reactions to associated triggers (such as visual cues) ranging from anxiety/fear, annoyance, and frustration– to heightened anger or marked disgust (Swedo et al., 2022). Retrospective survey studies indicate that misophonia often onsets during childhood or adolescence (Jager et al., 2020) and is associated with significant impairment and distress in many areas of life, including difficulty within social and familial relationships (Remmert et al., 2022), reduced life satisfaction (Rinaldi et al., 2022), and diminished quality of life (Möllmann et al., 2023). While relatively less studied in youth compared to adults, continued research efforts will undoubtedly facilitate further advances in classification, assessment, diagnosis, and treatment of misophonia across the lifespan.

Originally explicated within the discipline of audiology (Jastreboff & Jastreboff, 2002), the literature on misophonia from a psychological perspective has grown exponentially over the past decade, owing in part to the recognition of *neurobiological* (i.e., cortico-limbic-thalamic system connectivity) and *psychosocial* (i.e., cognitive, affective, behavioral) underpinnings of the condition in addition to its audiological features (Brout et al., 2018; Neacsiu et al., 2022). However, misophonia research is relatively nascent, most notably in regard to the classification status of misophonia within existing taxonomic systems (Taylor, 2017). Indeed, at the time of this writing, misophonia is not listed as a disorder in either the *Diagnostic and Statistical Manual-V-TR* (DSM-V-TR; American Psychiatric Association, 2022) or *International Classification of Diseases-11* (ICD-11; World Health Organization, 2019).

One of the earliest psychological accounts of misophonia (i.e., Schröder et al., 2013). suggested that it may be usefully conceptualized within the OCRD spectrum, owing to purported shared features with OCRDs in terms of preoccupation with specific stimuli (i.e., offending sounds) and concomitant avoidant-based reactivity functionally linked to triggers. Subsequent research demonstrating associations between misophonia and

DOI: 10.4324/9781003517429-12

OCD symptoms in both youth (e.g., Rinaldi et al., 2022; Siepsiak et al., 2023) and adults (e.g., Cavanna & Seri, 2015; Cusack et al., 2018; Wu et al., 2014), along with case studies of comorbid pediatric misophonia and OCD (e.g., Reid et al., 2016; Webber et al., 2014), have further perpetuated the debate concerning whether misophonia falls within the class of OCRDs. Alternatively, others have suggested that misophonia may be considered as either a symptom of another psychological disorder, an independent disorder in its own right, or a feature/subtype of a more generalized sensory or audiological sensitivity condition (Brout et al., 2018; McKay & Acevedo, 2020; Siepsiak et al., 2022; Taylor, 2017). As demonstrated by the inclusion of this chapter in a volume on OCRDs in childhood, resolution of the aforementioned debate and attainment of increased clarity regarding the classification status of misophonia are important priorities, with emerging evidence – as will be discussed – suggesting that it is not an OCRD.

However, caution is needed when attempting to conceptualize or classify misophonia from a particular diagnostic framework, as a consensus has yet to be reached on the aforementioned taxonomic issue (Clark & McKay, 2021; Taylor, 2017). Nevertheless, gaining further clarity on the classification status of misophonia is critical, as such a consensus will undoubtedly catalyze ongoing intervention development efforts; unify key stakeholders; and further legitimize misophonia within social and healthcare contexts (Swedo et al., 2022). In the present chapter, we work toward that end via the following objectives: (a) provide a psychological conceptualization and overview of misophonia; (b) briefly summarize the current state of the misophonia assessment and intervention literature, especially with children and adolescents; and (c) speculate on the most appropriate classification status for misophonia as it relates to transdiagnostic, etiological processes of change, rather than a reliance on topographically defined DSM disorders.

Conceptualization of misophonia

As conceptualizations of misophonia originated within the field of audiology, it is worth briefly mentioning some relevant audiological conditions distinct from misophonia in order to emphasize both the viability of misophonia as a psychological condition and also the importance of thorough audiological assessment for diagnostic purposes. As described in more detail elsewhere (Clark & McKay, 2021; Taylor, 2017), *tinnitus* is differentiated from misophonia in the sense that the former involves aversive reactions to alterations in auditory perception *irrespective* of external stimuli (e.g., disembodied, persistent ringing in the ears), while misophonia involves an aversive reaction to specific sounds perceived as originating from the *external* environment. While *hyperacusis* and misophonia share overlap in terms of sound sensitivity, they are distinguished by a sensitivity to certain acoustical properties (e.g., pitch, volume, timbre) spanning *broad* classes of sounds of ostensibly benign intensity in hyperacusis, contrasted with sensitivity to particular ordinary, repetitive, human-generated sounds in misophonia that are typically *context specific,* rather than linked to acoustical properties of the sound *per se* (Neacsiu et al., 2022).

Trigger sounds

In an effort to better understand misophonia, the literature is replete with studies explicating common trigger stimuli. In survey samples of adults with misophonia (e.g., Jager et al., 2020; Rouw & Erfanian, 2018; Wu et al., 2014), frequently endorsed auditory triggers include mouth-based or eating sounds, in addition to breathing, throat, or nasal sounds and repetitious mechanical tapping noises made by hand (e.g., pen or keyboard clicking). Visual triggers associated with, or independent of, trigger sounds, repetitious animal noises, or mechanically generated sounds (e.g., fans, cars, etc.) have also been described (Claiborn et al., 2020). Moreover, recent research suggests that youth with misophonia experience similar misophonia triggers as adults (Guzick et al., 2023), and that the majority of youth misophonia triggers involve family members (Siepsiak et al., 2023). The specific situation(s) in which the trigger occurs, its perceived controllability, and the idiosyncratic source of the trigger are also important contextual factors to consider in the assessment of misophonia.

Psychological dimensions

A review of relevant behavioral, cognitive, and affective processes underpinning misophonia can shed light on the psychological factors associated with this condition and prove useful for further elucidating its classification status.[1]

In terms of behavioral processes, misophonia can be usefully conceptualized from a *learning theory perspective* in which an aversive reaction to a given trigger is formed through classical conditioning principles. However, an open question remains as to why particular sounds that are ordinarily not found to be revulsive in the general population (i.e., unconditioned stimulus) initially become paired with aversive reactions in those with misophonia (Cowan et al., 2022). Some (i.e., McKay & Acevedo, 2020) speculate that pre-dispositional physiological and affective sensitivity to stress may play a role. However, more work is needed in this area to better understand vulnerability factors that contribute to the manifestation of misophonia in youth from a developmental psychopathology perspective. Irrespective of how the association is formed, behaviors that function to avoid or escape anticipated– or actual– misophonia trigger situations are maintained via negative reinforcement contingencies (i.e., experiential avoidance; Cowan et al., 2022). These operant principles further strengthen the salience of triggering stimuli, sensitizing the afflicted individual to more intense reactions in the future, along with a narrowing of flexible adaptive behavioral repertoires as avoidance predominates and quality of life decreases (Frank & McKay, 2019; Jager et al., 2020).

In terms of behavioral reactions to trigger situations, research has demonstrated that younger children were more likely to engage in socially disinhibited externalizing-based reactions (e.g., verbal aggression), while adolescents tended to engage in self-harm (Siepsiak et al., 2023).

One of the hallmark features of misophonia that distinguishes it from auditory processing disorders is the role of higher-order *attentional and cognitive functions* that are purported to mediate symptomology. More specifically, cognitive models of misophonia suggest that hypervigilant fixation toward potential and actual triggers at the expense of broad, flexible attention is a key psychopathological mechanism (Brout et al., 2018; Jastreboff & Jastreboff, 2014). Indeed, neurophysiological research suggests that adults with misophonia demonstrate sub-optimal attentional processes (a) when exposed to trigger situations (Daniels et al., 2020); and (b) on a generalized (i.e., trait-like) basis (Frank et al., 2020; Schröder et al., 2014). The former speaks to the role of diminished cognitive functioning during heightened states of arousal as a psychopathological process; the latter suggests that ongoing ruminative worry about future misophonia triggers may drain finite cognitive resources on a longer-term basis (McKay & Acevedo, 2020). Recent findings also suggest that individuals with misophonia tend to exhibit more rigid and inflexible attentional and cognitive processes compared to healthy controls (Eijsker et al., 2021; Simner et al., 2021; c.f. Murphy et al., in press, for a finding suggesting a notable lack of attentional difficulties in youth with misophonia relative to those with anxiety disorders). However, most research in this area to date has been conducted with adults, and thus more work is needed to explore these processes in youth with misophonia.

Affective reactions to triggers represent an additional noteworthy psychological dimension of misophonia. The complexity of this domain may have considerable implications for the classification status of misophonia, as the phenomenological experience of emotions in misophonia tends to vary more so than other fear/anxiety-based DSM disorders (e.g., phobias, generalized anxiety, OCD). That is, emotions characteristic of misophonia often range from fear/anxiety in response to future triggers, to more elevated emotions of panic, frustration, anger, or even disgust when triggered (Jager et al., 2020; Schröder et al., 2013). Relatedly, it has been suggested that disgust and anger are linked in terms of an interplay between cognitive interpretations and subjective experience of emotions (Eldesouky & Gross, 2019). In regard to misophonia, disgust may be initially elicited in response to oral/nasal or eating sounds (common misophonia triggers), perhaps owing to the evolutionary roots of disgust being linked to eating and bodily functions (McKay, 2017). Indeed, the emotions of moral disgust and anger often predominate in misophonia, especially to the extent that afflicted individuals interpret the trigger sound to be either a violation of socially appropriate behavior and/or within the volitional, conscious control of the offending party (McKay and Acevedo, 2020). Furthermore, the *perceived uncontrollability, unpredictability,* and *difficulty of escape/avoidance* of triggers also influence the degree of affective intensity of misophonic reactions (Brout et al., 2018). Uncontrollability of stressors in general has a long history of research that shows it provokes more intense affective reactions (i.e., Lazarus & Folkman, 1984), and is thus an unsurprising contributor to the strong emotional responses observed in misophonia sufferers.

Increased magnitude of emotional reactions within misophonia, especially those related to anger directed at offending parties, suggests that *affective dysregulation* may be an underlying diathesis (i.e., vulnerability factor). Research has shown that difficulties in emotion regulation are associated with misophonia symptom severity and intensity of reactions to triggers in adults (Guetta et al., 2022), in addition to youth– albeit on a more limited basis (Spencer et al., 2023). One unanswered question, however, concerns the degree to which *internalizing versus externalizing* features predominate in misophonia. More specifically, one of the first accounts of misophonia (i.e., Schröder et al., 2013) conceptualized it in terms of an "impulsive aversive physical reaction with irritability, disgust, and anger" (p. 4), which suggests the salience of externalizing features in the condition, including impulsivity, anger, and verbal aggression. However, a broad range of affective experiences within the internalizing spectra have been noted within misophonia, suggesting that considering anger to the exclusion of a range of other emotions may be untenable (Siepsiak et al., 2023). Aligned with this, recent deep phenotyping research on youth with misophonia found robust correlations between misophonia symptomology and internalizing symptoms (but not externalizing ones), and no differences in externalizing symptoms between youth with misophonia and anxious controls (Guzick et al., 2023).

Psychiatric Comorbidity. Phenotyping research of misophonia-confirmed samples in adults (e.g., Rosenthal et al., 2022; Rouw & Erfanian, 2018) and youth (e.g., Guzick et al., 2023; Siepsiak et al., 2023), as well as survey research involving community/university samples exploring misophonia symptomology dimensionally (e.g., McKay et al., 2018; Wu et al., 2014), have sought to examine potential overlap between misophonia and psychiatric conditions. While this work has provided some evidence of associations between misophonia and psychiatric conditions/symptoms, *no consistent patterns of comorbidity have emerged to date that would engender confidence in classifying misophonia under the umbrella of an existing psychiatric disorder.*

Indeed, evidence of psychiatric comorbidity in misophonia has been mixed. For example, Jager et al. (2020) found that 72 percent of their sample of 413 adults with misophonia did not exhibit any comorbidity. Observations among audiologists having treated over 800 patients with various decreased sound tolerance conditions also suggests minimal psychiatric comorbidity (Jastreboff & Jastreboff, 2023). In contrast to this, other studies have identified significant levels of concomitant psychopathology among adults (Rosenthal et al., 2022; Siepsiak et al., 2022). Aligned with this, Guzick et al. (2023) found high rates of comorbidity in a sample of 102 youth with misophonia, with 79 percent meeting criteria for a psychiatric disorder (depression and anxiety disorders were most common). Additionally, in a sample of 45 youth with misophonia, Siepsiak et al. (2023) observed elevated levels of anxiety, depression, and OCD symptoms. However, the extent to which such comorbid psychopathology represents distinct clinical phenomena or is better explained as sequalae of misophonia (e.g., hopelessness or generalized anxiety about the uncontrollably of future triggers), or alternatively extending from underlying, transdiagnostic vulnerabilities (e.g., affective dysregulation, internalizing psychopathology), is an important research question. It is also possible that youth with misophonia presenting to psychological studies experience a higher burden of psychopathology relative to those presenting to audiology clinics or not presenting for support at all, which underscores the need for community-based samples of youth with misophonia.

Additional caution is called for in understanding the relation between misophonia and OCRDs, as this particular purported comorbidity has historical and controversial roots. Such longstanding linkage between OCD and misophonia is likely a result of the seminal psychological conceptualization and assessment of misophonia originating from an OCD specialty clinic (i.e., Schröder et al., 2013), as well a preponderance of early case reports of treatments for comorbid misophonia and OCD (e.g., Reid et al., 2016; Webber et al., 2014). Survey research on the relation between misophonia and OCD is also equivocal. More specifically, some large-scale survey research indicates greater degree of overlap between these two phenomena in both adult (e.g., Cusack et al., 2018; Wu et al., 2014) and child (e.g., Siepsiak et al., 2023) samples, while other findings suggest that misophonia may actually be associated with *reduced* OCD symptoms (e.g., McKay et al., 2018).

In sum, misophonia may possess relations with a range of psychopathological processes underlying topographically diverse psychiatric conditions, but yet does not seem to reliably fall under the conceptual umbrella of any specific existing condition (McKay & Acevedo, 2020), including OCD. In further support of this, Neacsiu et al. (2022), in their review of neurobiological research on misophonia and related conditions, concluded that while some evidence exists of shared neural overlap between misophonia and related psychiatric conditions, *a distinct neu-robiological signature of misophonia does appear likely*. Additionally, evidence exists for associations between misophonia and generalized personality traits in adults (e.g., perfectionism; Jager et al., 2020, neuroticism; Cassiello-Robbins et al., 2020), in addition to broad internalizing symptoms in youth (Guzick et al., 2023; Siepsiak et al., 2023). Taken together, these findings suggest that conceptualizing misophonia in terms of transdiagnostic processes or spectra (e.g., HiTOP model of psychopathology; Conway et al., 2019) may hold more promise compared to a topographically defined DSM-based nosological framework, which possesses a number of salient limitations (Lilienfeld & Treadway, 2016).

Clinical approach to misophonia

Assessment. Despite a lack of current nosological clarity, several psycho-metric and measurement-related advances in misophonia have emerged as of late (e.g., Cervin et al., 2023; Rinaldi et al., 2022). However, given the nascent stage of misophonia research, there are no universal assessment guidelines at present, and considerable variability in assessment practices exists. Nevertheless, empirically supported assessment principles remain generally applicable. That is, assessors should comprehensively elucidate symptomology and functional impairment, and integrate data from clinician-administered and patient (or parent/caregiver)-report instruments to inform differential diagnosis and treatment planning.

Clinical Interview. Extant literature suggests that misophonia assessment should begin with a thorough diagnostic interview (McKay & Acevedo, 2020). Obtaining a clinical history is critical for understanding the patient's presenting concerns, verifying misophonia symptomology, and ruling out related conditions. This helps the clinician gather information on the onset and duration of symptoms, and also gain perspective on the patient's level of insight (Wiese et al., 2021). Such information can guide the clinical interview and selection of relevant nomothetic assessment instruments. Some areas to assess during the clinical interview include (a) history of presenting concerns; (b) symptom characteristics; (c) longitudinal progression of symptoms; (d) triggers/aversive stimuli; (e) emotional/behavioral responses; and (f) coping strategies (Ferrer-Torres & Giménez-Llort, 2022). Family history of misophonia symptoms should also be investigated (Guzick et al., 2023; Rouw & Erfanian, 2018). In the case of youth, family involvement and impairment in educational settings also require assessment. If possible, referrals to other healthcare professionals provides a comprehensive and interdisciplinary perspective, such as an audiological assessment to examine potentially related or overlapping conditions (e.g., hyperacusis).

Self-report instruments

To date, there exists self-report questionnaires designed to measure misophonia symptomology (Potgieter et al., 2019). These measures vary in function and scope, ranging from symptom checklists to inventories of auditory triggers, behavioral and emotional responses to triggers, functional impairment, owing to symptoms, and symptom severity. Despite the current lack of consensus on the classification status of misophonia, there are several self- or caregiver-report measures that can be useful clinical tools during the assessment process. However, variability in operational definitions of misophonia (Siepsiak et al., 2022), combined with a proliferation of novel measures without extensive psychometric evidence, has contributed to a lack of methodological clarity in the assessment of misophonia. While a comprehensive review of all available misophonia measures is beyond the scope of the present chapter, we highlight a few of the most commonly used instruments that have been psychometrically validated in youth populations here.

The *Amsterdam Misophonia Scale* (A-MISO-S; Schröder et al., 2013) is a self-report questionnaire adapted from the Yale-Brown Obsessive-Compulsive Scale (Y-BOCS; Goodman et al., 1989). The measure consists of six Likert scale items examining functional impairment, time taken by symptoms, emotional distress, avoidance, and control and resistance against symptoms. The A-MISO-S has demonstrated adequate psychometric properties among samples of adults (Naylor et al., 2021) and youth (Cervin et al., 2023).

The *Misophonia Assessment Questionnaire* (MAQ; Johnson, 2014) is a self-report questionnaire containing 21 Likert scale items designed to capture various features of misophonia, including recognition of difficulties, interference, and distress. Although originally developed in the context of applied clinical practice rather than an empirically derived psychometric process, the MAQ has recently been psychometrically validated with a youth sample with promising findings (Cervin et al., 2023).

The *Sussex Misophonia Scale for Adolescents* (SMS-A; Rinaldi et al., 2022) is a self-report questionnaire adapted from the SMS with developmentally appropriate language for adolescents. The SMS-A contains 109 items across two parts, with the first part involving a checklist of known misophonia triggers, and the latter part containing 39 Likert scale items examining frequency and intensity of responses to triggers. The SMS-A has demonstrated optimal psychometric properties, including convergent/divergent validity, with a youth sample (Rinaldi et al.).

Developmental considerations for assessment

Given the notable onset of misophonia in youth (Guzick et al., 2023), assessment with pediatric populations requires special consideration.

More specifically, children may not possess the vocabulary or communication skills to effectively articulate their experiences and emotional reactions to trigger sounds (Rinaldi et al., 2022). Therefore, clinicians should employ developmentally appropriate assessment practices to facilitate gathering reliable and valid information. Additionally, researchers often adapt commonly used measures originally developed with adults for child populations with rote linguistic modifications (e.g., simply substituting "work" for "school"). As a result, there is a paucity of psychometrically robust assessment tools specifically designed for pediatric misophonia (Cervin et al., 2023), and thus more work in this area is needed. Considering the developmental stage of the child is also essential, as misophonia symptoms may manifest differently in younger children compared to adolescents (Rinaldi et al., 2022; Siepsiak et al., 2023). For example, younger children may exhibit behavioral outbursts or tantrums in response to trigger sounds, whereas older children and adolescents may demonstrate more internalized emotional distress (Guzick et al., 2023), in addition to the possibility of self-harm (Siepsiak et al.). By tailoring the assessment process to account for these developmental considerations, clinicians can obtain a comprehensive understanding of a given child's misophonia to aid treatment planning.

Interventions

Given the lack of theoretical consensus and rapidly evolving conceptualizations of misophonia, there is considerable variability in extant treatment approaches. While much of the literature concerning misophonia treatment currently consists of case studies (e.g., Schneider & Arch, 2017; Petersen & Twohig, 2023), several more rigorous studies have emerged as of late (e.g., Jager et al., 2021; Schröder et al., 2017; see Mattson et al., 2023 for a review). Although there is no clear treatment consensus, advances in theoretical models for misophonia have generally taken place within a cognitive behavioral therapy (CBT) framework (Schröder et al., 2017).

Tinnitus retraining therapy

As described earlier in this chapter, Jastreboff and Jastreboff (2002) first conceptualized misophonia as a condition characterized by decreased sound tolerance. Based on this work, the Jastreboff's advanced Tinnitus Retraining Therapy (TRT), adapted for misophonia, as an early intervention approach (Jastreboff & Jastreboff, 2014). The main goal of TRT is to reduce emotional and physiological responses to trigger sounds via habituation and increased audiological tolerance. Treatment typically involves two main components: *sound therapy* and *general counseling* (e. g., psychoeducation and supportive therapy). Sound therapy utilizes a process called "sound enrichment," where soft, low-level background noise is paired with a hierarchy of triggers from least to most distressing to help desensitize the individual to trigger sounds. Over time, the volume of the background noise is gradually decreased, allowing the person to habituate to trigger sounds without experiencing intense emotional and physiological reactions. In this way, sound therapy appears to overlap with exposure therapy. To date, TRT has not been rigorously examined via RCT-based methodology.

CBT approaches

As mentioned above, much of the contemporary research on misophonia interventions has focused on CBT models of treatment (Lewin et al., 2021; Jager et al., 2021; Schröder et al., 2017). While loosely defined and often conceptualized differently across studies, CBT for misophonia generally aims to address the underlying *cognitive and behavioral patterns* that contribute to misophonia-related distress. The therapy focuses on identifying and challenging negative thoughts and beliefs associated with triggers, helping individuals develop healthier coping strategies and reducing overall distress and impairment (Jager et al.). Traditional CBT techniques, such as cognitive restructuring and relaxation training, are utilized to reframe perception of trigger sounds, manage emotional responses, and attain functional autonomy.

Case studies (Reid et al., 2016; Schneider & Arch, 2017; Webber et al., 2014), and randomized controlled trials (Jager et al., 2021; Schröder et al., 2017) have found CBT-based treatment to be moderately effective in reducing misophonia symptoms (for a review, see Mattson et al., 2023). While resounding evidence of efficacy and effectiveness has not fully crystallized to date, these preliminary findings are encouraging. For example, in a recent randomized controlled trial of CBT for misophonia, Jager et al. showed that participants who completed three months of group CBT demonstrated improvement in 56 percent of treatment completers. Additionally, Schröder et al. (2017) examined the use of group CBT for misophonia in a sample of 90 participants, with treatment involving a combination of cognitive restructuring, relaxation techniques, and exposure therapy. Results revealed that nearly half of the sample endorsed significant reduction in misophonia symptoms and improvements in functioning following the CBT intervention. While these findings are promising, further research with larger sample sizes and component and moderator analyses are needed to more definitively establish treatment efficacy. It is also worth noting that CBT approaches for misophonia described in the literature are often *heterogeneous in nature* – that is, possibly involving a multidisciplinary approach or incorporating techniques from other therapeutic modalities.

While much of the research on treatments for misophonia has been conducted with adults, CBT has also preliminarily been found to be an effective treatment approach for youth. For example, Dover and McGuire (2023) have recently developed a *family-based CBT protocol for youth with misophonia*, which includes habit reversal training, parent management training, and exposure therapy, and note promising findings in an initial case study. Additionally, Lewin et al. (2021) provide preliminary evidence for the efficacy of the *Unified Protocol for Transdiagnostic Treatment of Emotional Disorders in Children and Adolescents*, adapted for misophonia, although early reports of a follow-up randomized controlled trial suggest minimal differences between this protocol and a relaxation control condition (Lewin, 2022).

Exposure-based approaches

Based on extant behavioral conceptualizations of misophonia, principles of exposure are often included in extant CBT treatments for misophonia to a greater or lesser degree (Lewin et al., 2021; Rabasco & McKay, 2021). Exposure aims to reduce negative affect associated with trigger sounds and build distress tolerance by gradually exposing the individual to trigger stimuli in a controlled and systematic manner. However, owing to heterogeneity within the affective response in misophonia (which differs from the decidedly more homogeneous fear response in phobias and anxiety disorders), traditional exposure models predicated on habituation may be less applicable in misophonia. As a result, the *inhibitory learning model (ILT)* has been identified as a promising guide for maximally tailoring exposure for misophonia (Frank & McKay, 2019). An ILT application to misophonia involves (a) building distress tolerance and stress management skills; (b) generating novel and flexible contexts in which triggers can be experienced (e.g., humor instead of hypervigilant tension); and (c) postulating unique considerations for hierarchy development in light of differences between misophonia and classic fear/anxiety disorders. In essence, an ILT approach emphasizes new learning when confronted with previously avoided stimuli rather than a sole emphasis on habituation.

Treatment considerations for youth

As described above, there is a paucity of research concerning child and adolescent treatment for misophonia despite the early age of onset. However, aligned with the burgeoning lines of work in this area (e.g., Dover & McGuire, 2023; Lewin et al., 2021) and based on general pediatric CBT principles, several key considerations for providing treatment to youth with misophonia can be gleaned. Here, treatment often involves a combination of therapeutic approaches, depending on the child's age, developmental stage, and individual needs. More specifically, CBT techniques, including psychoeducation and problem-solving, can help children understand misophonia, develop coping skills, and manage their emotional reactions to triggers. Therapists may draw from family-based CBT, depending on the child's age and child and family member preferences (Dover & McGuire, 2023), in addition to principles from acceptance and commitment therapy (Petersen & Twohig, 2023). A CBT approach to misophonia can also help children understand and modify their thoughts, emotions, and behaviors related to trigger sounds. Several key components include: (a) psychoeducation; (b) trigger identification and awareness; (c) cognitive restructuring; (d) exposure practice; (e) relaxation techniques; (f) coping skills and regulation; and (g) parental support (Dover & McGuire; Rappoldt et al., 2023).

Parental and family support is a critical component of misophonia treatment in children and adolescents. Given the significant degree of family involvement in misophonia-related coping and avoidance, as well as the role of parents in participating in children's treatment, incorporation of parents in treatment seems especially important. In general, treatment may initially involve providing psychoeducation about misophonia and relevant maintaining factors. As treatment progresses, focus may shift to empowering parents to learn and practice strategies for appropriately managing trigger sounds at home without engaging in maladaptive family accommodation, responding calmly and consistently to the child's distress, and encouraging and reinforcing their child's use of coping skills learned in therapy (Dover & McGuire, 2023). Finally, directly addressing *maladaptive* family accommodation while identifying potentially adaptive, supportive accommodations is important for generalizing treatment principles to diverse contexts of the child's life, including familial and academic domains.

Classification status of misophonia

A lingering question exists concerning the proper classification status of misophonia. To that end, some researchers have conceptualized misophonia as a putative member of the OCRDs (see Cavanna & Seri, 2015 and Taylor, 2017 for extended discussions). Understandably, much of the perpetuation of the misophonia-OCRD linkage is likely due to the seminal nature of the Schröder et al. (2013) account and corresponding A-MISO-S measure, along with several early case studies describing comorbid misophonia and OCD. Historical context aside, a greater understanding of the conceptual logic behind psychiatric classification may shed light on challenges in conceptualizing misophonia as an OCRD. That is, the rationale for the argument concerning the classification of misophonia as a member of the OCRDs appears to rest on general assumptions concerning how a condition becomes a member of a larger class of disorders. We address these assumptions in turn.

Psychiatric comorbidity equals member of the same disorder class

The conceptual foundations and early research that informed the current OCRDs (formerly the obsessive-compulsive spectrum, OCS; Hollander, 1993) was based on the idea that two or more disorders are part of the same class of conditions if they commonly co-occurred. The reasoning behind this conceptual model asserts that two or more conditions that typically co-occur means each shares a *common underlying diathesis* (i.e., generalized psychopathological process). While this seems a reasonable foundation for the development of a class of conditions, subsequent research did not bear out for the common diathesis assumption in the realm of OCRDs (Abramowitz et al., 2009). Thus, until common mechanisms are identified between misophonia and OCRDs, it is premature to conclude that they are part of the same class of conditions. Identification of such common mechanisms seems especially unlikely considering the current state of the neurobiological misophonia literature, which suggests that misophonia possesses an overlapping yet distinct neural signature compared to commonly co-occurring psychiatric conditions (Neacsiu et al., 2022).

Topographically similar symptom expressions are members of same disorder class

This argument also emerged in the genesis of the OCRDs– namely, that any condition marked by repetitive behaviors or persistent intrusive thoughts were members of the same disorder class. This assumes that repetitive behaviors occur in response to the same stimuli or a consequence of the same neurobiological circuit. In earlier critical analyses, this was likewise demonstrated to be insufficient based on available evidence for other candidate OCS conditions (Abramowitz et al., 2009; McKay et al., 2008; Storch et al., 2008). In the development of the OCRDs, even the most enthusiastic supporters of a broader class of conditions conceptualized as based on a common thread of behavioral excesses narrowed the scope considerably on the basis of insufficient neurobiological support for many previous candidate disorders (Hollander et al., 2008).

Based on descriptive research on misophonia symptomology, the criterion of topographically similar symptoms is not met. Individuals with misophonia primarily avoid particular sounds and react to or avoid situations that might be associated with these trigger sounds. While many individuals with OCD avoid situations that might provoke obsessions or compulsions, *that is but one symptom of a broader syndrome.* Conversely, there are numerous other psychiatric conditions marked by a similar emotional response to specific situations and/or marked avoidance of distressing inner states (i.e., experiential avoidance; EA; Hayes et al., 1996), such as anxiety disorders, substance abuse, and PTSD. Moreover, it has been argued that EA represents a *generalized, transdiagnostic process of psychopathology* (Chawla & Ostafin, 2007). The scope of a construct such as EA presents challenges for developing a taxonomic system with descriptive precision and clinical utility based solely on topographical features of conditions (Hayes & Hofmann, 2020). It also weakens the argument that misophonia should be classified as an OCRD based on the shared feature of EA (Cowan et al., 2022). Thus, until further research demonstrates that there is a *specific* common underlying mechanism for emotional reactions and learned situational avoidance shared between misophonia and OCRDs that distinguishes this pair from other disorders in which EA predominates, such a classification remains untenable.

Conditions with shared treatment models are part of same disorder class

Again, drawing parallels with the earlier argument for an OCS, the basis for this assumption proceeds as follows: if condition X responds to treatment Y, and OCD also responds to treatment Y, then condition X is part of the OCS. Unfortunately, to date, there is limited support for common psychosocial interventions in the treatment of OCRDs and misophonia. Indeed, as described earlier in this chapter, a CBT model of misophonia intervention development (similar in some ways to the CBT framework underpinning interventions for OCRDs) has demonstrated promise. However, the extent to which CBT principles require substantial adaptation for misophonia, coupled with the relatively nascent phase of misophonia treatment development research, suggest that *any conclusion concerning shared class status based on shared treatment models is premature at this time.* Furthermore, while exposure-based treatments have been examined (discussed in Rabasco & McKay, 2021), there has been primarily case series support for this, or the use of exposure as part of more comprehensive treatment programs (Potgieter et al., 2019). Additionally, anecdotal clinical evidence suggests that the habituation response commonly found in exposure treatment for more fear-based psychiatric conditions is less likely to manifest in misophonia. However, such anecdotal clinical evidence requires further empirical examination.

Summary of shared feature criteria

Thus far, there appears to be quite limited evidence supporting the classification of misophonia under the taxonomic umbrella of OCRDs. While research on misophonia across the lifespan is nascent, the evidence to date appears to suggest that misophonia could just as plausibly be considered a member of several other disorder classes, or an independent condition (Taylor, 2017). The current problem in placing misophonia in the OCRDs is similar to the historical issue faced by putative members of the OCS. Moreover, the classification criteria enumerated above demands showing that conditions are *similar*, which is antithetical to most statistical methodologies. Demonstrating similarity is often a low statistical power affair and can lead to troublesome conclusions, such as mistaking null findings for equivalence (Tryon, 2008). To date, there have not been any taxometric tests to demonstrate misophonia should be in the OCRDs, such as the application of statistical equivalence testing or cluster analysis (McKay & Neziroglu, 2009). As a result, it would be premature to consider misophonia an OCRD, and classification research would need to rule out numerous other possible disorder classes to identify the correct placement of the condition.

Misophonia: an emerging taxonomic story

Whether misophonia is ultimately classified as a member of the OCRDs, determined to be part of some other class of disorders, or stands alone as a unique condition, the classification approach researchers have taken is often marked by DSM-based clinical assumptions rather than an *etiologically based, theoretically informed, nosological approach* (Hayes et al., 1996). This is unsurprising, as the tradition in psychiatry has been to articulate descriptive phenomenological commonalities (i.e., topographical features) as a means for classifying disorders (Lilienfeld & Treadway, 2016). Conversely, other– more mature– branches of science classify based on robust theoretical (i.e., etiological) models that permit robust prediction and a priori categorization. Indeed, this discrepancy has been identified as an area of growth for clinical psychological science writ large (Hayes et al., 2020).

If psychiatry had a unifying theoretical model that would allow for such a priori categorization, the entire discussion of where to place misophonia would likely be moot. To that end, some researchers (i.e., Conway et al., 2019; Hayes & Hofmann, 2020) have postulated that a psychiatric classification system predicated on transdiagnostic, etiologically based psychopathological processes may hold promise for improving the understanding and amelioration of human suffering, including misophonia. This focus on generalized processes of change is further buttressed by findings suggesting *internalizing symptoms* in youth (Guzick et al., 2023), along with *sound sensitivity* (McKay & Acevedo, 2020) and *emotion regulation difficulties* (Guetta et al., 2022) in adults, as candidate vulnerability factors in misophonia from a developmental perspective.

Conclusion

Misophonia is a condition characterized by decreased tolerance and intense adverse reactions to contextually specific sounds. Due, in part, to known onset in childhood, a developmental perspective on misophonia seems especially relevant (Guzick et al., 2023; Siepsiak et al., 2023), including nuanced adaptations to assessment and intervention practices. While misophonia research efforts are growing, and CBT-based treatments continue to demonstrate promise– especially for youth (e.g., Dover & McGuire, 2023; Petersen & Twohig, 2023), more research is clearly needed to further elucidate misophonia in terms of conceptual boundaries from other psychiatric and audiological conditions. Obtaining further clarity on the classification status of misophonia, especially in regard to existing psychiatric taxonomic systems, is an important research priority moving forward. While the classification of misophonia as an OCRD may have initially held promise, findings to date suggest otherwise, and that considering a range of underlying processes beyond topographically defined DSM diagnoses, including internalizing symptoms, generalized sensory sensitivity, and experiential avoidance, represents a more tenable approach to understanding, and ultimately treating, this debilitating condition.

Note

1 Editor's note: We again emphasize that although this psychological perspective is invaluable, particularly as it related to OCRD classification, this does not minimize the contribution of other meaningful domains of research, including neurobiology.

References

Abramowitz, J. S., Storch, E. A., McKay, D., Taylor, S., & Asmundson, G. J. G. (2009). The obsessive-compulsive spectrum: A critical review. In D. McKay, J. S. Abramowitz, S. Taylor, & G. J. G. Asmundson (Eds), *Current perspectives on anxiety disorders: Implications for DSM-V and beyond* (pp. 329–352). New York: Springer.

American Psychiatric Association. (2022). *Diagnostic and statistical manual of mental disorders* (5th Ed., text rev.). doi:10.1176/appi.books.9780890425787.

Brout, J. J., Edelstein, M., Erfanian, M., Mannino, M., Miller, L. J., Rouw, R., Kumar, S., & Rosenthal, M. Z. (2018). Investigating misophonia: A review of the empirical literature, clinical implications, and a research agenda. *Frontiers in Neuroscience,* doi:10.3389/fnins.2018.00036.

Cassiello-Robbins, C., Anand, D., McMahon, K., Guetta, R., Trumbell, J., Kelley, L., & Rosenthal, M. Z. (2020). The mediating role of emotion regulation within the relationship between neuroticism and misophonia: A preliminary investigation. *Frontiers in Psychiatry.* doi:10.3389/fpsyt.2020.00847.

Cavanna, A. E. & Seri, S. (2015). Misophonia: Current perspectives. *Neuropsychiatric Disease and Treatment*, 18(11), 2117–2123. doi:10.2147/NDT. S81438.

Cervin, M., Guzick, A. G., Clinger, J., Smith, E., Draper, I. A., Goodman, W. K., Lijffift, M., ... & Storch, E. A. (2023). Measuring misophonia in youth: A psychometric evaluation of child and parent measures. *Journal of Affective Disorders*, 338(1), 180–186. doi:10.1016/j.jad.2023.05.093.

Chawla, N. & Ostafin, B. (2007). Experiential avoidance as a functional dimensional approach to psychopathology: An empirical review. *Journal of Clinical Psychology*, 63(9), 871–890. doi:10.1002/jclp.20400.

Claiborn, J. M., Dozier, T. H., Hart, S. L., & Lee, J. (2020). Self-identified misophonia phenomenology, impact, and clinical correlates. *Psychological Thought*, 13(2), 349–375. doi:10.37708/psyct.v13i2.454.

Clark, L. & McKay, D. (2021). Misophonia: An obsessive-compulsive disorder? In E. A. Storch et al. (Eds), *Complexities in obsessive compulsive and related disorders: Advances in conceptualization and treatment*. Oxford University Press. doi:10.1093/med-psych/9780190052775.003.0006.

Conway, C. C., Forbes, M. K., Forbush, K. T., Fried, E. I., Hallquist, M. N., Kotov, R., Mullins-Sweatt, S. N.,..., & Eaton, N. R. (2019). A hierarchical taxonomy of psychopathology can transform mental health research. *Perspectives on Psychological Science*, 14(3), 419–436. doi:10.1177/1745691618810696.

Cowan, E. N., Marks, D. R., & Pinto, A. (2022). Misophonia: A psychological model and proposed treatment. *Journal of Obsessive-compulsive and Related Disorders*, 32. doi:10.1016/j.jocrd.2021.100691.

Cusack, S. E., Cash, T. V., & Vrana, S. R. (2018). An examination of the relationship between misophonia, anxiety sensitivity, and obsessive-compulsive symptoms. *Journal of Obsessive-Compulsive and Related Disorders*, 18, 67–72. doi:10.1016/j.jocrd.2018.06.004.

Daniels, E. C., Rodriguez, A., & Zabelina, D. L. (2020). Severity of misophonia symptoms is associated with worse cognitive control when exposed to misophonia trigger sounds. *PLoS One*, 15(1), e0227118. doi:10.1371/journal. pone.0227118.

Dover, N., & McGuire, J. F. (2023). Family-based cognitive behavioral therapy for youth with misophonia: A case report. *Cognitive and Behavioral Practice*, 30(1), 169–176. doi:10.1016/j.cbpra.2021.05.005.

Eijsker, N., Schröder, A., Smit, D. J., van Wingen, G., & Denys, D. (2021). Structural and functional brain abnormalities in misophonia. *European Neuropsychopharmacology*, 52, 62–71. doi:10.1016/j.euroneuro.2021.05.013.

Eldesouky, L. & Gross, J. J. (2019). Emotion regulation goals: An individual difference perspective. *Social and Personality Psychology Compass*, 13(9), e12493. doi:10.1111/spc3.12493.

Ferrer-Torres, A. & Giménez-Llort, L. (2022). Misophonia: A systematic review of current and future trends in this emerging clinical field. *International Journal of Environmental Research and Public Health*, 19(11), 6790. doi:10.3390/ijerph19116790.

Frank, B. & McKay, D. (2019). The suitability of an inhibitory learning approach in exposure when habituation fails: A clinical application to misophonia. *Cognitive and Behavioral Practice*, 26, 130–142. doi:10.1016/j.cbpra.2018.04.003.

Frank, B., Roszyk, M., Hurley, L., Drejaj, L., & McKay, D. (2020). Inattention in misophonia: Difficulties achieving and maintaining alertness. *Journal of Clinical and Experimental Neuropsychology*, 42(1), 66–75. doi:10.1080/13803395.2019.1666801.

Goodman, W. K., Price, L. H., Rasmussen, S. A., Mazure, C., Fleishmann, R. L., Hill, C. L., Heninger, G. R., & Charney, D. S. (1989). The Yale-Brown obsessive compulsive scale. 1. Development, use, and reliability. *Archives of General Psychiatry*, 46(11), 1006–1011. doi:10.1001/archpsyc.1989.01810110048007.

Guetta, R. E., Cassiello-Robbins, C., Trumbull, J., Anand, D., & Rosenthal, M. Z. (2022). Examining emotional functioning in misophonia: The role of affective instability and difficulties with emotion regulation. *PLoS One*, 17(2), e0263230. doi:10.1371/journal.pone.0263230.

Guzick, A. G., Cervin, M., Smith, E. E. A., Clinger, J., Draper, I., Goodman, W. K., Lijffijt, M., ... & Storch, E. A. (2023). Clinical characteristics, impairment, and psychiatric morbidity in 102 youth with misophonia. *Journal of Affective Disorders*, 1, 395–402. doi:10.1016/j.jad.2022.12.083.

Hayes, S. C., Wilson, K. G., Gifford, E. V., Follette, V. M., & Strosahl, K. (1996). Experiential avoidance and behavioral disorders: A functional dimensional approach to diagnosis and treatment. *Journal of Consulting and Clinical Psychology*, 64(6), 1152–1168.

Hayes, S. C. & Hofmann, S. G. (Eds). (2020). *Beyond the DSM: Toward a process-based alternative for diagnosis and mental health treatment*. New Harbinger Publications.

Hollander, E. (1993). Obsessive-compulsive spectrum disorders: An overview. *Psychiatric Annals*, 23, 355–358.

Hollander, E., Braun, A., & Simeon, D. (2008). Should OCD leave the anxiety disorders in DSM-V? The case for obsessive compulsive related disorders. *Depression & Anxiety*, 25, 317–329.

Jager, I. J., de Koning, P., Bost, T., Denys, D., & Vulink, N. (2020). Misophonia: Phenomenology, comorbidity, and demographics in a large sample. *PLoS ONE*, 15(4), e0231390. doi:10.1371/journal.pone.0231390.

Jager, I. J., Vulink, N. C., Bergfeld, I. O., van Loon, J., & Denys, D. (2021). Cognitive behavioral therapy for misophonia: A randomized clinical trial. *Depression and Anxiety*, 38(7), 708–718. doi:10.1002/da.23127.

Jastreboff, M. M. & Jastreboff, P. J. (2002). Decreased sound tolerance and tinnitus retraining therapy (TRT). *Australian and New Zealand Journal of Audiology*, 24 (2), 74–84. doi:10.1375/audi.24.2.74.31105.

Jastreboff, P. J. & Jastreboff, M. M. (2014). Treatments for decreased sound tolerance (hyperacusis and misophonia). *Seminars in Hearing*, 35(2), 105–120. doi:10.1055/s-0034-1372527.

Jastreboff, P. J. & Jastreboff, M. M. (2023). The neurophysiological approach to misophonia: Theory and treatment. *Frontiers in Neuroscience*, 17, 895574. doi:10.3389/fnins.2023.895574.

Johnson, M. (2014). *50 cases of Misophonia using the MMP. Paper presented at the Misophonia Conference of the Tinnitus Practitioners Association*. Atlanta, GA.

Lazarus, R. S. & Folkman, S. (1984). *Stress, appraisal and coping*. New York: Springer.

Lewin, A. B. (2022). Transdiagnostic CBT for youth with misophonia: A randomized controlled trial. 2022 Meeting of the Misophonia Research Fund.

Lewin, A. B., Dickinson, S., Kudryk, K., Karlovich, A. R., Harmon, S. L., Phillips, D. A., ..., & Ehrenreich-May, J. (2021). Transdiagnostic cognitive behavioral therapy for misophonia in youth: Methods for a clinical trial and four pilot cases. *Journal of Affective Disorders*, 291, 400–408. doi:10.1016/j.jad.2021.04.027.

Lilienfeld, S. O. & Treadway, M. T. (2016). Clashing diagnostic approaches: DSM-ICD versus RDoC. *Annual Review of Clinical Psychology*, 12, 435–463. doi:10.1146/annurev-clinpsy-021815-093122.

Mattson, S. A., D'Souza, J., Wojcik, K. D., Guzick, A. G., Goodman, W. K., & Storch, E. A. (2023). A systematic review of treatments for misophonia. *Personalized Medicine in Psychiatry*, 39–40, 100104. doi:10.1016/j.pmip.2023.100104.

McKay, D. (2017). Presidential address: Embracing the repulsive: the case for disgust as a functionally central emotional state in the theory, practice, and dissemination of cognitive-behavior therapy. *Behavior Therapy*, 48, 731–738.

McKay, D., Abramowitz, J.S., & Taylor, S. (2008). How should we conceptualize the Obsessive-Compulsive Spectrum? In J.S. Abramowitz, D. McKay, & S. Taylor (Eds), *Obsessive-Compulsive Disorder: Subtypes and Spectrum Conditions (pp. 287–300)*. Oxford: Elsevier.

McKay, D. & Acevedo, B. P. (2020). Clinical characteristics of misophonia and its relation to sensory processing sensitivity: A critical analysis. In *The highly sensitive brain: Research, assessment, and treatment of sensory processing sensitivity* (pp. 165–185). Academic Press.

McKay, D., Kim, S. K., Mancusi, L., Storch, E. A., & Spankovich, C. (2018). Profile Analysis of Psychological Symptoms Associated With Misophonia: A Community Sample. *Behavior therapy, 49*(2), 286–294. https://doi.org/10.1016/j.beth.2017.07.002.

McKay, D. & Neziroglu, F. (2009). Methodological issues in the obsessive-compulsive spectrum. *Psychiatry Research*, 170, 61–65.

Möllmann, A., Heinrichs, N., Illies, L., Potthast, N., & Kley, H. (2023). The central role of symptom severity and associated characteristics for functional impairment in misophonia. *Frontiers in Psychiatry*, 14, 1112472. doi:10.3389/fpsyt.2023.1112472.

Murphy, N., Lijffijt, M., Guzick, A. G., Cervin, M., Clinger, J., Smith, E. A., Draper, I., ... & Storch, E. A. (under review). Alterations in attentional processing in youth with misophonia: A phenotypical cross-comparison with anxiety patients.

Naylor, J., Caimino, C., Scutt, P., Hoare, D. J., & Baguley, D. M. (2021). The prevalence and severity of misophonia in a UK undergraduate medical student population and validation of the Amsterdam Misophonia Scale. *Psychiatric Quarterly*, 92, 609–619. doi:10.1007/s11126-020-09825-3.

Neacsiu, A. D., Szymkiewicz, V., Galla, J. T., Li, B., Kulkarni, Y., & Spector, C. W. (2022). The neurobiology of misophonia and implications for novel, neuroscience-driven interventions. *Frontiers in Neuroscience*, 16:893903. doi:10.3389/fnins.2022.893903.

Petersen, J. M. & Twohig, M. P. (2023). Acceptance and commitment therapy for a child with misophonia: A case study. *Clinical Case Studies*, 22(3), 211–223. doi:10.1177/15346501221126136.

Potgieter, I., MacDonald, C., Partridge, L., Cima, R., Sheldrake, J., & Hoare, D.J. (2019). Misophonia: A scoping review of research. *Journal of Clinical Psychology*, 75, 1203–1218. doi:10.1002/jclp.22771.

Rabasco, A. & McKay, D. (2021). Exposure therapy for misophonia: Concepts and procedures. *Journal of Cognitive Psychotherapy*, 35(3), 156–166. doi:10.1891/JCPSY-D-20-00042.

Rappoldt, L. R., van der Pol, M. M., de Wit, C., Slaghekke, S., Houben, C., Sondaar, T., ... & Utens, E. M. (2023). Effectiveness of an innovative treatment protocol for misophonia in children and adolescents: Design of a randomized controlled trial. *Contemporary Clinical Trials Communications*, 33, 101105. doi:10.1016/j.conctc.2023.101105.

Reid, A. M., Guzick, A. G., Gernand, A., & Olsen, B. (2016). Intensive cognitive-behavioral therapy for comorbid misophonia and obsessive-compulsive symptoms: A systematic case study. *Journal of Obsessive-Compulsive and Related Disorders*, 10, 1–9. doi:10.1016/j.jocrd.2016.04.009.

Remmert, N., Jebens, A., Gruzman, R., Gregory, J., & Vitoratou, S. (2022). A nomological network for misophonia in two German samples using the S-Five model for misophonia. *Frontiers in Psychology*, 13, 902807. doi:10.3389/fpsyg.2022.902807.

Rinaldi, L. J., Smees, R., Ward, J., & Simner, J. (2022). Poorer well-being in children with misophonia: Evidence from the Sussex Misophonia Scale for adolescents. *Frontiers in Psychology*, 13, 808379. doi:10.3389/fpsyg.2022.808379.

Rosenthal, M. Z., McMahon, K., Greenleaf, A. S., Cassiello-Robbins, C., Guetta, R., Trumbull, J., Anand, D., Frazer-Abel, E. S., & Kelley, L. (2022). Phenotyping misophonia: Psychiatric disorders and medical health corelates. *Frontiers in Psychology*, 13, 941898. doi:10.3389/fpsyg.2022.941898.

Rouw, R. & Erfanian, M. (2018). A large-scale study of misophonia. *Journal of Clinical Psychology*, 74(3), 453–479. doi:10.1002/jclp.22500.

Schneider, R. L. & Arch, J. J. (2017). Case study: A novel application of mindfulness- and acceptance-based components to treat misophonia. *Journal of Contextual Behavioral Science*, 6(2), 221–225. doi:10.1016/j.jcbs.2017.04.003.

Schröder, A., van Diepen, R., Mazaheri, A., Petropoulos-Petalas, D., Soto de Amesti, V., Vulink, N., & Denys, D. (2014). Diminished n1 auditory evoked potentials to oddball stimuli in misophonia patients. *Frontiers in Behavioral Neuroscience*, 8, 123. doi:10.3389/fnbeh.2014.00123.

Schröder, A., Vulink, N., & Denys, D. (2013). Misophonia: Diagnostic criteria for a new psychiatric disorder. *PLoS One* 8(1), e54706. doi:10.1371/journal.pone.0054706.

Schröder, A., Vulink, N., van Loon, A. J., & Denys, D. (2017). Cognitive behavioral therapy is effective in misophonia: An open trial. *Journal of Affective Disorders*, 217, 289–294. doi:10.1016/j.jad.2017.04.017.

Siepsiak, M., Rosenthal, M. Z., Raj-Koziak, D., & Dragan, W. (2022). Psychiatric and audiologic features of misophonia: Use of a clinical control group with auditory over-responsivity. *Journal of Psychosomatic Research*, 156, 110777. doi:10.1016/j.jpsychores.2022.110777.

Siepsiak, M., Turek, A., Michalowska, M., Gambin, M., & Dragan, W. (2023). Misophonia in children and adolescents: Age differences, risk factors, psychiatric and psychological correlates: A pilot study with mothers' involvement. *Child Psychiatry & Human Development.* doi:10.1007/s10578-023-01593-y.

Simner, J., Koursarou, S., Rinaldi, L. J., & Ward, J. (2021). Attention, flexibility, and imagery in misophonia: Does attention exacerbate everyday disliking of sound?. *Journal of Clinical and Experimental Neuropsychology*, 43(10), 1006–1017. doi:10.1080/13803395.2022.2056581.

Spencer, S. D., Guzick, A. G., Cervin, M., & Storch, E. A. (2023). Mindfulness and cognitive emotion regulation in pediatric misophonia. *Journal of Contextual Behavioral Science*, 29, 182–191. doi:10.1016/j.jcbs.2023.07.005.

Storch, E. A., Abramowitz, J., & Goodman, W. K. (2008). Where does obsessive-compulsive disorder belong in DSM-V? *Depression and Anxiety, 25(4)*, 336–347. https://doi.org/10.1002/da.20488.

Storch, E. A., Guzick, A. G., D'Souza, J., Clinger, J., Cervin, M., Rork, C., Smith, E., ..., & Goodman, W. K. (under review). Family accommodation in children and adolescents with misophonia.

Swedo, S. E., Baguley, D. M., Denys, D., Dixon, L. J., Erfanian, M., Fioretti, A., Jastreboff, P. J., Kumar, S., ... & Raver, S. M. (2022). Consensus definition of misophonia: A Delphi study. *Frontiers in Neuroscience*, 16, (1–16),841816. doi:10.3389/fnins.2022.841816.

Taylor, S. (2017). Misophonia: A new mental disorder? *Medical Hypotheses*, 103, 109–117. doi:10.1016/j.mehy.2017.05.003.

Tryon, W.W. (2008). Statistical equivalence. In D. McKay (Ed.), *Handbook of Research Methods in Abnormal and Clinical Psychology (pp. 309–316).* Newbury Park, CA: Sage Publications.

Webber, T. A., Johnson, P. L., & Storch, E. A. (2014). Pediatric misophonia with comorbid obsessive-compulsive spectrum disorders. *General Hospital Psychiatry*, 36(2), 231.e1–231.e2. doi:10.1016/j.genhosppsych.2013.10.018.

Wiese, A. D., Wojcik, K. D., & Storch, E. A. (2021). Assessment and intervention for individuals with misophonia. *Journal of Health Service Psychology*, 47(1), 51–60. doi:10.1007/s42843-021-00025-6.

World Health Organization. (2019). *International statistical classification of diseases and related health problems* (11th Ed.). https://icd.who.int.

Wu, M. S., Lewin, A. B., Murphy, T. K., & Storch, E. A. (2014). Misophonia: Incidence, phenomenology, and clinical correlates in an undergraduate student sample. *Journal of Clinical Psychology*, 70(10), 994–1007. doi:10.1002/jclp.22098.

13 Inflammation and OCD

Sydenham chorea, PANS/PANDAS, and other inflammatory conditions relating to OCD and other psychiatric comorbidities

Allison Vreeland, Noelle Schlenk, Emily Mendoza, Meiqian Ma, Theresa A. Willett and Jennifer Frankovich

Acknowledgements: Support for the infrastructure of our research program was provided by: National Institute of Mental Health, Lucile Packard Foundation for Children's Health, Neuroimmune Foundation, Brain Inflammation Collaborative, The Brain Foundation, O'Sullivan Foundation, Stanford MCHRI, Stanford SPARK, Tara and Dave Dollinger PANS Biomarker Discovery Core, PANDAS Physician Network, and Oxnard Foundation.

Introduction

Evidence supporting a link between obsessive-compulsive symptoms and inflammatory pathophysiology continues to mount. The current research model for investigations of post-infectious autoimmunity leading to neuropsychiatric symptoms stems from Sydenham's chorea (SC), a neurologic disorder that while initially controversial has become a widely accepted and treatable condition (Dean & Singer, 2017). The working model of SC posits that anti-neuronal antibodies cross-react (through molecular mimicry) with neuronal antigens. In a similar fashion, research on pediatric acute-onset neuropsychiatric syndrome (PANS) and pediatric autoimmune disorder associated with streptococcus (PANDAS) provide evidence for a related postinfectious pathogenic mechanism (Cutforth et al., 2016; Vreeland et al., 2023). The psychiatric symptoms (e.g., obsessions, compulsions, behavior outbursts) associated with SC and PANS/PANDAS can improve with standard evidence-based psychiatric interventions (e.g., cognitive behavioral therapy) and with treatment of the underlying infection and inflammation (Swedo et al., 2017). This chapter provides a review of the current clinical diagnostic criteria, recommended evaluation pathways, and treatment recommendations for SC and PANS/PANDAS. Additionally, we outline research examining associations between inflammation and symptoms of SC and PANS/PANDAS. Lastly,

DOI: 10.4324/9781003517429-13

we provide a summary of known connections between other autoimmune conditions and psychiatric symptoms (e.g., systemic lupus erythematosus, Sjögren's syndrome, Beçhet's disease).

Sydenham Chorea

Sydenham chorea (SC) is the most common form of childhood chorea (Dean & Singer, 2017; Zomorrodi & Wald, 2006) and is known to be a post-streptococcal neurologic manifestation of acute rheumatic fever (ARF) (Dajani et al., 1992; Taranta & Stollerman, 1956). A wide variety of psychiatric symptoms (e.g., anxiety, restlessness, irritability, aggression, sleep disturbances) are associated with SC, the most common of which are obsessive-compulsive symptoms; up to 80 percent of patients with SC exhibit obsessive-compulsive symptoms (Asbahr et al., 1998; Maia et al., 2005; Swedo et al., 1993). In addition to psychiatric symptoms, SC may be accompanied by migratory joint pain, carditis, erythema marginatum, and subcutaneous nodules (Zomorrodi & Wald, 2006). While these other features are supportive, they are not necessary for the diagnosis (Cardoso, 2011). Thus, treatment of SC targets both the chorea and the additional psychological and cardiological sequelae (Dean & Singer, 2017; Vasconcelos et al., 2019).

Table 13.1 Diagnostic Criteria for PANDAS and PANS

PANDAS Criteria (Swedo et al., 1998)	*PANS Criteria (Swedo, 2012)*
1. Presence of diagnosis of OCD and/or tic disorder	1. Abrupt, dramatic onset of OCD or severely restricted food intake
2. Pediatric onset	2. Concurrent presence of additional neuropsychiatric symptoms, (with similarly severe and acute onset), from at least two of the following seven categories

3. Episodic course	A. Anxiety
	    B. Emotional lability and/or depression
	    C. Irritability, aggression, and/or severely oppositional behaviors
	    D. Behavioral (developmental) regression
	    E. Deterioration in school performance
	    F. Sensory or motor difficulties
	    G. Somatic signs or symptoms, including sleep disturbances, enuresis, or urinary frequency

4. Temporal association with GAS infection	3. Symptoms are not better explained by a known neurologic or medical disorder, such as Sydenham chorea, systemic lupus erythematosus, Tourette syndrome, or others
5. Association with neurologic abnormalities	

Diagnosis

SC is characterized by involuntary, brief, random, and irregular move-ments of the limbs and face that often first present sub-acutely (Dajani et al., 1992). The onset of SC is generally within 4–12 weeks (but can present up to 8 months) following a group A streptococcal (GAS) infection (Cardoso et al., 2006; Dean & Singer, 2017; Garvey & Swedo, 1997). There are no reliable diagnostic markers for SC, and while confirmation of GAS is helpful, proof of infection is not necessary (particularly if the window for detecting GAS has past). Thus, it is important for clinicians to consider broader differential diagnoses including Huntington's disease (the most common inherited cause of chorea), systemic lupus erythematosus (SLE), antiphospholipid antibody syndrome, and Wilson's disease (Cardoso, 2011). It is recommended that clinicians complete a thorough medical exam to assess for features of ARF including arthritis, carditis, erythema marginatum, subcutaneous nodules, fever, elevated erythrocyte sedimenta-tion rate (ESR) or C-reactive protein (CRP), and prolonged PR interval on electrocardiogram (Gewitz et al., 2015). In addition, it is important that clinicians assessing for SC complete a comprehensive review of the patient's medical history, including a review of medications, as some medications (e.g., neuroleptics, antiepileptics, oral contraceptives, central nervous system stimulants) have known associations with chorea (Cardoso, 2011).

Pathophysiology and research

It is posited that SC results from an autoimmune process in which GAS-induced antibodies disrupt the cortico-basal ganglia-thalamo-cortical (CBGTC) circuities through molecular mimicry (Bronze & Dale, 1993; Cunningham, 2019; Dale et al., 2001; Husby et al., 1976; Kirvan et al., 2003; Kirvan, Swedo, Kurahara, et al., 2006). In one study, sera taken from a patient with active post-GAS chorea successfully induced CaM kinase II (CaMKII) activity in neuronal cells, while sera from post-strep patients without chorea did not (Kirvan et al., 2003). Furthermore, ongo-ing animal model and imaging studies continue to provide evidence link-ing post-GAS basal ganglia inflammation and SC (Vreeland et al., 2023). Current research continues to investigate the different pathways involved in the immunogenesis of GAS-reactive neuropsychiatric infections, with many focusing on mechanisms associated with inflammation of the basal ganglia (Vasconcelos et al., 2023).

Prevalence

SC occurs in 25 percent of ARF cases, with the average age of onset between 9.2 and 11.7 years and has a well-established female predominance (approximately 3:1) (Kirvan et al., 2003; Cardoso et al., 1997; Faustino et al., 2003; Orsini et al., 2022). Although chorea can often self-resolve, as many as 50 percent of patients have recurrent attacks (Cardoso, 2011). In addition, women with a history of SC or other auto-immune disorder are more likely to develop chorea during pregnancy (Hermann & Walker, 2015).

While the prevalence of SC has decreased, owing to changes in hygienic practices, the development of antibiotics, and the advancement of health-care, in areas of the world where access to health care is limited and household crowding is common, SC is seen more frequently (Cardoso, 2011).

Treatment

Some patients with SC have a spontaneous resolution of symptoms within months of onset (Jordan & Singer, 2003), while others have moderate to severe chorea and/or behavioral impairments warranting intervention. Up to 50 percent of patients with SC have persistent symptoms for more than two years (Cardoso et al., 1999). Treatment for SC includes eliminating infection in the patient and home (e.g., family members, close contacts), immunomodulatory therapy, and psychiatric care. While the efficacy of immunomodulation and/or antibiotics for SC has not been established via randomized controlled trials, these remain the recommended treatments for moderate to severe cases (Ben-Pazi et al., 2012; Gilbert, 2022; Teixeira et al., 2021; Vasconcelos et al., 2019). Penicillin or equivalent prophylaxis is recommended to reduce the risk of re-infection and new ARF episodes and can reduce both the severity of chorea and the accompanying cardiac complications (Dean & Singer, 2017; Gurkas et al., 2016). In cases where antibiotics are not effective for symptom control, corticosteroids and intravenous immunoglobulin (IVIG) have been suggested as effective alternative treatments for patients with SC (Cardoso et al., 2003). Finally, antipsychotic and anticonvulsant medications have been used in conjunc-tion with antibiotics to address significant chorea symptoms (Dean & Singer, 2017).

PANS/PANDAS

Diagnosis

Similar to SC, PANS/PANDAS are proposed to be post-infectious, immune-mediated syndromes that are characterized by an abrupt and severe symptom onset, a relapsing and remitting course, and specific comorbid symptoms. Although PANS/PANDAS have diagnostic criteria (see Table 13.1), they continue to be provisional diagnoses with provi-sional treatments. By definition, PANDAS is temporally associated with

GAS infection. However, like SC, patients often present after the window of opportunity to diagnose GAS. Thus, the PANS criteria is preferred as it is agnostic to any identifiable preceding infection. Data supporting neuroinflammation in SC strongly overlap with data in PANS/PANDAS, including a similar autoantibody profile and imaging data showing alterations in the basal ganglia (Vreeland et al., 2023). However, reliable clinically available imaging and molecular tools are still being developed.

Since there are no clinically available diagnostic markers for PANS/PANDAS (as is the case of SC), PANS/PANDAS requires a comprehensive diagnostic workup in order to rule out other psychiatric and medical conditions (K. Chang et al., 2015). History and physical examination aid in refining differential diagnosis, ruling out other medical conditions (e.g., Sydenham chorea, autoimmune encephalitis, neuropsychiatric lupus), and other neuropsychiatric conditions (e.g., anorexia nervosa, Tourette syndrome). Collecting a family history provides important clues to psychiatric, medical, and genetic susceptibilities (K. Chang et al., 2015). Laboratory evaluations and physical exam may uncover inflammatory markers suggesting a defined inflammatory disease (e.g. celiac disease, systemic lupus, JIA); however, the absence of standard inflammatory markers does not preclude an early inflammatory process or brain specific process (Turina et al., 2017). Brain magnetic resonance imaging and cerebral spinal fluid evaluation may be indicated when certain neurologic signs and symptoms are present (e.g., focal neurologic symptoms, chorea, encephalopathy, epilepsy, marked headaches, gait disturbances, cognitive deterioration, memory impairment, or psychosis) or when other conditions are suspected (e.g., lupus, autoimmune encephalitis) (K. Chang et al., 2015).

Pathophysiology and Research

The prevailing model of PANS/PANDAS posits that symptoms result from an aberrant immune response to an infectious trigger. Specifically, it is thought that cortico-basal ganglia-thalamo-cortical (CBGTC) circuities become disrupted by poly-reactive antibodies. These antibodies, which are generated to fight the infectious trigger, cross-react with CNS targets and breach a compromised blood-brain barrier; they then bind to non-neuronal and neuronal cells and neurotransmitter receptors, primarily within the basal ganglia, leading to the resultant symptoms. Currently, there are no specific, reliable diagnostic and predictive biomarkers. Nevertheless, antibody studies (Brimberg et al., 2012; Chain et al., 2020; Cox et al., 2015; Hoffman et al., 2004; Kirvan, Swedo, Snider, et al., 2006; Xu et al., 2021), imaging studies (Cabrera et al., 2019; Giedd et al., 2000; Kumar et al., 2015; Zheng et al., 2020), and response to immunomodulation (Perlmutter et al., 1999) support this proposed pathogenic model.

Elevated levels of autoantibodies have been reported in several studies. Specifically, antineuronal autoantibodies and CaMKII activation in both

Table 13.2 Examples of systemic autoimmune diseases, arthritis, and co-morbid psychiatric manifestations

Disease	Autoimmune Disease Manifestations	Reported Psychiatric, Behavioral, and Cognitive Manifestations
Antiphospholipid Antibody Syndrome (APS) (Lim, 2009; Petri, 2000)	Characterized by: antiphospholipid antibodies increased risk of blood clot formation (arterial or venous), thrombocytopenia, miscarriage Age of onset: most often adulthood and in conjunction with lupus (including childhood-onset) (Wincup & Ioannou, 2018) Additional findings (variably present): • migraines • memory loss/dementia • seizures • chorea Suspected infectious triggers: Multiple viral and bacterial pathogens but no definitive links (Blank et al., 2004; Zinger et al., 2009)	Cognitive impairment[++], depression[++], psychosis[++] (Hallab et al., 2018; Panopoulos et al., 2021)
Behçet's Disease (Alpsoy et al., 2007)	Characterized by: recurrent oral and/or genital ulcers; vasculitis of small, medium, large vessels of arteries and veins Age of onset: most often early adulthood, childhood-onset is subtle and often missed Additional findings (variably present): • headaches, aseptic meningitis or meningoencephalitis, seizures, palsies, stroke. • occular disease including uveitis and retinal vasculitis • myocarditis, endocarditis, aneurysm • gastrointestinal ulcers, pain, anorexia, diarrhea • arthralgia or transient arthritis • cutaneous lesions (erythema nodosum, pseudofolliculitius, and acneiform nodules, and others) • pathergy	Anxiety[++], bipolar disorder[+++], depression[+++], **obsessive-compulsive symptoms**, personality changes, sleep disorder[++] (Calikoglu et al., 2001; Dursun et al., 2007; Talarico et al., 2018)

Disease	Autoimmune Disease Manifestations	Reported Psychiatric, Behavioral, and Cognitive Manifestations
Celiac Disease (Fasano, 2005; Green et al., 2005; Lubrano et al., 1996; Pastore et al., 2007)	Characterized by: gluten-triggered enteropathy presenting as diarrhea, constipation, abdominal distention/bloating Age of onset: most often early childhood and middle adulthood Additional findings (variably present): <ul><li>mucocutaneous symptoms (dermatitis herpetiformis, oral lesions, and atrophic glossitis)</li><li>arthritis</li><li>anemia</li><li>delayed growth</li><li>osteopenia</li></ul>Suspected infectious triggers: Enterovirus (Kahrs et al., 2019), adenovirus and hepatitis C (Plot & Amital, 2009)	Pediatrics: Anorexia, depression, **obsessive-compulsive symptoms**, schizophrenia Adults: Depression[+++] (Ciacci et al., 1998; Efe & Tok, 2023; Fasano, 2005; Kalaydjian et al., 2006)
Inflammatory Bowel Disease (IBD), including Crohns disease and ulcerative colitis (Seyedian et al., 2019)	Characterized by: episodic or chronic inflammation of the gastrointestinal tract presenting as abdominal pain/cramping, alternating constipation and diarrhea, bloody stools, fecal urgency Age of onset: childhood or adulthood Additional findings (variably present): <ul><li>oral or rectal ulcers</li><li>anemia</li><li>growth failure</li><li>arthritis, sacralillitis, back pain</li><li>cutaneous lesions (erythema nodosum or pyoderma gangrenosum).</li></ul>Suspected infectious triggers: no definitive infections linked with disease onset, although commensal microbe changes are noted (Mann & Saeed, 2012)	Anxiety[++], bipolar disorder[+], depression[++], schizophrenia[+] (Bernstein et al., 2019; Kao et al., 2019; Sung et al., 2022; Tribbick et al., 2015)

Disease	Autoimmune Disease Manifestations	Reported Psychiatric, Behavioral, and Cognitive Manifestations
Juvenile Idiopathic Arthritis (JIA) (Armstrong & Read, 2020; Ravelli & Martini, 2007; Weiss et al., 2012)	JIA encompasses all forms of juvenile arthritis. Characterization of subtypes include: • Enthesitis-related arthritis (ERA) and spondyloarthritis: arthritis, enthesitis, sacroiliac joint tenderness, inflammatory back pain, uveitis, HLA B27 • Psoriatic arthritis: arthritis, patient or first-degree relative with psoriatic rash, dactylitis, nail pitting • Oligoarthritis or polyarthritis: positive or negative rheumatoid factor [RF] • Systemic arthritis: arthritis, daily fever, evanescent rash, serositis, lymphadenopathy, hepato- or splenomegaly, high ferritin Age of onset: before age 16 years Suspected infectious triggers: no specific infections identified, although seasonality in diagnoses has been noted (Mellins et al., 2011)	Anxiety[+], depression[+], **obsessive-compulsive symptoms[+]**, PANS, psychotic disorders[+], somatic disturbances/disorders[+] (Fair et al., 2019; Kyllönen et al., 2021; Hanns et al., 2018; McHugh et al., 2022; Ma et al., 2023)
Psoriasis (Armstrong & Read, 2020; Raychaudhuri et al., 2014)	Characterized by: dry, raised skin patches covered with silver scales with varying patterns (e.g., plaque, pustular, erythrodermic, inverse, and guttate) Age of onset: all Additional findings (variably present): • nail pitting, onycholysis, nail discoloration and thickening • arthritis, enthesitis, dactylitis • increased risk for inflammatory bowel disease, cardiovascular disease Suspected infectious triggers: guttate psoriasis, GAS, or respiratory infection. (Fry & Baker, 2007)	Alcohol dependence[++], anxiety[++], bipolar disorder[+], depression[+++], schizophrenia[+], somatic disturbances/disorders[+] (Ferreira et al., 2016; Kimball et al., 2012)

Disease	Autoimmune Disease Manifestations	Reported Psychiatric, Behavioral, and Cognitive Manifestations
Rheumatoid Arthritis (RA) (Grassi et al., 1998)	Characterized by: insidious onset of joint pain, stiffness, swelling, and tenderness (primarily hands, feet, wrists, ankles) Age of onset: 16 years and up, primarily middle adulthood Additional findings (variably present): • fever, fatigue, weight loss • anemia • vasculitis (cutaneous ulcers, necrosis, scleritis, neuropathy/ mononeuritis multiplex) • cardiopulmonary disease (e.g., pericarditis, myocarditis, interstitial lung disease) • rheumatoid nodules • Raynaud's phenomenon (blood flow restriction in fingertips and/or toes) Suspected infectious triggers: mycobacteria and EBV (Bo et al., 2020)	Anxiety[++], depression[++], **obsessive-compulsive symptoms**[+], schizophrenia[+] (Dickens et al., 2002; Hyphantis et al., 2006; Lok et al., 2010)
Sarcoidosis (Costabel, 2001; Sève et al., 2021)	Characterized by: granulomas (clusters of immune cells) on organs. Commonly, this involves the mediastinal lymph nodes and lungs (diffuse interstitial lung disease). Age of onset: childhood and adulthood Additional findings (variably present): • lesions of the skin, eye, or brain • arrhythmia, conduction abnormalities, heart failure • constitutional symptoms including fatigue, malaise, fever, and weight loss • cough, dyspnea, chest pain Suspected infectious triggers: *M. tuberculosis* (Starshinova et al., 2020)	Anxiety[+], bipolar disorder[+], depression[++], **obsessive-compulsive symptoms**[+] (Goracci et al., 2008)

Disease	Autoimmune Disease Manifestations	Reported Psychiatric, Behavioral, and Cognitive Manifestations
Scleroderma (Ferreli et al., 2017; Gabrielli et al., 2009)	Characterized by: thickening and hardening of skin on the fingers and face, which can spread to the arms, trunk, and legs. Age of onset: primarily 20–50 years Additional findings (variably present): • Raynaud's phenomenon • fibrosis, which can affect organs (heart, esophagus, kidneys, and lungs). • diarrhea, intestinal pseudo-obstruction • nailfold capillary changes Suspected infectious triggers: parvovirus B19, human herpesvirus-6, CMV, and SarsCoV-2 (Ferri et al., 2021)	Anxiety, depression[+++], obsessive-compulsive symptoms, somatic disturbances/disorders (Angelopoulos et al., 2001)
Sjögren's Syndrome (Delalande et al., 2004; Mori et al., 2005; Skopouli et al., 2000).	Characterized by: inflammation of salivary and lacrimal glands, also impacting the kidneys, liver, lungs, and skin Age of onset: most often early (<35 yr) and late (>65 yr) adulthood Additional findings (variably present): • dry mouth and dry eyes (most common symptoms) • autonomic dysfunction • proximal muscle weakness • fatigue, fever • arthritis, arthralgia, myalgia • Raynaud's phenomenon • peripheral neuropathies • interstitial lung disease, dry cough Suspected infectious triggers: Epstein Barr, hepatitis C, and coxsackie viruses (Igoe & Scofield, 2013)	Anxiety[+++], depression[+++], psychosis, sleep disorders[+++], somatic disturbances/disorders (Goulabchand et al., 2022; Hammett et al., 2020)

Disease	Autoimmune Disease Manifestations	Reported Psychiatric, Behavioral, and Cognitive Manifestations
Spondyloar-thritis (Dougados & Baeten, 2011)	Characterized by: back or neck pain worse in morning and/or with stationary positions, alternating buttock pain Age of onset: most often teens to early adulthood Additional findings (variably present): • arthritis of large joints (hips, knees, ankles, shoulders) • enthesitis • uveitis (eye inflammation) • psoriasis • inflammatory bowel disease (IBD) • association with HLA-B27 Suspected infectious triggers: *Yersinia, Salmonella, Campylobacter,* and *Chlamydia* species, as well as HIV and Hepatitis C (Cristea et al., 2019)	Anger/hostility, anxiety, depression, **obsessive-compulsive symptoms**, PANS, self-harm, sleep disturbances[+++], somatic disturbances/disorders, self-harm. (Durmus et al., 2015; Li et al., 2012; Frankovich, Thienemann, Pearlstein, et al., 2015; McHugh et al., 2022)
Sydenham Chorea (SC) (Cardoso, 2011; Dale & Brilot, 2012; Gewitz et al., 2015)	Characterized by: random, irregular, brief, involuntary movements of limbs/face, truncal hypotonia, emotional disturbances, psychiatric symptoms Age of onset: 5–15 years Additional findings (variably present): • migratory joint pain • carditis • erythema marginatum • subcutaneous nodules • fever • elevated ESR/CRP • prolonged PR interval on EKG Suspected infectious triggers: GAS	ADD, anxiety[++], depression[++], **obsessive-compulsive symptoms**[+++], schizophrenia (Casanova et al., 1995; Dale & Brilot, 2012; Moreira et al., 2014)

Disease	Autoimmune Disease Manifestations	Reported Psychiatric, Behavioral, and Cognitive Manifestations
Systemic Lupus Erythematosus (SLE) & Neuropsychiatric Lupus (Fayyaz et al., 2015; Kivity et al., 2015)	Characterized by: autoantibodies, immune complex deposition, small vessel vasculitis, and heterogeneous, multisystem involvement Age of onset: late adolescence and young adulthood Additional findings (variably present): • arthritis, fatigue, fever • nonpainful ulcer on hard palate or in nose • rash (malar, discoid, photosensitive rash, etc.) • diffuse hair loss • serositis (pleural effusions, pericardial effusions) • renal disorders (microscopic proteinuria and/or hematuria) • cytopenias (anemia, leukopenia, thrombocytopenia, hemolytic anemia). • autoantibodies (dsDNA, Smith, RNP, antiphospholipid antibody) • headaches, seizures, stroke • psychosis and other psychiatric • vasculitis (brain and other organs) • transverse myelitis • neuropathies Suspected infectious triggers: Epstein–Barr virus, parvovirus B19, and cytomegalovirus (Illescas-Montes et al., 2019)	SLE without meeting criteria for Neuropsychiatric Lupus: Anxiety[+++], cognitive impairment, depression[++ +], **obsessive-compulsive symptoms+**, somatic disturbances/disorders[+] (Carlomagno et al., 2000; Palagini et al., 2013; Tench et al., 2000; Slattery et al., 2004; Bachen et al., 2009; Nery et al., 2008) Neuropsychiatric Lupus: Anxiety[+++], cognitive impairment[+++], depression[+++], psychosis[+] (Kivity et al., 2015; Pego-Reigosa & Isenberg, 2008)

the sera and CSF of patients in the early-acute phase of PANS/PANDAS are elevated compared to controls (Chain et al., 2020). Serum samples from patients with PANS/PANDAS exhibit elevated titers of dopamine D1 and D2 receptor autoantibodies (D1R, D2R) (Cox et al., 2015), lysoganglioside (Cox et al., 2015; Fallon et al., 2020), and tubulin (Kirvan, Swedo, Snider, et al., 2006); importantly, these studies have been difficult to replicate (Dale et al., 2012).

Table 13.3 Examples of Primary Inflammatory brain diseases, symptoms, and psychiatric manifestations

Disease	Inflammatory Brain Disease Manifestations	Reported Psychiatric, Behavioral, and Cognitive Manifestations
Anti-NMDA (N-methyl-D-aspartic acid) Receptor Encephalitis (Chapman & Vause, 2011)	Autoimmune encephalitis associated with autoantibodies against NMDA glutamate receptors in the brain. Symptoms may include: • headache • dyskinesia • autonomic dysfunction • seizures within three months of onset of psychiatric symptoms (typical)	Aggression[+++], anxiety[++], depression[++], hallucinations, memory deficits[+++], psychosis[+++], schizophrenia, somatic disturbances/disorders (Chapman & Vause, 2011; W. Wang et al., 2020)
Basal Ganglia Encephalitis (Dale & Brilot, 2012)	Basal ganglia inflammation resulting in movement abnormalities and psychiatric symptoms. Symptoms may include: • dystonia • choreiform movements • parkinsonism	ADD, emotional lability, psychosis (Dale & Brilot, 2012)
Primary Small vessel vasculitis of the Central Nervous System (CNS) (Salvarani et al., 2007)	Inflammation of small vessels of the brain resulting in non-specific white matter lesions on MRI, meningeal inflammation. Symptoms may include: • headaches • behavior changes • +/- fever	Pediatrics: Cognitive impairment[+++], personality changes[++] Adults: Cognitive impairment[+++] (Benseler et al., 2006; Salvarani et al., 2007; Twilt & Benseler, 2016)
Steroid Responsive Encephalitis associated with Thyroiditis (Schiess & Pardo, 2008)	Waxing and waning psychiatric disorder progressing to seizures which is strongly responsive to steroids and associated with elevated thyroid antibodies but typically normal thyroid function. Symptoms may include: • headache • sleep disturbance • seizures • ataxia • thyroid dysfunction	Bipolar disorder[++], dementia[++], depression[++], hallucinations, psychosis[++], schizophrenia[+], sleep disturbance (Menon et al., 2017; Schiess & Pardo, 2008)

Disease	Inflammatory Brain Disease Manifestations	Reported Psychiatric, Behavioral, and Cognitive Manifestations
Multiple Sclerosis (MS) (Dobson & Giovannoni, 2019; Soldan & Lieberman, 2023)	Relapsing-remitting inflammatory brain disease which targets myelin and results in progressive accumulation of demyelinating lesions in the brain. Epstein-Barr virus is a likely trigger. Symptoms include: • optic neuritis • ataxia • brain or spinal cord lesions visible on MRI	Fatigue, Bipolar disorder[++], cognitive impairment[+++], depression[+++], hallucinations[+++], psychosis[+++], schizophrenia[++], suicidal ideation[++] (Camara-Lemarroy et al., 2017; Feinstein, 2004)
Neuromyelitis Optica (NMO) (Wingerchuk et al., 2007)	Inflammation resulting in damage to the optic nerve and/or spinal cord. Symptoms include: • optic neuritis/vision loss • contiguous spinal segments of myelitis • paraplegia • bladder dysfunction	Anxiety, depression[+++], **obsessive-compulsive symptoms**, suicidal ideation[+++] (Moore et al., 2016)
Pediatric Acute-onset Neuropsychiatric Syndrome (PANS) (Swedo, 2012)	Abrupt-onset **OCD** or eating restriction, accompanied by additional neuropsychiatric symptoms. See Table 13.1 for symptoms.	Anxiety[+++], depression[+++], eating restriction[++], emotional lability[+++], **obsessive-compulsive symptoms**[+++], sensory abnormalities[+++], sleep disturbances[+++], suicidal ideation[+++] (Swedo, 2012)
Pediatric Autoimmune Neuropsychiatric Disorder Associated with Streptococcal Infections (PANDAS) (Swedo, 2012)	Acute-onset **OCD** or tic disorder associated with a GAS infection; in addition to psychiatric symptoms, patients may also develop neurologic symptoms such as choreiform movements or tics. See Table 13.1 for symptoms.	ADD, anxiety[+++], **obsessive-compulsive symptoms**[+++], sensory abnormalities[+++], sleep disturbances[+++], tics[+++] (Dale & Brilot, 2012; Swedo, 2012; Swedo et al., 2015)

Neuroimaging studies further implicate CGBTC circuits in the pathophysiology of PANS/PANDAS, with the most prominent findings being alterations in the basal ganglia. Importantly, studies examining volumetric differences between PANS/PANDAS and control groups are mixed, owing to differences in the subjects' stage and duration of illness.

Initial changes to organs affected by inflammation involve swelling or edema (e.g., nephritis secondary to SLE), while chronic disease is associated with atrophy. Consistent with this, an initial study that limited enrollment to recent-onset PANDAS subjects reported higher volumes of the caudate, putamen, and globus pallidus in patients compared to age- and sex-matched controls (Giedd et al., 2000). On the other hand, a second study that enrolled patients with a range of symptom duration and stage (recent onset [35 percent], chronic [21 percent], flare on chronic [44 percent]) did not find statistically significant volumetric differences, although the range of basal ganglia volumes was greater in the PANS group compared to the controls (Zheng et al., 2020). The link between PANS/PANDAS and neural inflammation is further supported by additional MRI, positron emission tomography (PET), and diffusion weighted imaging studies (Cabrera et al., 2019; Kumar et al., 2015). While neuroimaging techniques are not currently efficacious in aiding the diagnosis or treatment of PANS/PANDAS patients, continued research in this area can enrich our understanding of the pathophysiologic model and may ultimately guide the creation of diagnostic biomarkers.

Prevalence

Abrupt-onset OCD is thought to represent 5 percent of pediatric OCD, which has a child-population prevalence of 1–4 percent (Frick et al., 2018). However, since PANS also includes abrupt-onset restrictive eating, the actual prevalence of PANS is likely higher. Demographic data from several PANS cohorts reveal a slight male predominance and an average age of onset in the range of 6 to 8.5 years (Frankovich, Thienemann, Pearlstein, et al., 2015; Gromark et al., 2019; M. Johnson et al., 2019; Murphy et al., 2007; Swedo et al., 2015). Comorbid autoimmune and/or inflammatory disease include inflammatory back pain, reactive or persistent arthritis, and other immune deficiencies (Calaprice et al., 2017; Frankovich, Thienemann, Pearlstein, et al., 2015) Enthesitis related arthritis has also been reported in patients with PANS/PANDAS (Ma et al., 2023).

Patients with PANS have families with remarkably high incidences of both autoimmune disorders (67–80 percent) and psychiatric disorders (51–78 percent) (Chan et al., 2020; Frankovich, Thienemann, Pearlstein, et al., 2015; Gagliano et al., 2020; Gromark et al., 2019; M. Johnson et al., 2019; Lougee et al., 2000; Murphy et al., 2010), suggesting an inherited vulnerability (Chan et al., 2020; Lougee et al., 2000). Specifically, siblings of patients with PANS have a higher rate of immune disorders compared to controls (Chan et al., 2020), and other first-degree relatives have up to a ten-fold increase in rates of OCD, tic disorders, and acute rheumatic fever (Chan et al., 2020; Lougee et al., 2000).

Treatment

Treatment for PANS/PANDAS is based on the proposed pathophysiology and focuses on three important target areas. First, clinicians should treat confirmed or strongly suspected active infection(s) (e.g., impetigo, ecthyma, GAS pharyngitis, peri-anal GAS, vaginal GAS, sinusitis, otitis media, abscesses, ingrown toenails) and attempt to clear GAS from the home. In addition, clinicians should treat postinfectious inflammation (e. g., corticosteroids, NSAIDS, IVIG) and psychiatric symptoms (e.g., cognitive behavioral therapy [CBT], psychotropic medication) using standard evidence-based interventions (Cooperstock et al., 2017; Frankovich et al., 2017; Nadeau et al., 2015; Storch et al., 2006; Swedo et al., 2017; Thienemann et al., 2017). CBT has been shown to be effective in reducing OCD symptoms in patients with PANS/PANDAS (Nadeau et al., 2015; Storch et al., 2006). While standard evidence-based psychotropic medications are recommended, children with PANS/PANDAS may tolerate lower than typical doses of psychotropic medications (Thienemann et al., 2021).

Autoimmunity, Infection, and OCD

In the past few decades, research examining the link between OCD and autoimmunity has grown, with many studies documenting an association between OCD and well-established autoimmune conditions like systemic lupus erythematosus (SLE) (Bachen et al., 2009; Maciel et al., 2016; Slattery et al., 2004), Sjörgen's syndrome (Y.-J. Chang et al., 2021; Ong et al., 2017), and dermatomyositis (L.-Y. Wang et al., 2019). Individuals with OCD are more likely than unaffected individuals to develop an autoimmune disorder (Mataix-Cols et al., 2018), and there are a number of studies suggesting a link between maternal autoimmune disorders and childhood OCD/tics (Mataix-Cols et al., 2018; Murphy et al., 2010).

We outline several well-established autoimmune disorders and their associated neuropsychiatric symptoms in Table 13.2. Many of these disorders have dermatological and rheumatological presentations, which we also briefly describe. It is possible that patients presenting with obsessive-compulsive and other psychiatric symptoms carry an underlying autoimmune disease(s). Treatment of underlying inflammatory disorders will improve the general health of patients and possibly the psychiatric symptoms. Therefore, it is crucial for these conditions to be considered upon patient intake and re-evaluations.

Symptoms indicated with + are prevalent in <10 percent (+), 10–29 percent (++), or >30 percent (+++) of affected individuals. The absence of + indicates a lack of available data.

In SC and PANS/PANDAS, it is apparent that GAS infections have the capacity to trigger a variety of health complications, including obsessive-compulsive symptoms as well as other neuropsychiatric symptoms. Studies of school-aged children with repeated GAS infections show an increased risk for the development of behavioral, movement, and psychiatric symptoms (Murphy et al., 2007; Orlovska et al., 2017).

In addition to GAS, other pathogens have been associated with new onset or worsened psychiatric symptoms. Non-GAS throat infections have been linked with the development of mental disorders and OCD, but not tics (Orlovska et al., 2017). Supporting this finding are a range of case studies and reports concerning the onset of OCD and tics following *Mycoplasma pneumoniae* (Frankovich, Thienemann, Rana, et al., 2015; Kim et al., 2016) and, more recently, SARS-CoV-2 (COVID-19) (Pavone et al., 2021). It has been estimated that as many as 46.8 percent of COVID-19-affected individuals developed neuropsychiatric sequelae, with the most common being headache, sleep disruption/fatigue, anxiety, mood changes, and memory/attention difficulties (Méndez et al., 2022; Nalleballe et al., 2020; Taquet et al., 2021). One case report describes two pediatric patients who developed acute-onset obsessive-compulsive symptoms within two weeks of infection by COVID-19 (Pavone et al., 2021). It is posited that such symptoms result from virus-triggered neuroinflammation (Vanderheiden & Klein, 2022). These same neuroinflammatory processes are suspected to contribute to the worsening of obsessions and compulsions in COVID-19-affected individuals with preexisting OCD, which has been reported since the early stages of the pandemic (Davide et al., 2020). Together, these observations suggest a link between neuropsychiatric symptoms (including OCD) and post-infectious neuroinflammatory conditions.

A list of inflammatory brain diseases, their symptoms, and their psychiatric manifestations is outlined in Table 13.3. As with Table 13.2, patients with these conditions benefit from early identification and treatment of the underlying inflammation as late diagnosis is associated with long term sequelae (Broadley et al., 2019). The provider should also consider infection history as part of patient intake, especially in cases where the patient reports an abrupt or atypical onset of symptoms, as their symptoms may be related to inflammation.

Symptoms indicated with + are prevalent in <10 percent (+), 10–29 percent (++), or >30 percent (+++) of affected individuals. The absence of + indicates a lack of available data.

Evaluating, diagnosing, and treating infection and autoimmune diseases

Given the association of multiple psychiatric syndromes with inflammation and autoimmunity, it is essential that clinicians consider inflammation as part of the clinical intake with intermittent re-evaluation if signs and symptoms suggest an evolving inflammatory disease. Patients overwhelmed by severe psychiatric symptoms, such as OCD, may not spontaneously report symptoms of inflammation (i.e. arthritis) or infection (i.e. sinusitis) (Ma et al., 2023). Thus, it is important for clinicians to consider these factors during evaluation. Identification and intervention at the early stages of illness will likely result in better outcomes. While some tests for infection and inflammation may be ordered and collected at any laboratory (e.g., blood tests, urine tests), other assays will require the provider to perform an appropriate collection (e.g., throat, nasopharyngeal, and perianal/perivaginal swabs). When infection is considered as part of a patient's illness, the psychiatrist/psychologist should partner with the patient's primary care provider to facilitate a comprehensive infection evaluation. For suspected autoimmune or rheumatologic conditions, the patient and his/her team will benefit from the input of a rheumatologist.

Recognizing Infection

Neuropsychiatric responses to infection have been observed after exposure to a variety of pathogens, the most well-established of which is streptococcus. Streptococcal infection is implicated in SC, PANS/ PANDAS, psoriasis, Behçet's, and other autoimmune diseases. Streptococcal infections, particularily GAS, can present in many forms such as sinusitis, perianal dermatitis, impetigo, ecthyma, and most commonly, pharyngitis.

GAS pharyngitis – or "strep throat" – is characterized by acute-onset sore throat, swallowing difficulties, and throat redness, in the absence of cough or nasal congestion (Cooperstock et al., 2017; Gerber et al., 2009). Palatal petechiae and scarlatiniform rash are 95 percent and 98 percent specific (respectively) for the diagnosis of GAS pharyngitis (Shaikh et al., 2012). The diagnosis of GAS pharyngitis requires either streptococcal rapid antigen testing, culture, or PCR of the throat swab, the collection of which should consist of vigorous swabbing of both tonsils and the posterior pharynx (Cooperstock et al., 2017; Shulman, Bisno, Clegg, Gerber, Kaplan, Lee, Martin, & Van Beneden, 2012). Approximately 15 percent of GAS pharyngeal infections are missed during rapid testing, so negative rapid testing should prompt secondary PCR or culture (Lean et al., 2014). In some cases, GAS infections occur in the absence of clinical symptoms (D. R. Johnson et al., 2010), but more commonly, the psychiatric symptoms present weeks after the GAS infection has resolved. Resolution of GAS infections may be spontaneous which has led many pediatricians to elect to not treat. The concept of asymptomatic carriers of pharyngeal GAS describes a subset of patients who test positive for GAS but have low to no risk of developing suppurtive or non-suppurtive complications and have low likelihood of transmitting infection (Shulman, Bisno, Clegg, Gerber, Kaplan, Lee, Martin, Van Beneden, et al., 2012). However, it may be reasonable to consider any confirmed GAS as a potential contributing factor in patients with neuropsychiatric symptoms even if they have no associated pharyngeal symptoms.

Non-streptococcal infections would be identified by a variety of means depending on the pathogen. Infections that may be detected via rapid or culture swab include staphylococcal infections (like methicillin-resistant staphylococcus aureus), mycoplasma pneumoniae, and viral respiratory pathogens (like COVID-19). Most blood testing for the presence of an infection detects a patient's immune response to a recent or more distant past pathogen exposure (IgM and IgG serology, respectively), and must be interpreted with some caution when attempting to assess causation. Common infections confirmed via serology tests include Epstein Barr virus, borrelia burgdorferi (Lyme), and mycoplasma pneumonia. Recognizing an active infection in a timely manner via examination or testing allows for appropriate antimicrobial treatment, which in turn, may or may not impact the course of illness. Positive serology may reflect a passed, already resolved infection that does not need treatment.

Patients who have unusually frequent recurrent or severe infections including sinopulmonary infections, recurrent skin infections, or infections requiring hospital admission or prolonged antibiotic courses may need an immunodeficiency evaluation or metabolic/mitochondrial evaluation, which can be facilitated through an immunologist.

Physical Examination

As is noted in Table 13.2, several autimmune conditions physically manifest on the skin and in the musculoskeletal system. Distinctive skin lesions may require dermatologic evaluation to help with diagnosis (e.g., SLE, Behçet's disease, sarcoidosis, psoriasis) (Alpsoy et al., 2007; Costabel, 2001; Kaneko et al., 1985; Sève et al., 2021). The most common of these conditions is psoriasis, which is characterized and differentiated into types by lesion appearance and location. The most common type is plaque psoriasis which is characterized by red, scaly patches or plaques on the elbows, knees, scalp, gluteal fold, trunk, behind the ears, and umbilicus (Armstrong & Read, 2020). Patients with psoriasis should also be evaluated for musculoskeletal inflammation, as they are at increased risk for arthritis, including axial (chest, spine, and pelvis), dactylitis (inflammation of fingers/toes), and enthesitis (ligaments and tendons) (Armstrong & Read, 2020). If a patient is suspected to have one of these autoimmune conditions, a thorough dematologic and/or rheumatologic history and examination may identify an underlying disorder and guide treatment. Because autoimmune diseases may present later in life, it is important for providers to consider these conditions throughout the course of their time with the patient, even if autoimmune disease was not evident from initial screenings.

Treatment

Most autoimmune conditions and their associated symptoms are managed by treating immune dysregulation. However, as evidenced in SC and PANS/PANDAS, treatment of underlying inflammation and infection may also improve the psychiatric symptoms.

For SC and post-GAS PANS/PANDAS, treatment involves standard antibiotics targeting GAS infections (e.g., penicillin V, amoxicillin) (Gerber et al., 2009). For individuals with recurring GAS infections or history of GAS-reactive conditions like SC/rheumatic fever and PANS/PANDAS, continued antibiotic prophylaxis is recommended (Cooperstock et al., 2017; Gerber et al., 2009). Duration of prophylaxis depends on patient history, case severity, and communal living situation. For children attending school, it is possible to stop treatment during the summer and resume in the fall. Recurring GAS infections in PANS/PANDAS are known to exacerbate psychiatric symptoms after initial onset, so extended prophylaxis should be considered for patients with suspected ongoing GAS exposures and patients with a history of recurrent GAS infections (Cooperstock et al., 2017).

In the case of other autoimmune neuropsychiatric conditions, there are a range of both bacterial (*Mycoplasma pneumoniae, Lyme borreliosis*) and viral (COVID-19, Epstein-Barr virus) triggers (Cooperstock et al., 2017; Soldan & Lieberman, 2023). Providers should follow standard treatment recommendations upon recognition of any of these infections in association with the onset of psychiatric symptoms; however, most cases may present after resolution of the infection, and thus treatment of the infection may not be needed.

Patients exhibiting repeated or prolonged neuropsychiatric deteriorations (or "flares") may benefit from other treatments as well. NSAIDS and corticosteroids are reported to reduce symptoms and duration of flares (K. Brown et al., 2017; K. D. Brown et al., 2017), but randomized trials are lacking. IVIG can be used as second-line treatment and have been reported to contribute to resolution of symptoms (Hajjari et al., 2022; Melamed et al., 2021), but randomized control trials are conflicting in PANS (Perlmutter et al., 1999; Williams et al., 2016) and lacking in SC. When comorbid inflammatory or autoimmune disorders are identified, immunomodulatory therapies should be based on standard practice for those disorders. Antimicrobial or immune modulation interventions may be considered concurrently with cognitive-behavioral therapy and psychotropic medications. Patients with suspected autoimmune conditions with dermatologic symptoms (e.g., psoriasis) should be referred to a dermatologist for potential topical or systemic therapies and long-term management. Upon suspicion of any of the autoimmune conditions listed in Table 13.2 a referral to rheumatology should be considered for additional evaluation and treatment, as these disorders are multisystemic and chronic.

Patients with suspected encephalitis should be referred for an expedited neurology assessment (MRI, EEG, lumbar puncture), and they may have rapid progression to seizures.

Conclusion

A link between obsessive-compulsive symptoms and inflammatory pathophysiology is supported by research in SC, PANS/PANDAS, as well as other autoimmune conditions. It is important to consider inflammation/autoimmunity during evaluation of OCD in patients, especially if the OCD is unusually severe, atypical, or co-morbid with other findings (rash, joint pains, stiffness, headaches). Severe cases would benefit from a multidisciplinary team assessment in order to expedite and treatment evaluation and treatment.

References

Alpsoy, E., Zouboulis, C. C., & Ehrlich, G. E. (2007). Mucocutaneous lesions of Behcet's disease. *Yonsei Medical Journal*, 48(4), 573–585. doi:10.3349/ymj.2007.48.4.573.

Angelopoulos, N. V., Drosos, A. A., & Moutsopoulos, H. M. (2001). Psychiatric symptoms associated with scleroderma. *Psychotherapy and Psychosomatics*, 70 (3), 145–150. doi:10.1159/000056240.

Armstrong, A. W. & Read, C. (2020). Pathophysiology, Clinical Presentation, and Treatment of Psoriasis: A Review. *JAMA*, 323(19), 1945–1960. doi:10.1001/jama.2020.4006.

Asbahr, F. R., Negrão, A. B., Gentil, V., Zanetta, D. M. T., da Paz, J. A., Marques-Dias, M. J., & Kiss, M. H. (1998). Obsessive-Compulsive and Related Symptoms in Children and Adolescents With Rheumatic Fever With and Without Chorea: A Prospective 6-Month Study. *American Journal of Psychiatry*, 155(8), 1122–1124. doi:10.1176/ajp.155.8.1122.

Bachen, E. A., Chesney, M. A., & Criswell, L. A. (2009). Prevalence of mood and anxiety disorders in women with systemic lupus erythematosus. *Arthritis and Rheumatism*, 61(6), 822–829. doi:10.1002/art.24519.

Ben-Pazi, H., Kroyzer, N., & Hashkes, P. J. (2012). Sydenham's chorea: Long-term immunosuppression for psychiatric symptoms. *Journal of Pediatric Neurology*, 10(3), 211–214. doi:10.3233/JPN-2012-0561.

Benseler, S. M., Silverman, E., Aviv, R. I., Schneider, R., Armstrong, D., Tyrrell, P. N., & deVeber, G. (2006). Primary central nervous system vasculitis in children. *Arthritis & Rheumatism*, 54(4), 1291–1297. doi:10.1002/art.21766.

Bernstein, C. N., Hitchon, C. A., Walld, R., Bolton, J. M., Sareen, J., Walker, J. R., Graff, L. A., Patten, S. B., Singer, A., Lix, L. M., El-Gabalawy, R., Katz, A., Fisk, J. D., Marrie, R. A., & CIHR Team in Defining the Burden and Managing the Effects of Psychiatric Comorbidity in Chronic Immunoinflammatory Disease. (2019). Increased Burden of Psychiatric Disorders in Inflammatory Bowel Disease. *Inflammatory Bowel Diseases*, 25(2), 360–368. doi:10.1093/ibd/izy235.

Blank, M., Asherson, R. A., Cervera, R., & Shoenfeld, Y. (2004). Antiphospholipid Syndrome Infectious Origin. *Journal of Clinical Immunology*, 24(1), 12–23. doi:10.1023/B:JOCI.0000018058.28764.ce.

Bo, M., Jasemi, S., Uras, G., Erre, G. L., Passiu, G., & Sechi, L. A. (2020). Role of Infections in the Pathogenesis of Rheumatoid Arthritis: Focus on Mycobacteria. *Microorganisms*, 8(10), 1459. doi:10.3390/microorganisms8101459.

Brimberg, L., Benhar, I., Mascaro-Blanco, A., Alvarez, K., Lotan, D., Winter, C., Klein, J., Moses, A. E., Somnier, F. E., Leckman, J. F., Swedo, S. E., Cunningham, M. W., & Joel, D. (2012). Behavioral, Pharmacological, and Immunological Abnormalities after Streptococcal Exposure: A Novel Rat Model of Sydenham Chorea and Related Neuropsychiatric Disorders. *Neuropsychopharmacology*, 37(9), Article 9. doi:10.1038/npp.2012.56.

Broadley, J., Seneviratne, U., Beech, P., Buzzard, K., Butzkueven, H., O'Brien, T., & Monif, M. (2019). Prognosticating autoimmune encephalitis: A systematic review. *Journal of Autoimmunity*, 96, 24–34. https://doi.org/10.1016/j.jaut.2018.10.014.

Bronze, M. S. & Dale, J. B. (1993). Epitopes of streptococcal M proteins that evoke antibodies that cross-react with human brain. *The Journal of Immunology*, 151 (5), 2820–2828. doi:10.4049/jimmunol.151.5.2820.

Brown, K. D., Farmer, C., Freeman, G. M., Spartz, E. J., Farhadian, B., Thienemann, M., & Frankovich, J. (2017). Effect of Early and Prophylactic Nonsteroidal Anti-Inflammatory Drugs on Flare Duration in Pediatric Acute-Onset Neuropsychiatric Syndrome: An Observational Study of Patients Followed by an Academic Community-Based Pediatric Acute-Onset Neuropsychiatric Syndrome Clinic. *Journal of Child and Adolescent Psychopharmacology*, 27(7), 619–628. doi:10.1089/cap.2016.0193.

Brown, K., Farmer, C., Farhadian, B., Hernandez, J., Thienemann, M., & Frankovich, J. (2017). Pediatric Acute-Onset Neuropsychiatric Syndrome Response to Oral Corticosteroid Bursts: An Observational Study of Patients in an Academic Community-Based PANS Clinic. *Journal of Child and Adolescent Psychopharmacology*, 27(7), 629–639. doi:10.1089/cap.2016.0139.

Cabrera, B., Romero-Rebollar, C., Jiménez-Ángeles, L., Genis-Mendoza, A. D., Flores, J., Lanzagorta, N., Arroyo, M., de la Fuente-Sandoval, C., Santana, D., Medina-Bañuelos, V., Sacristán, E., & Nicolini, H. (2019). Neuroanatomical features and its usefulness in classification of patients with PANDAS. *CNS Spectrums*, 24(5), 533–543. doi:10.1017/S1092852918001268.

Calaprice, D., Tona, J., Parker-Athill, E. C., & Murphy, T. K. (2017). A Survey of Pediatric Acute-Onset Neuropsychiatric Syndrome Characteristics and Course. *Journal of Child and Adolescent Psychopharmacology*, 27(7), 607–618. doi:10.1089/cap.2016.0105.

Calikoglu, E., Onder, M., Cosar, B., & Candansayar, S. (2001). Depression, anxiety levels and general psychological profile in Behçet's disease. *Dermatology (Basel, Switzerland)*, 203(3), 238–240. doi:10.1159/000051756.

Camara-Lemarroy, C. R., Ibarra-Yruegas, B. E., Rodriguez-Gutierrez, R., Berrios-Morales, I., Ionete, C., & Riskind, P. (2017). The varieties of psychosis in multiple sclerosis: A systematic review of cases. *Multiple Sclerosis and Related Disorders*, 12, 9–14. doi:10.1016/j.msard.2016.12.012.

Cardoso, F. (2011). Chapter 14—Sydenham's chorea. In W. J. Weiner & E. Tolosa (Eds), *Handbook of Clinical Neurology* (Vol. 100, pp. 221–229). Elsevier. doi:10.1016/B978-0-444-52014-2.00014-8.

Cardoso, F., Eduardo, C., Silva, A. P., & Mota, C. C. C. (1997). Chorea in fifty consecutive patients with rheumatic fever. *Movement Disorders*, 12(5), 701–703. doi:10.1002/mds.870120512.

Cardoso, F., Maia, D., Cunningham, M. C. Q. S., & Valença, G. (2003). Treatment of Sydenham chorea with corticosteroids. *Movement Disorders*, 18(11), 1374–1377. doi:10.1002/mds.10521.

Cardoso, F., Seppi, K., Mair, K. J., Wenning, G. K., & Poewe, W. (2006). Seminar on choreas. *The Lancet Neurology*, 5(7), 589–602. doi:10.1016/S1474-4422(06)70494-X.

Carlomagno, S., Migliaresi, S., Ambrosone, L., Sannino, M., Sanges, G., & Di Iorio, G. (2000). Cognitive impairment in systemic lupus erythematosus: A follow-up study. *Journal of Neurology*, 247(4), 273–279. doi:10.1007/s004150050583.

Casanova, M. F., Crapanzano, K. A., Mannheim, G., & Kruesi, M. (1995). Sydenham's chorea and schizophrenia: A case report. *Schizophrenia Research*, 16(1), 73–76. doi:10.1016/0920-9964(95)00004-00006.

Chain, J. L., Alvarez, K., Mascaro-Blanco, A., Reim, S., Bentley, R., Hommer, R., Grant, P., Leckman, J. F., Kawikova, I., Williams, K., Stoner, J. A., Swedo, S. E., & Cunningham, M. W. (2020). Autoantibody Biomarkers for Basal Ganglia Encephalitis in Sydenham Chorea and Pediatric Autoimmune Neuropsychiatric Disorder Associated With Streptococcal Infections. *Frontiers in Psychiatry*, 11, 564. doi:10.3389/fpsyt.2020.00564.

Chan, A., Phu, T., Farhadian, B., Willett, T., Thienemann, M., & Frankovich, J. (2020). Familial Clustering of Immune-Mediated Diseases in Children with Abrupt-Onset Obsessive Compulsive Disorder. *Journal of Child and Adolescent Psychopharmacology*, 30(5), 345–346. doi:10.1089/cap.2019.0167.

Chang, K., Frankovich, J., Cooperstock, M., Cunningham, M. W., Latimer, M. E., Murphy, T. K., Pasternack, M., Thienemann, M., Williams, K., Walter, J., Swedo, S. E., & PANS Collaborative Consortium. (2015). Clinical evaluation of youth with pediatric acute-onset neuropsychiatric syndrome (PANS): Recommendations from the 2013 PANS Consensus Conference. *Journal of Child and Adolescent Psychopharmacology*, 25(1), 3–13. https://doi.org/10.1089/cap.2014.0084.

Chang, Y.-J., Tseng, J.-C., Leong, P.-Y., Wang, Y.-H., & Wei, J. C.-C. (2021). Increased Risk of Sjögren's Syndrome in Patients with Obsessive-Compulsive Disorder: A Nationwide Population-Based Cohort Study. *International Journal of Environmental Research and Public Health*, 18(11), 5936. doi:10.3390/ijerph18115936.

Chapman, M. R. & Vause, H. E. (2011). Anti-NMDA Receptor Encephalitis: Diagnosis, Psychiatric Presentation, and Treatment. *American Journal of Psychiatry*, 168(3), 245–251. doi:10.1176/appi.ajp.2010.10020181.

Ciacci, C., Iavarone, A., Mazzacca, G., & De Rosa, A. (1998). Depressive symptoms in adult coeliac disease. *Scandinavian Journal of Gastroenterology*, 33(3), 247–250. doi:10.1080/00365529850170801.

Cooperstock, M. S., Swedo, S. E., Pasternack, M. S., & Murphy, T. K. (2017). Clinical Management of Pediatric Acute-Onset Neuropsychiatric Syndrome:

Part III—Treatment and Prevention of Infections. *Journal of Child and Adolescent Psychopharmacology*, 27(7), 594–606. doi:10.1089/cap.2016.0151.

Costabel, U. (2001). Sarcoidosis: Clinical update. *European Respiratory Journal*, 18 (32 suppl), 56S–68S. doi:10.1183/09031936.01.18s320056.

Cox, C. J., Zuccolo, A. J., Edwards, E. V., Mascaro-Blanco, A., Alvarez, K., Stoner, J., Chang, K., & Cunningham, M. W. (2015). Antineuronal Antibodies in a Heterogeneous Group of Youth and Young Adults with Tics and Obsessive-Compulsive Disorder. *Journal of Child and Adolescent Psychopharmacology*, 25 (1), 76–85. doi:10.1089/cap.2014.0048.

Cristea, D., Trandafir, M., Bojinca, V. C., Ciontea, A. S., Andrei, M. M., Popa, A., Lixandru, B. E., Militaru, C. M., Nascutiu, A. M., Predeteanu, D., Ionescu, R., Popescu, C., Cotar, A. I., Popa, M. I., Spandidos, D. A., & Codita, I. (2019). Usefulness of complex bacteriological and serological analysis in patients with spondyloarthritis. *Experimental and Therapeutic Medicine*, 17(5), 3465–3476. doi:10.3892/etm.2019.7336.

Cunningham, M. W. (2019). Molecular Mimicry, Autoimmunity, and Infection: The Cross-Reactive Antigens of Group A Streptococci and their Sequelae. *Microbiology Spectrum*, 7(4), 7. 4. 20. doi:10.1128/microbiolspec.GPP3-0045-2018.

Cutforth, T., DeMille, M. M., Agalliu, I., & Agalliu, D. (2016). CNS autoimmune disease after Streptococcus pyogenes infections: Animal models, cellular mechanisms and genetic factors. *Future Neurology*, 11(1), 63–76. doi:10.2217/fnl.16.4.

Dajani, A. S., Ayoub, E., Bierman, F. Z., Bisno, A. L., Denny, F. W., Durack, D. T., Ferrieri, P., Freed, M., Gerber, M., Kaplan, E. L., Karchmer, A. W., Markowitz, M., Rahimtoola, S. H., Shulman, S. T., Stollerman, G., Takahashi, M., Taranta, A., Taubert, K. A., Wilson, W., & Durack. (1992). Guidelines for the Diagnosis of Rheumatic Fever: Jones Criteria, 1992 Update. *JAMA*, 268(15), 2069–2073. doi:10.1001/jama.1992.03490150121036.

Dale, R. C. & Brilot, F. (2012). Autoimmune Basal Ganglia Disorders. *Journal of Child Neurology*, 27(11), 1470–1481. doi:10.1177/0883073812451327.

Dale, R. C., Church, A. J., Cardoso, F., Goddard, E., Cox, T. C., Chong, W. K."Kling," Williams, A., Klein, N. J., Neville, B. G., Thompson, E. J., & Giovannoni, G. (2001). Poststreptococcal acute disseminated encephalomyelitis with basal ganglia involvement and auto-reactive antibasal ganglia antibodies. *Annals of Neurology*, 50(5), 588–595. doi:10.1002/ana.1250.

Dale, R. C., Merheb, V., Pillai, S., Wang, D., Cantrill, L., Murphy, T. K., Ben-Pazi, H., Varadkar, S., Aumann, T. D., Horne, M. K., Church, A. J., Fath, T., & Brilot, F. (2012). Antibodies to surface dopamine-2 receptor in autoimmune movement and psychiatric disorders. *Brain*, 135(11), 3453–3468. doi:10.1093/brain/aws256.

Davide, P., Andrea, P., Martina, O., Andrea, E., Davide, D., & Mario, A. (2020). The impact of the COVID-19 pandemic on patients with OCD: Effects of contamination symptoms and remission state before the quarantine in a preliminary naturalistic study. *Psychiatry Research*, 291, 113213. https://doi.org/10.1016/j.psychres.2020.113213.

Dean, S. L. & Singer, H. S. (2017). Treatment of Sydenham's Chorea: A Review of the Current Evidence. *Tremor and Other Hyperkinetic Movements*, 7, 456. doi:10.7916/D8W95GJ2.

Delalande, S., de Seze, J., Fauchais, A.-L., Hachulla, E., Stojkovic, T., Ferriby, D., Dubucquoi, S., Pruvo, J.-P., Vermersch, P., & Hatron, P.-Y. (2004). Neurologic manifestations in primary Sjögren syndrome: A study of 82 patients. *Medicine*, 83(5), 280–291. doi:10.1097/01.md.0000141099.53742.16.

Dickens, C., McGowan, L., Clark-Carter, D., & Creed, F. (2002). Depression in rheumatoid arthritis: A systematic review of the literature with meta-analysis. *Psychosomatic Medicine*, 64(1), 52–60. doi:10.1097/00006842-200201000-00008.

Dobson, R. & Giovannoni, G. (2019). Multiple sclerosis—A review. *European Journal of Neurology*, 26(1), 27–40. doi:10.1111/ene.13819.

Dougados, M. & Baeten, D. (2011). Spondyloarthritis. *The Lancet*, 377(9783), 2127–2137. doi:10.1016/S0140-6736(11)60071–60078.

Durmus, D., Sarisoy, G., Alayli, G., Kesmen, H., Çetin, E., Bilgici, A., Kuru, O., & Ünal, M. (2015). Psychiatric symptoms in ankylosing spondylitis: Their relationship with disease activity, functional capacity, pain and fatigue. *Comprehensive Psychiatry*, 62, 170–177. doi:10.1016/j.comppsych.2015.07.016.

Dursun, R., Uguz, F., Kaya, N., Savas Cilli, A., & Endogru, H. (2007). Psychiatric disorders in patients with Behçet's disease. *International Journal of Psychiatry in Clinical Practice*, 11(1), 16–20. doi:10.1080/13651500600811438.

Efe, A. & Tok, A. (2023). Obsessive–Compulsive Symptomatology and Disgust Propensity in Disordered Eating Behaviors of Adolescents with Celiac Disease. *International Journal of Behavioral Medicine*. doi:10.1007/s12529-023-10163-4.

Fair, D. C., Rodriguez, M., Knight, A. M., & Rubinstein, T. B. (2019). Depression And Anxiety In Patients With Juvenile Idiopathic Arthritis: Current Insights And Impact On Quality Of Life, A Systematic Review. *Open Access Rheumatology: Research and Reviews*, 11, 237–252. doi:10.2147/OARRR.S174408.

Fallon, B. A., Strobino, B., Reim, S., Stoner, J., & Cunningham, M. W. (2020). Anti-lysoganglioside and other anti-neuronal autoantibodies in post-treatment Lyme Disease and Erythema Migrans after repeat infection. *Brain, Behavior, & Immunity – Health*, 2, 100015. doi:10.1016/j.bbih.2019.100015.

Fasano, A. (2005). Clinical presentation of celiac disease in the pediatric population. *Gastroenterology*, 128(4 Suppl 1), S68–73. doi:10.1053/j.gastro.2005.02.015.

Faustino, P. C., Terreri, M. T. R. A., da Rocha, A. J., Zappitelli, M. C., Lederman, H. M., & Hilário, M. O. E. (2003). Clinical, laboratory, psychiatric and magnetic resonance findings in patients with Sydenham chorea. *Neuroradiology*, 45(7), 456–462. doi:10.1007/s00234-003-0999-8.

Fayyaz, A., Igoe, A., Kurien, B. T., Danda, D., James, J. A., Stafford, H. A., & Scofield, R. H. (2015). Haematological manifestations of lupus. *Lupus Science & Medicine*, 2(1), e000078. doi:10.1136/lupus-2014-000078.

Feinstein, A. (2004). The Neuropsychiatry of Multiple Sclerosis. *The Canadian Journal of Psychiatry*, 49(3), 157–163. doi:10.1177/070674370404900302.

Ferreira, B. I. R. C., Abreu, J. L. P. D. C., Reis, J. P. G. D., & Figueiredo, A. M. D. C. (2016). Psoriasis and Associated Psychiatric Disorders: A Systematic Review on Etiopathogenesis and Clinical Correlation. *The Journal of Clinical and Aesthetic Dermatology*, 9(6), 36–43.

Ferreli, C., Gasparini, G., Parodi, A., Cozzani, E., Rongioletti, F., & Atzori, L. (2017). Cutaneous Manifestations of Scleroderma and Scleroderma-Like Disorders: A Comprehensive Review. *Clinical Reviews in Allergy & Immunology*, 53(3), 306–336. doi:10.1007/s12016-017-8625-4.

Ferri, C., Arcangeletti, M.-C., Caselli, E., Zakrzewska, K., Maccari, C., Calderaro, A., D'Accolti, M., Soffritti, I., Arvia, R., Sighinolfi, G., Artoni, E., & Giuggioli, D. (2021). Insights into the knowledge of complex diseases: Environmental infectious/toxic agents as potential etiopathogenetic factors of systemic sclerosis. *Journal of Autoimmunity*, 124, 102727. doi:10.1016/j.jaut.2021.102727.

Frankovich, J., Swedo, S., Murphy, T., Dale, R. C., Agalliu, D., Williams, K., Daines, M., Hornig, M., Chugani, H., Sanger, T., Muscal, E., Pasternack, M., Cooperstock, M., Gans, H., Zhang, Y., Cunningham, M., Bernstein, G., Bromberg, R., Willett, T., ... Thienemann, M. (2017). Clinical Management of Pediatric Acute-Onset Neuropsychiatric Syndrome: Part II—Use of Immunomodulatory Therapies. *Journal of Child and Adolescent Psychopharmacology*, 27 (7), 574–593. doi:10.1089/cap.2016.0148.

Frankovich, J., Thienemann, M., Pearlstein, J., Crable, A., Brown, K., & Chang, K. (2015). Multidisciplinary Clinic Dedicated to Treating Youth with Pediatric Acute-Onset Neuropsychiatric Syndrome: Presenting Characteristics of the First 47 Consecutive Patients. *Journal of Child and Adolescent Psychopharmacology*, 25(1), 38–47. doi:10.1089/cap.2014.0081.

Frankovich, J., Thienemann, M., Rana, S., & Chang, K. (2015). Five Youth with Pediatric Acute-Onset Neuropsychiatric Syndrome of Differing Etiologies. *Journal of Child and Adolescent Psychopharmacology*, 25(1), 31–37. doi:10.1089/cap.2014.0056.

Frick, L. R., Rapanelli, M., Jindachomthong, K., Grant, P., Leckman, J. F., Swedo, S., Williams, K., & Pittenger, C. (2018). Differential binding of antibodies in PANDAS patients to cholinergic interneurons in the striatum. *Brain, Behavior, and Immunity*, 69, 304–311. doi:10.1016/j.bbi.2017.12.004.

Fry, L. & Baker, B. S. (2007). Triggering psoriasis: The role of infections and medications. *Clinics in Dermatology*, 25(6), 606–615. doi:10.1016/j.clindermatol.2007.08.015.

Gabrielli, A., Avvedimento, E. V., & Krieg, T. (2009). Scleroderma. *New England Journal of Medicine*, 360(19), 1989–2003. doi:10.1056/NEJMra0806188.

Gagliano, A., Galati, C., Ingrassia, M., Ciuffo, M., Alquino, M. A., Tanca, M. G., Carucci, S., Zuddas, A., & Grossi, E. (2020). Pediatric Acute-Onset Neuropsychiatric Syndrome: A Data Mining Approach to a Very Specific Constellation of Clinical Variables. *Journal of Child and Adolescent Psychopharmacology*, 30(8), 495–511. doi:10.1089/cap.2019.0165.

Garvey, M. A., & Swedo, S. E. (1997). Sydenham's Chorea Clinical and Therapeutic Update. In T. Horaud, A. Bouvet, R. Leclercq, H. de Montclos, & M. Sicard (Eds), *Streptococci and the Host* (pp. 115–120). Springer US. doi:10.1007/978-1-4899-1825-3_28.

Gerber, M. A., Baltimore, R. S., Eaton, C. B., Gewitz, M., Rowley, A. H., Shulman, S. T., & Taubert, K. A. (2009). Prevention of Rheumatic Fever and Diagnosis and Treatment of Acute Streptococcal Pharyngitis. *Circulation*, 119 (11), 1541–1551. doi:10.1161/CIRCULATIONAHA.109.191959.

Gewitz, M. H., Baltimore, R. S., Tani, L. Y., Sable, C. A., Shulman, S. T., Carapetis, J., Remenyi, B., Taubert, K. A., Bolger, A. F., Beerman, L., Mayosi, B. M., Beaton, A., Pandian, N. G., Kaplan, E. L., & American Heart Association Committee on Rheumatic Fever, Endocarditis, and Kawasaki Disease of the Council on Cardiovascular Disease in the Young. (2015). Revision of the Jones

Criteria for the diagnosis of acute rheumatic fever in the era of Doppler echo-cardiography: A scientific statement from the American Heart Association. *Circulation*, 131(20), 1806–1818. doi:10.1161/CIR.0000000000000205.

Giedd, J. N., Rapoport, J. L., Garvey, M. A., Perlmutter, S., & Swedo, S. E. (2000). MRI assessment of children with obsessive-compulsive disorder or tics associated with streptococcal infection. *The American Journal of Psychiatry*, 157(2), 281–283. doi:10.1176/appi.ajp.157.2.281.

Gilbert, D. L. (2022). Sydenham chorea. In M. C. Patterson, S. L. Kaplan, & R. Sundel (Eds), *UptoDate*. www.uptodate.com/contents/sydenham-chorea?search= sydenham%20chorea&source=search_result&selectedTitle=1~12&usage_type= default&display_rank=1#H8.

Goracci, A., Fagiolini, A., Martinucci, M., Calossi, S., Rossi, S., Santomauro, T., Mazzi, A., Penza, F., Fossi, A., Bargagli, E., Pieroni, M. G., Rottoli, P., & Castrogiovanni, P. (2008). Quality of life, anxiety and depression in sarcoidosis. *General Hospital Psychiatry*, 30(5), 441–445. doi:10.1016/j. genhosppsych.2008.04.010.

Goulabchand, R., Castille, E., Navucet, S., Etchecopar-Etchart, D., Matos, A., Maria, A., Gutierrez, L. A., Le Quellec, A., de Champfleur, N. M., Gabelle, A., & Guilpain, P. (2022). The interplay between cognition, depression, anxiety, and sleep in primary Sjogren's syndrome patients. *Scientific Reports*, 12(1), Article 1. doi:10.1038/s41598-022-17354-1.

Grassi, W., De Angelis, R., Lamanna, G., & Cervini, C. (1998). The clinical features of rheumatoid arthritis. *European Journal of Radiology, 27 Suppl* 1, S18–24. doi:10.1016/s0720-048x(98)00038-00032.

Green, P. H. R., Rostami, K., & Marsh, M. N. (2005). Diagnosis of coeliac disease. *Best Practice & Research. Clinical Gastroenterology*, 19(3), 389–400. doi:10.1016/j.bpg.2005.02.006.

Gromark, C., Harris, R. A., Wickström, R., Horne, A., Silverberg-Mörse, M., Serlachius, E., & Mataix-Cols, D. (2019). Establishing a Pediatric Acute-Onset Neuropsychiatric Syndrome Clinic: Baseline Clinical Features of the Pediatric Acute-Onset Neuropsychiatric Syndrome Cohort at Karolinska Institutet. *Journal of Child and Adolescent Psychopharmacology*, 29(8), 625–633. doi:10.1089/ cap.2018.0127.

Gurkas, E., Karalok, Z. S., Taskin, B. D., Aydogmus, U., Guven, A., Degerliyurt, A., Bektas, O., & Yilmaz, C. (2016). Predictors of recurrence in Sydenham's chorea: Clinical observation from a single center. *Brain and Development*, 38(9), 827–834. doi:10.1016/j.braindev.2016.04.010.

Hajjari, P., Oldmark, M. H., Fernell, E., Jakobsson, K., Vinsa, I., Thorsson, M., Monemi, M., Stenlund, L., Fasth, A., Furuhjelm, C., Johnels, J. Å., Gillberg, C., & Johnson, M. (2022). Paediatric Acute-onset Neuropsychiatric Syndrome (PANS) and intravenous immunoglobulin (IVIG): Comprehensive open-label trial in ten children. *BMC Psychiatry*, 22(1), 535. doi:10.1186/s12888-022-04181-x.

Hallab, A., Naveed, S., Altibi, A., Abdelkhalek, M., Ngo, H. T., Le, T. P., Hirayama, K., & Huy, N. T. (2018). Association of psychosis with antiphospholipid antibody syndrome: A systematic review of clinical studies. *General Hospital Psychiatry*, 50, 137–147. doi:10.1016/j.genhosppsych.2017.11.005.

Hammett, E. K., Fernandez-Carbonell, C., Crayne, C., Boneparth, A., Cron, R. Q., & Radhakrishna, S. M. (2020). Adolescent Sjogren's syndrome presenting as psychosis: A case series. *Pediatric Rheumatology*, 18(1), 15. doi:10.1186/s12969-020-0412-8.

Hanns, L., Cordingley, L., Galloway, J., Norton, S., Carvalho, L. A., Christie, D., Sen, D., Carrasco, R., Rashid, A., Foster, H., Baildam, E., Chieng, A., Davidson, J., Wedderburn, L. R., Hyrich, K., Thomson, W., & Ioannou, Y. (2018). Depressive symptoms, pain and disability for adolescent patients with juvenile idiopathic arthritis: Results from the Childhood Arthritis Prospective Study. *Rheumatology (Oxford, England)*, 57(8), 1381–1389. doi:10.1093/rheumatology/key088.

Hermann, A. & Walker, R. H. (2015). Diagnosis and Treatment of Chorea Syndromes. *Current Neurology and Neuroscience Reports*, 15(2), 1. https://doi.org/10.1007/s11910-014-0514-0.

Hoffman, K. L., Hornig, M., Yaddanapudi, K., Jabado, O., & Lipkin, W. I. (2004). A murine model for neuropsychiatric disorders associated with group A beta-hemolytic streptococcal infection. *The Journal of Neuroscience: The Official Journal of the Society for Neuroscience*, 24(7), 1780–1791. doi:10.1523/JNEUROSCI.0887-03.2004.

Husby, G., van de Rijn, I., Zabriskie, J. B., Abdin, Z. H., & Williams, R. C., Jr. (1976). Antibodies reacting with cytoplasm of subthalamic and caudate nuclei neurons in chorea and acute rheumatic fever. *Journal of Experimental Medicine*, 144(4), 1094–1110. doi:10.1084/jem.144.4.1094.

Hyphantis, T. N., Bai, M., Siafaka, V., Georgiadis, A. N., Voulgari, P. V., Mavreas, V., & Drosos, A. A. (2006). Psychological distress and personality traits in early rheumatoid arthritis: A preliminary survey. *Rheumatology International*, 26(9), 828–836. doi:10.1007/s00296-005-0086-z.

Igoe, A. & Scofield, R. H. (2013). Autoimmunity and infection in Sjögren's syndrome. *Current Opinion in Rheumatology*, 25(4), 480–487. doi:10.1097/BOR.0b013e32836200d2.

Illescas-Montes, R., Corona-Castro, C. C., Melguizo-Rodríguez, L., Ruiz, C., & Costela-Ruiz, V. J. (2019). Infectious processes and systemic lupus erythematosus. *Immunology*, 158(3), 153–160. doi:10.1111/imm.13103.

Johnson, D. R., Kurlan, R., Leckman, J., & Kaplan, E. L. (2010). The human immune response to streptococcal extracellular antigens: Clinical, diagnostic, and potential pathogenetic implications. *Clinical Infectious Diseases: An Official Publication of the Infectious Diseases Society of America*, 50(4), 481–490. doi:10.1086/650167.

Johnson, M., Fernell, E., Preda, I., Wallin, L., Fasth, A., Gillberg, C., & Gillberg, C. (2019). Paediatric acute-onset neuropsychiatric syndrome in children and adolescents: An observational cohort study. *The Lancet. Child & Adolescent Health*, 3(3), 175–180. doi:10.1016/S2352-4642(18)30404-30408.

Jordan, L. C. & Singer, H. S. (2003). Sydenham chorea in children. *Current Treatment Options in Neurology*, 5(4), 283–290. doi:10.1007/s11940-003-0034-8.

Kahrs, C. R., Chuda, K., Tapia, G., Stene, L. C., Mårild, K., Rasmussen, T., Rønningen, K. S., Lundin, K. E. A., Kramna, L., Cinek, O., & Størdal, K. (2019). Enterovirus as trigger of coeliac disease: Nested case-control study within prospective birth cohort. *BMJ (Clinical Research Ed.)*, 364, l231. doi:10.1136/bmj.l231.

Kalaydjian, A. E., Eaton, W., Cascella, N., & Fasano, A. (2006). The gluten connection: The association between schizophrenia and celiac disease. *Acta Psychiatrica Scandinavica*, 113(2), 82–90. doi:10.1111/j.1600-0447.2005.00687.x.

Kaneko, F., Takahashi, Y., Muramatsu, Y., & Miura, Y. (1985). Immunological studies on aphthous ulcer and erythema nodosum-like eruptions in Behcet's disease. *The British Journal of Dermatology*, 113(3), 303–312. doi:10.1111/j.1365-2133.1985.tb02082.x.

Kao, L.-T., Lin, H.-C., & Lee, H.-C. (2019). Inflammatory bowel disease and bipolar disorder: A population-based cross-sectional study. *Journal of Affective Disorders*, 247, 120–124. doi:10.1016/j.jad.2019.01.014.

Kim, Y., Ko, T.-S., Yum, M.-S., Jung, A. Y., & Kim, H.-W. (2016). Obsessive-Compulsive Disorder Related to Mycoplasma-Associated Autoimmune Encephalopathy with Basal Ganglia Involvement. *Journal of Child and Adolescent Psychopharmacology*, 26(4), 400–402. doi:10.1089/cap.2015.0080.

Kimball, A. B., Wu, E. Q., Guérin, A., Yu, A. P., Tsaneva, M., Gupta, S. R., Bao, Y., & Mulani, P. M. (2012). Risks of developing psychiatric disorders in pediatric patients with psoriasis. *Journal of the American Academy of Dermatology*, 67 (4), 651–657.e2. doi:10.1016/j.jaad.2011.11.948.

Kirvan, C. A., Swedo, S. E., Heuser, J. S., & Cunningham, M. W. (2003). Mimicry and autoantibody-mediated neuronal cell signaling in Sydenham chorea. *Nature Medicine*, 9(7), Article 7. doi:10.1038/nm892.

Kirvan, C. A., Swedo, S. E., Kurahara, D., & Cunningham, M. W. (2006). Streptococcal mimicry and antibody-mediated cell signaling in the pathogenesis of Sydenham's chorea. *Autoimmunity*, 39(1), 21–29. doi:10.1080/08916930500484757.

Kirvan, C. A., Swedo, S. E., Snider, L. A., & Cunningham, M. W. (2006). Antibody-mediated neuronal cell signaling in behavior and movement disorders. *Journal of Neuroimmunology*, 179(1–2),173–179. doi:10.1016/j.jneuroim.2006.06.017.

Kivity, S., Agmon-Levin, N., Zandman-Goddard, G., Chapman, J., & Shoenfeld, Y. (2015). Neuropsychiatric lupus: A mosaic of clinical presentations. *BMC Medicine*, 13(1), 43. doi:10.1186/s12916-015-0269-8.

Kumar, A., Williams, M. T., & Chugani, H. T. (2015). Evaluation of basal ganglia and thalamic inflammation in children with pediatric autoimmune neuropsychiatric disorders associated with streptococcal infection and tourette syndrome: A positron emission tomographic (PET) study using 11C-[R]-PK11195. *Journal of Child Neurology*, 30(6), 749–756. doi:10.1177/0883073814543303.

Kyllönen, M. S., Ebeling, H., Kautiainen, H., Puolakka, K., & Vähäsalo, P. (2021). Psychiatric disorders in incident patients with juvenile idiopathic arthritis—A case-control cohort study. *Pediatric Rheumatology*, 19(1), 105. doi:10.1186/s12969-021-00599-x.

Lean, W. L., Arnup, S., Danchin, M., & Steer, A. C. (2014). Rapid diagnostic tests for group A streptococcal pharyngitis: A meta-analysis. *Pediatrics*, 134(4), 771–781. doi:10.1542/peds.2014-1094.

Li, Y., Zhang, S., Zhu, J., Du, X., & Huang, F. (2012). Sleep disturbances are associated with increased pain, disease activity, depression, and anxiety in ankylosing spondylitis: A case-control study. *Arthritis Research & Therapy*, 14 (5), R215. doi:10.1186/ar4054.

Lim, W. (2009). Antiphospholipid antibody syndrome. *Hematology. American Society of Hematology. Education Program*, 233–239. https://doi.org/10.1182/asheducation-2009.1.233.

Lok, E. Y. C., Mok, C. C., Cheng, C. W., & Cheung, E. F. C. (2010). Prevalence and determinants of psychiatric disorders in patients with rheumatoid arthritis. *Psychosomatics*, 51(4), 338–338.e8. doi:10.1176/appi.psy.51.4.338.

Lougee, L., Perlmutter, S. J., Nicolson, R., Garvey, M. A., & Swedo, S. E. (2000). Psychiatric disorders in first-degree relatives of children with pediatric autoimmune neuropsychiatric disorders associated with streptococcal infections (PANDAS). *Journal of the American Academy of Child and Adolescent Psychiatry*, 39(9), 1120–1126. doi:10.1097/00004583-200009000-00011.

Lubrano, E., Ciacci, C., Ames, P. R., Mazzacca, G., Oriente, P., & Scarpa, R. (1996). The arthritis of coeliac disease: Prevalence and pattern in 200 adult patients. *British Journal of Rheumatology*, 35(12), 1314–1318. doi:10.1093/rheumatology/35.12.1314.

Ma, M., Sandberg, J., Farhadian, B., Silverman, M., Xie, Y., Thienemann, M., & Frankovich, J. (2023). Arthritis in children with psychiatric deteriorations: A case series. *Developmental Neuroscience*, 1. doi:10.1159/000530854.

Maciel, R. O. H., Ferreira, G. A., Akemy, B., & Cardoso, F. (2016). Executive dysfunction, obsessive–compulsive symptoms, and attention deficit and hyperactivity disorder in Systemic Lupus Erythematosus: Evidence for basal ganglia dysfunction? *Journal of the Neurological Sciences*, 360, 94–97. doi:10.1016/j.jns.2015.11.052.

Maia, D. P., Teixeira, A. L., Quintão Cunningham, M. C., & Cardoso, F. (2005). Obsessive compulsive behavior, hyperactivity, and attention deficit disorder in Sydenham chorea. *Neurology*, 64(10), 1799–1801. doi:10.1212/01.WNL.0000161840.62090.0E.

Mann, E. A. & Saeed, S. A. (2012). Gastrointestinal infection as a trigger for inflammatory bowel disease. *Current Opinion in Gastroenterology*, 28(1), 24. doi:10.1097/MOG.0b013e32834c453e.

Mataix-Cols, D., Frans, E., Pérez-Vigil, A., Kuja-Halkola, R., Gromark, C., Isomura, K., Fernández de la Cruz, L., Serlachius, E., Leckman, J. F., Crowley, J. J., Rück, C., Almqvist, C., Lichtenstein, P., & Larsson, H. (2018). A total-population multigenerational family clustering study of autoimmune diseases in obsessive-compulsive disorder and Tourette's/chronic tic disorders. *Molecular Psychiatry*, 23(7), 1652–1658. doi:10.1038/mp.2017.215.

McHugh, A., Chan, A., Herrera, C., Park, J. M., Balboni, I., Gerstbacher, D., Hsu, J. J., Lee, T., Thienemann, M., & Frankovich, J. (2022). Profiling Behavioral and Psychological Symptoms in Children Undergoing Treatment for Spondyloarthritis and Polyarthritis. *The Journal of Rheumatology*, 49(5), 489–496. doi:10.3899/jrheum.210489.

Melamed, I., Kobayashi, R. H., O'Connor, M., Kobayashi, A. L., Schechterman, A., Heffron, M., Canterberry, S., Miranda, H., & Rashid, N. (2021). Evaluation of Intravenous Immunoglobulin in Pediatric Acute-Onset Neuropsychiatric Syndrome. *Journal of Child and Adolescent Psychopharmacology*, 31(2), 118–128. doi:10.1089/cap.2020.0100.

Mellins, E. D., Macaubas, C., & Grom, A. A. (2011). Pathogenesis of systemic juvenile idiopathic arthritis: Some answers, more questions. *Nature Reviews Rheumatology*, 7(7), Article 7. doi:10.1038/nrrheum.2011.68.

Méndez, R., Balanzá-Martínez, V., Luperdi, S. C., Estrada, I., Latorre, A., González-Jiménez, P., Bouzas, L., Yépez, K., Ferrando, A., Reyes, S., & Menéndez, R. (2022). Long-term neuropsychiatric outcomes in COVID-19 survivors: A 1-year longitudinal study. *Journal of Internal Medicine*, 291(2), 247–251. doi:10.1111/joim.13389.

Menon, V., Subramanian, K., & Thamizh, J. S. (2017). Psychiatric Presentations Heralding Hashimoto's Encephalopathy: A Systematic Review and Analysis of Cases Reported in Literature. *Journal of Neurosciences in Rural Practice*, 8(2), 261–267. doi:10.4103/jnrp.jnrp_440_16.

Moore, P., Methley, A., Pollard, C., Mutch, K., Hamid, S., Elsone, L., & Jacob, A. (2016). Cognitive and psychiatric comorbidities in neuromyelitis optica. *Journal of the Neurological Sciences*, 360, 4–9. doi:10.1016/j.jns.2015.11.031.

Moreira, J., Kummer, A., Harsányi, E., Cardoso, F., & Teixeira, A. L. (2014). Psychiatric disorders in persistent and remitted Sydenham's chorea. *Parkinsonism & Related Disorders*, 20(2), 233–236. doi:10.1016/j.parkreldis.2013.10.029.

Mori, K., Iijima, M., Koike, H., Hattori, N., Tanaka, F., Watanabe, H., Katsuno, M., Fujita, A., Aiba, I., Ogata, A., Saito, T., Asakura, K., Yoshida, M., Hirayama, M., & Sobue, G. (2005). The wide spectrum of clinical manifestations in Sjögren's syndrome-associated neuropathy. *Brain: A Journal of Neurology*, 128 (Pt 11), 2518–2534. doi:10.1093/brain/awh605.

Murphy, T. K., Snider, L. A., Mutch, P. J., Harden, E., Zaytoun, A., Edge, P. J., Storch, E. A., Yang, M. C. K., Mann, G., Goodman, W. K., & Swedo, S. E. (2007). Relationship of Movements and Behaviors to Group A Streptococcus Infections in Elementary School Children. *Biological Psychiatry*, 61(3), 279–284. doi:10.1016/j.biopsych.2006.08.031.

Murphy, T. K., Storch, E. A., Turner, A., Reid, J. M., Tan, J., & Lewin, A. B. (2010). Maternal History of Autoimmune Disease in Children Presenting with Tics and/or Obsessive-Compulsive Disorder. *Journal of Neuroimmunology*, 229 (1–2), 243–247. doi:10.1016/j.jneuroim.2010.08.017.

Nadeau, J. M., Jordan, C., Selles, R. R., Wu, M. S., King, M. A., Patel, P. D., Hanks, C. E., Arnold, E. B., Lewin, A. B., Murphy, T. K., & Storch, E. A. (2015). A pilot trial of cognitive-behavioral therapy augmentation of antibiotic treatment in youth with pediatric acute-onset neuropsychiatric syndrome-related obsessive-compulsive disorder. *Journal of Child and Adolescent Psychopharmacology*, 25(4), 337–343. doi:10.1089/cap.2014.0149.

Nalleballe, K., Reddy Onteddu, S., Sharma, R., Dandu, V., Brown, A., Jasti, M., Yadala, S., Veerapaneni, K., Siddamreddy, S., Avula, A., Kapoor, N., Mudassar, K., & Kovvuru, S. (2020). Spectrum of neuropsychiatric manifestations in COVID-19. *Brain, Behavior, and Immunity*, 88, 71–74. doi:10.1016/j.bbi.2020.06.020.

Nery, F. G., Borba, E. F., Viana, V. S. T., Hatch, J. P., Soares, J. C., Bonfá, E., & Neto, F. L. (2008). Prevalence of depressive and anxiety disorders in systemic lupus erythematosus and their association with anti-ribosomal P antibodies. *Progress in Neuro-Psychopharmacology & Biological Psychiatry*, 32(3), 695–700. doi:10.1016/j.pnpbp.2007.11.014.

Ong, L. T. C., Galambos, G., & Brown, D. A. (2017). Primary Sjogren's Syndrome Associated With Treatment-Resistant Obsessive–Compulsive Disorder. *Frontiers in Psychiatry*, 8, 124. doi:10.3389/fpsyt.2017.00124.

Orlovska, S., Vestergaard, C. H., Bech, B. H., Nordentoft, M., Vestergaard, M., & Benros, M. E. (2017). Association of Streptococcal Throat Infection With Mental Disorders: Testing Key Aspects of the PANDAS Hypothesis in a Nationwide Study. *JAMA Psychiatry*, 74(7), 740–746. doi:10.1001/jamapsychiatry.2017.0995.

Orsini, A., Foiadelli, T., Magistrali, M., Carli, N., Bagnasco, I., Dassi, P., Verrotti, A., Marcotulli, D., Canavese, C., Nicita, F., Capuano, A., Marra, C., Fetta, A., Nosadini, M., Sartori, S., Papa, A., Viri, M., Greco, F., Pavone, P., ... Savasta, S. (2022). A nationwide study on Sydenham's chorea: Clinical features, treatment and prognostic factors. *European Journal of Paediatric Neurology*, 36, 1–6. doi:10.1016/j.ejpn.2021.11.002.

Palagini, L., Mosca, M., Tani, C., Gemignani, A., Mauri, M., & Bombardieri, S. (2013). Depression and systemic lupus erythematosus: A systematic review. *Lupus*, 22(5), 409–416. doi:10.1177/0961203313477227.

Panopoulos, S., Thomas, K., Georgiopoulos, G., Boumpas, D., Katsiari, C., Bertsias, G., Drosos, A. A., Boki, K., Dimitroulas, T., Garyfallos, A., Papagoras, C., Katsimbri, P., Tziortziotis, A., Adamichou, C., Kaltsonoudis, E., Argyriou, E., Vosvotekas, G., Sfikakis, P. P., Vassilopoulos, D., & Tektonidou, M. G. (2021). Comparable or higher prevalence of comorbidities in antiphospholipid syndrome vs rheumatoid arthritis: A multicenter, case-control study. *Rheumatology*, 60(1), 170–178. doi:10.1093/rheumatology/keaa321.

Pastore, L., Lo Muzio, L., & Serpico, R. (2007). Atrophic glossitis leading to the diagnosis of celiac disease. *The New England Journal of Medicine*, 356(24), 2547. doi:10.1056/NEJMc070200.

Pavone, P., Ceccarelli, M., Marino, S., Caruso, D., Falsaperla, R., Berretta, M., Rullo, E. V., & Nunnari, G. (2021). SARS-CoV-2 related paediatric acute-onset neuropsychiatric syndrome. *The Lancet Child & Adolescent Health*, 5(6), e19–e21. doi:10.1016/S2352-4642(21)00135-00138.

Pego-Reigosa, J. M. & Isenberg, D. A. (2008). Psychosis due to systemic lupus erythematosus: Characteristics and long-term outcome of this rare manifestation of the disease. *Rheumatology (Oxford, England)*, 47(10), 1498–1502. doi:10.1093/rheumatology/ken260.

Perlmutter, S. J., Leitman, S. F., Garvey, M. A., Hamburger, S., Feldman, E., Leonard, H. L., & Swedo, S. E. (1999). Therapeutic plasma exchange and intravenous immunoglobulin for obsessive-compulsive disorder and tic disorders in childhood. *The Lancet*, 354(9185), 1153–1158. doi:10.1016/S0140-6736(98)12297-12293.

Petri, M. (2000). Epidemiology of the Antiphospholipid Antibody Syndrome. *Journal of Autoimmunity*, 15(2), 145–151. doi:10.1006/jaut.2000.0409.

Plot, L. & Amital, H. (2009). Infectious associations of Celiac disease. *Autoimmunity Reviews*, 8(4), 316–319. doi:10.1016/j.autrev.2008.10.001.

Ravelli, A. & Martini, A. (2007). Juvenile idiopathic arthritis. *The Lancet*, 369 (9563), 767–778. doi:10.1016/S0140-6736(07)60363-60368.

Raychaudhuri, S. K., Maverakis, E., & Raychaudhuri, S. P. (2014). Diagnosis and classification of psoriasis. *Autoimmunity Reviews*, 13(4–5), 490–495. doi:10.1016/j.autrev.2014.01.008.

Salvarani, C., Brown Jr, R. D., Calamia, K. T., Christianson, T. J. H., Weigand, S. D., Miller, D. V., Giannini, C., Meschia, J. F., Huston III, J., & Hunder, G. G.

(2007). Primary central nervous system vasculitis: Analysis of 101 patients. *Annals of Neurology*, 62(5), 442–451. doi:10.1002/ana.21226.

Schiess, N. & Pardo, C. A. (2008). Hashimoto's Encephalopathy. *Annals of the New York Academy of Sciences, 1142*(1), 254–265doi:10.1196/annals.1444.018.

Sève, P., Pacheco, Y., Durupt, F., Jamilloux, Y., Gerfaud-Valentin, M., Isaac, S., Boussel, L., Calender, A., Androdias, G., Valeyre, D., & El Jammal, T. (2021). Sarcoidosis: A Clinical Overview from Symptoms to Diagnosis. *Cells*, 10(4), 766. https://doi.org/10.3390/cells10040766.

Seyedian, S. S., Nokhostin, F., & Malamir, M. D. (2019). A review of the diagnosis, prevention, and treatment methods of inflammatory bowel disease. *Journal of Medicine and Life*, 12(2), 113–122. doi:10.25122/jml-2018-0075.

Shaikh, N., Swaminathan, N., & Hooper, E. G. (2012). Accuracy and precision of the signs and symptoms of streptococcal pharyngitis in children: A systematic review. *The Journal of Pediatrics*, 160(3), 487–493.e3. doi:10.1016/j.jpeds.2011.09.011.

Shulman, S. T., Bisno, A. L., Clegg, H. W., Gerber, M. A., Kaplan, E. L., Lee, G., Martin, J. M., & Van Beneden, C. (2012). Clinical Practice Guideline for the Diagnosis and Management of Group A Streptococcal Pharyngitis: 2012 Update by the Infectious Diseases Society of America. *Clinical Infectious Diseases*, 55(10), e86–e102. doi:10.1093/cid/cis629.

Shulman, S. T., Bisno, A. L., Clegg, H. W., Gerber, M. A., Kaplan, E. L., Lee, G., Martin, J. M., Van Beneden, C., & Infectious Diseases Society of America. (2012). Clinical practice guideline for the diagnosis and management of group A streptococcal pharyngitis: 2012 update by the Infectious Diseases Society of America. *Clinical Infectious Diseases: An Official Publication of the Infectious Diseases Society of America*, 55(10), e86–102. doi:10.1093/cid/cis629.

Skopouli, F. N., Dafni, U., Ioannidis, J. P., & Moutsopoulos, H. M. (2000). Clinical evolution, and morbidity and mortality of primary Sjögren's syndrome. *Seminars in Arthritis and Rheumatism*, 29(5), 296–304. doi:10.1016/s0049-0172 (00)80016-80015.

Slattery, M. J., Dubbert, B. K., Allen, A. J., Leonard, H. L., Swedo, S. E., & Gourley, M. F. (2004). Prevalence of obsessive-compulsive disorder in patients with systemic lupus erythematosus. *The Journal of Clinical Psychiatry*, 65(3), 301–306. doi:10.4088/jcp.v65n0303.

Soldan, S. S., & Lieberman, P. M. (2023). Epstein–Barr virus and multiple sclerosis. *Nature Reviews Microbiology*, 21(1), Article 1. doi:10.1038/s41579-022-00770-5.

Starshinova, A. A., Malkova, A. M., Basantsova, N. Y., Zinchenko, Y. S., Kudryavtsev, I. V., Ershov, G. A., Soprun, L. A., Mayevskaya, V. A., Churilov, L. P., & Yablonskiy, P. K. (2020). Sarcoidosis as an Autoimmune Disease. *Frontiers in Immunology*, 10. www.frontiersin.org/articles/10.3389/fimmu.2019.02933.

Storch, E. A., Murphy, T. K., Geffken, G. R., Mann, G., Adkins, J., Merlo, L. J., Duke, D., Munson, M., Swaine, Z., & Goodman, W. K. (2006). Cognitive-behavioral therapy for PANDAS-related obsessive-compulsive disorder: Findings from a preliminary waitlist controlled open trial. *Journal of the American Academy of Child and Adolescent Psychiatry*, 45(10), 1171–1178. doi:10.1097/01. chi.0000231973.43966.a0.

Sung, K.-Y., Zhang, B., Wang, H. E., Bai, Y.-M., Tsai, S.-J., Su, T.-P., Chen, T.-J., Hou, M.-C., Lu, C.-L., Wang, Y.-P., & Chen, M.-H. (2022). Schizophrenia and risk of new-onset inflammatory bowel disease: A nationwide longitudinal study. *Alimentary Pharmacology & Therapeutics*, 55(9), 1192–1201. doi:10.1111/apt.16856.

Swedo, S. E. (2012). From Research Subgroup to Clinical Syndrome: Modifying the PANDAS Criteria to Describe PANS (Pediatric Acute-onset Neuropsychiatric Syndrome). *Pediatrics & Therapeutics*, 02(02). doi:10.4172/2161-0665.1000113.

Swedo, S. E., Frankovich, J., & Murphy, T. K. (2017). Overview of Treatment of Pediatric Acute-Onset Neuropsychiatric Syndrome. *Journal of Child and Adolescent Psychopharmacology*, 27(7), 562–565. doi:10.1089/cap.2017.0042.

Swedo, S. E., Leonard, H. L., Casey, B. J., Mannheim, G. B., Lenane, M. C., Rettew, D. C., & Schapiro, M. B. (1993). Sydenham's Chorea: Physical and Psychological Symptoms of St Vitus Dance. *Pediatrics*, 91(4), 706–713. doi:10.1542/peds.91.4.706.

Swedo, S. E., Leonard, H. L., Garvey, M., Mittleman, B., Allen, A. J., Perlmutter, S., Dow, S., Zamkoff, J., Dubbert, B. K., & Lougee, L. (1998). Pediatric Autoimmune Neuropsychiatric Disorders Associated With Streptococcal Infections: Clinical Description of the First 50 Cases. *American Journal of Psychiatry*, 155 (2), 264–271. doi:10.1176/ajp.155.2.264.

Swedo, S. E., Seidlitz, J., Kovacevic, M., Latimer, M. E., Hommer, R., Lougee, L., & Grant, P. (2015). Clinical presentation of pediatric autoimmune neuropsychiatric disorders associated with streptococcal infections in research and community settings. *Journal of Child and Adolescent Psychopharmacology*, 25 (1), 26–30. doi:10.1089/cap.2014.0073.

Talarico, R., Palagini, L., Elefante, E., Ferro, F., Tani, C., Gemignani, A., Bombardieri, S., & Mosca, M. (2018). Behçet's syndrome and psychiatric involvement: Is it a primary or secondary feature of the disease? *Clinical and Experimental Rheumatology*, 36(6 Suppl 115), 125–128.

Taquet, M., Geddes, J. R., Husain, M., Luciano, S., & Harrison, P. J. (2021). 6-month neurological and psychiatric outcomes in 236 379 survivors of COVID-19: A retrospective cohort study using electronic health records. *The Lancet Psychiatry*, 8(5), 416–427. doi:10.1016/S2215-0366(21)00084–00085.

Taranta, A., & Stollerman, G. H. (1956). The relationship of Sydenham's chorea to infection with group A streptococci. *The American Journal of Medicine*, 20(2), 170–175. doi:10.1016/0002-9343(56)90186–90183.

Teixeira, A. L., Vasconcelos, L. P., do Carmo Pereira Nunes, M., & Singer, H. (2021). Sydenham's chorea: From pathophysiology to therapeutics. *Expert Review of Neurotherapeutics*, 21(8), 913–922. doi:10.1080/14737175.2021.1965883.

Tench, C. M., McCurdie, I., White, P. D., & D'Cruz, D. P. (2000). The prevalence and associations of fatigue in systemic lupus erythematosus. *Rheumatology*, 39 (11), 1249–1254. doi:10.1093/rheumatology/39.11.1249.

Thienemann, M., Murphy, T., Leckman, J., Shaw, R., Williams, K., Kapphahn, C., Frankovich, J., Geller, D., Bernstein, G., Chang, K., Elia, J., & Swedo, S. (2017). Clinical Management of Pediatric Acute-Onset Neuropsychiatric Syndrome: Part I-Psychiatric and Behavioral Interventions. *Journal of Child and Adolescent Psychopharmacology*, 27(7), 566–573. doi:10.1089/cap.2016.0145.

Thienemann, M., Park, M., Chan, A., & Frankovich, J. (2021). Patients with abrupt early-onset OCD due to PANS tolerate lower doses of antidepressants and antipsychotics. *Journal of Psychiatric Research*, 135, 270–278. doi:10.1016/j.jpsychires.2021.01.022.

Tribbick, D., Salzberg, M., Ftanou, M., Connell, W. R., Macrae, F., Kamm, M. A., Bates, G. W., Cunningham, G., Austin, D. W., & Knowles, S. R. (2015). Prevalence of mental health disorders in inflammatory bowel disease: An Australian outpatient cohort. *Clinical and Experimental Gastroenterology*, 8, 197–204. doi:10.2147/CEG.S77567.

Turina, M. C., Yeremenko, N., van Gaalen, F., van Oosterhout, M., Berg, I. J., Ramonda, R., Lebre, C. (M C., Landewé, R., & Baeten, D. (2017). Serum inflammatory biomarkers fail to identify early axial spondyloarthritis: Results from the SpondyloArthritis Caught Early (SPACE) cohort. *RMD Open*, 3(1), e000319. https://doi.org/10.1136/rmdopen-2016-000319.

Twilt, M. & Benseler, S. M. (2016). Chapter 16—Central nervous system vasculitis in adults and children. In S. J. Pittock & A. Vincent (Eds), *Handbook of Clinical Neurology* (Vol. 133, pp. 283–300). Elsevier. doi:10.1016/B978-0-444-63432-0.00016-5.

Vanderheiden, A. & Klein, R. S. (2022). Neuroinflammation and COVID-19. *Current Opinion in Neurobiology*, 76, 102608. doi:10.1016/j.conb.2022.102608.

Vasconcelos, L. P. B., Vasconcelos, M. C., do Carmo Pereira Nunes, M., & Teixeira, A. L. (2023). Chapter 18—Rheumatic chorea. In N. Rezaei (Ed.), *Translational Autoimmunity* (pp. 373–387). Academic Press. doi:10.1016/B978-0-323-85831-1.00018-8.

Vasconcelos, L. P. B., Vasconcelos, M. C., do Carmo Pereira Nunes, M., & Teixeira, A. L. (2019). Sydenham's chorea: An update on pathophysiology, clinical features and management. *Expert Opinion on Orphan Drugs*, 7(11), 501–511. doi:10.1080/21678707.2019.1684259.

Vreeland, A., Thienemann, M., Cunningham, M., Muscal, E., Pittenger, C., & Frankovich, J. (2023). Neuroinflammation in Obsessive-Compulsive Disorder: Sydenham Chorea, Pediatric Autoimmune Neuropsychiatric Disorders Associated with Streptococcal Infections, and Pediatric Acute Onset Neuropsychiatric Syndrome. *Psychiatric Clinics*, 46(1), 69–88. doi:10.1016/j.psc.2022.11.004.

Wang, L.-Y., Chen, S.-F., Chiang, J.-H., Hsu, C.-Y., & Shen, Y.-C. (2019). Systemic autoimmune diseases are associated with an increased risk of obsessive–compulsive disorder: A nationwide population-based cohort study. *Social Psychiatry and Psychiatric Epidemiology*, 54(4), 507–516. doi:10.1007/s00127-018-1622-y.

Wang, W., Zhang, L., Chi, X.-S., He, L., Zhou, D., & Li, J.-M. (2020). Psychiatric Symptoms of Patients With Anti-NMDA Receptor Encephalitis. *Frontiers in Neurology*, 10, 1330. doi:10.3389/fneur.2019.01330.

Weiss, P. F., Beukelman, T., Schanberg, L. E., Kimura, Y., Colbert, R. A., & CARRA Registry Investigators. (2012). Enthesitis-related arthritis is associated with higher pain intensity and poorer health status in comparison with other categories of juvenile idiopathic arthritis: The Childhood Arthritis and Rheumatology Research Alliance Registry. *The Journal of Rheumatology*, 39(12), 2341–2351. https://doi.org/10.3899/jrheum.120642.

Williams, K. A., Swedo, S. E., Farmer, C. A., Grantz, H., Grant, P. J., D'Souza, P., Hommer, R., Katsovich, L., King, R. A., & Leckman, J. F. (2016). Randomized, Controlled Trial of Intravenous Immunoglobulin for Pediatric Autoimmune Neuropsychiatric Disorders Associated With Streptococcal Infections. *Journal of the American Academy of Child and Adolescent Psychiatry*, 55(10), 860–867.e2. doi:10.1016/j.jaac.2016.06.017.

Wincup, C. & Ioannou, Y. (2018). The Differences Between Childhood and Adult Onset Antiphospholipid Syndrome. *Frontiers in Pediatrics*, 6. www.frontiersin. org/articles/10.3389/fped.2018.00362.

Wingerchuk, D. M., Lennon, V. A., Lucchinetti, C. F., Pittock, S. J., & Weinshenker, B. G. (2007). The spectrum of neuromyelitis optica. *The Lancet. Neurology*, 6(9), 805–815. doi:10.1016/S1474-4422(07)70216–70218.

Xu, J., Liu, R.-J., Fahey, S., Frick, L., Leckman, J., Vaccarino, F., Duman, R. S., Williams, K., Swedo, S., & Pittenger, C. (2021). Antibodies From Children With PANDAS Bind Specifically to Striatal Cholinergic Interneurons and Alter Their Activity. *The American Journal of Psychiatry*, 178(1), 48–64. doi:10.1176/appi. ajp.2020.19070698.

Zheng, J., Frankovich, J., McKenna, E. S., Rowe, N. C., MacEachern, S. J., Ng, N. N., Tam, L. T., Moon, P. K., Gao, J., Thienemann, M., Forkert, N. D., & Yeom, K. W. (2020). Association of Pediatric Acute-Onset Neuropsychiatric Syndrome With Microstructural Differences in Brain Regions Detected via Diffusion-Weighted Magnetic Resonance Imaging. *JAMA Network Open*, 3(5), e204063. https://doi.org/10.1001/jamanetworkopen.2020.4063.

Zinger, H., Sherer, Y., Goddard, G., Berkun, Y., Barzilai, O., Agmon-Levin, N., Ram, M., Blank, M., Tincani, A., Rozman, B., Cervera, R., & Shoenfeld, Y. (2009). Common infectious agents prevalence in antiphospholipid syndrome. *Lupus*, 18(13), 1149–1153. doi:10.1177/0961203309345738.

Zomorrodi, A. & Wald, E. R. (2006). Sydenham's Chorea in Western Pennsylvania. *Pediatrics*, 117(4), e675–e679. doi:10.1542/peds.2005-1573.

14 Early Onset and Tic-Related OCD

Madison Fitzpatrick and Brian A. Zaboski

Introduction

Obsessive-compulsive disorder (OCD) is characterized by distressing unwanted or intrusive thoughts, images, or urges (obsessions) and repetitive behaviors/mental actions done to assuage distress or anxiety caused by obsessions (compulsions; American Psychiatric Association, 2022). OCD has a bimodal age of onset, with a childhood age of onset around age nine to ten and another onset in the early 20s (Geller et al., 2000; Rasmussen & Eisen, 1992). Early-onset OCD is defined somewhat inconsistently, e.g., before age 15, starting at age ten, before the age of 18 (Millet et al., 2004; Tükel et al., 2005; Sobin et al., 2000). In this chapter we use the term *early onset* broadly to describe onset prior to age 18. Despite evidence that individuals with early onset OCD possess a distinct demographic, genetic, and comorbidity profile from later onset OCD, there is no recognized subtype for this disorder (Geller et al., 2021). Nevertheless, clinicians and researchers recognize that early onset OCD warrants special consideration.

Epidemiology

OCD prevalence ranges from 1 percent–4 percent percent in the general population (Kessler et al., 2012; Ruscio et al., 2010); however, early-onset OCD ranges from 0.25 percent-2 percent percent in epidemiological studies (Flament et al., 1988; Heyman et al., 2001) with 50 percent-80 percent of all OCD cases being considered early-onset based on retrospective self-report (Millet et al., 2004). Of note, pediatric prevalence is subject to extensive error. For instance, children are often unable to recognize their symptoms and frequently hide them, owing to shame or embarrassment (Geller et al., 2021). Furthermore, varying remission rates also add to error as early-onset cases may achieve remission before patients reach adulthood. For instance, in a long-term follow-up study, 78 percent of an early-onset OCD sample (*n* = 46) achieved full/partial remission for three years following an initial intake (Mancebo et al., 2014) compared to 46

DOI: 10.4324/9781003517429-14

percent of an adult sample (*n* = 221). Lastly, while OCD cases have been reported as early as age 3 (Hollingsworth et al., 1980; Zohar, 1999), these are often excluded from general analyses of early-onset OCD. This may be because OCD scales are typically developed for children older than age eight, leaving an open question about the construct validity of scores from younger children (Garcia et al., 2009).

Demographics

Early onset OCD may be more common in boys than girls (do Rosario-Campos et al., 2005; Geller et al., 2000), although ongoing research has challenged this through cohort studies. Data from the Danish Psychiatric Central Register show 55 percent of the children hospitalized or treated in psychiatric centers for early onset-OCD are female (Nissen et al., 2017). Male-biased prevalence may result from higher comorbidities between OCD and male-prevalent disorders that often demand clinical attention like attention-deficit/hyperactivity disorder (ADHD), autism spectrum disorder, and/or tic disorders (Geller et al., 2021). Of note, even the male preponderance for ADHD, autism, and tic-disorders in children may be inaccurate as boys often display secondary externalizing or disruptive behaviors than girls that result in diagnosis (Garcia-Delgar et al., 2022; Murray et al., 2019; Werling & Geschwind, 2013).

By contrast to cisgender males and females, the current point prevalence of OCD within adult transgender female populations is 9.8 percent and 7.6 percent in adult transgender males (Millet et al., 2017). There are no current studies examining transgender youth populations, but the rates in adult populations may suggest an elevated prevalence. More research is needed to understand early-onset OCD in these underrepresented populations (see Chapter 17 – Sexual and Gender Minority Considerations in OCD Treatment).

A notable caveat for all these data is warranted: samples in most investigations have been predominantly White. Across epidemiological examinations of adult psychiatric populations, OCD rates are comparable across non-Hispanic white (0.5 percent), and non-Hispanic Black (0.6 percent) individuals (Breslau et al., 2006). Similar investigations have not been conducted for pediatric populations. It is essential to include diverse samples in examinations of OCD, as ethnic and cultural identity can affect OCD presentation through differing value systems (Ching & Williams, 2019; Williams et al., 2012). Because minoritized populations have also been systematically excluded or alienated from many scientific investigations, inclusion of diverse samples can help better illustrate the demographic picture of early-onset OCD and ensure that people of all races are included in research-driven examinations of this disorder.

Developmental considerations

The presentation of early-onset OCD is like its late-onset counterpart, but with additional developmental considerations. In children, symptoms must be distinguished from developmentally appropriate rituals. Rituals are important to the developing child, as they provide comfort and structure to the child's day (e.g., bedtime rituals, or the organization of special stuffed animals; Geller et al., 2021). When the routines become so elaborate or excessive that they become disruptive, or the disruption of these routines causes distressing behavioral outbursts, early-onset obsessive compulsive disorder might be considered. Magical thinking, or the connection of thoughts/ideas to actions that are not causally related, is also developmentally appropriate for children younger than 8, as their conception of how reality operates has not been fully formed (Garcia et al., 2009; Geller et al., 2021). For children younger than 8, obsessions encompass multiple domains, but studies have shown that contamination and catastrophe (i.e. family members dying while they are away from the child) were the most common followed by washing and checking compulsions (Garcia et al., 2009). A larger meta-analysis corroborated these findings in children ages 5–18, with symmetry (ordering, arranging, repeating), taboo obsessions (aggressive, sexual), contamination, and hoarding as the most common obsessions and compulsions (Bloch et al., 2008). Additionally, younger children have higher rates of "tic-like" compulsions, such as touching, tapping, or rubbing that are often done repetitively or ritualistically to achieve a just right feeling. These rituals may require further assessment for tic-disorders.

Younger children will often have trouble articulating their concerns, so much of the onus of recognizing symptoms will fall on parents/guardians. Older children and adolescents experiencing OCD symptoms are typically able to verbalize what they are feeling and may be more likely to express their concerns to loved ones, friends, or trusted adults (i.e., teachers, school counselors). Providers should acquire a full diagnostic history from an adolescent patient and their parents/guardians, as their symptoms may have emerged early in childhood, before the child had the ability to describe their symptoms (Thomsen, 2013). Compared to children and adults, adolescents with OCD have higher risk for scrupulosity and sexual obsessions, as these typically start to cause moral conflict and anxiety during and after puberty (Geller et al., 2021). Overestimation of responsibility and thought suppression strategies may also become more common in adolescents with OCD, thereby exacerbating symptoms (Farrell & Barrett, 2006). Additionally, associated comorbidities in adolescents resemble adults, with significantly higher rates of depression in adults (62 percent) than in children (38 percent) (Geller, 2006).

Comorbidity

As in late-onset OCD, comorbidity is common. As high as 86 percent of individuals with early-onset OCD will present with a concomitant psychiatric disorder (Farrell et al., 2012; Tanidir et al., 2015). However, the profile of comorbid disorders in early-onset OCD differs from its late-onset counterpart. Adults have a higher preponderance toward mood and anxiety disorder comorbidity, but in children/adolescents with OCD, there is a higher chance for ADHD and tic disorders (Geller et al., 2021); for example, rates of comorbid ADHD appear higher in pediatric populations (19 percent) compared to adults (9 percent; Abramovitch et al., 2015). Also compared to adults, comorbid tics were higher in early-onset OCD populations (30 percent vs. 12.5 percent; do Rosario-Campos et al., 2005; Lochner et al., 2014). Comorbid psychiatric conditions with OCD can decrease quality of life and complicate treatment, so it is important that potential comorbid conditions are thoroughly assessed (Zaboski et al., 2019).

Genetics

Heritability estimates for OCD range from 25 percent–30 percent (Arnold et al., 2018); however, heritability for late-onset OCD is lower (12 percent) than early-onset OCD (26 percent; Nestadt et al., 2000). While there is clearly a genetic and heritability component involved in early-onset OCD, environmental factors complicate gene expression. In monozygotic twin studies, OCD has been found to have a 50 percent concordance rate (van Grootheest et al., 2005). The unexplained 50 percent of the variability may be related to events during gestation, psychosocial stress, and infection during childhood (Geller et al., 2021). Owing to the complexity of OCD, a meta-analytic review over 128 studies attempting to identify environmental stressors (i.e., perinatal complication, family dynamics, traumatic events, infection, etc.) for OCD have been unable to find any causal events (Brander et al., 2021). However, the authors noted that future research into this area should employ broader sampling strategies and take the heterogeneity of OCD into consideration when designing subsequent studies.

Treatment considerations

Cognitive Behavioral Therapy with Exposure and Response Prevention (CBT ERP)

Cognitive behavioral therapy with exposure and response prevention (CBT ERP) uses exposure to feared stimuli to encourage children to confront obsession-inducing stimuli to challenge distress-based cognitions (e.g., "If I hold these scissors, then I'll hurt my mom.") while resisting or reducing compulsions (e.g., not checking mom for scratches), thereby developing new neural connections that inhibit existing obsession-related pathways. Several meta-analyses have supported the use of this technique in early-onset populations. An early meta-analysis of randomized controlled trials for youth found a large overall effect size (Hedge's g = 1.45), with effect sizes attenuated by between-study variability and whether the studies were tested against an active treatment control (Watson & Rees, 2008). A subsequent meta-analysis with 13 pediatric studies found a pre-post weighted mean difference on the Children's Yale-Brown Obsessive Compulsive Scale (Goodman et al., 1991) between 11 and 12 points before and after CBT (Wu et al., 2016).

Insight

Insight is a crucial factor for treatment efficacy and engagement. In early onset OCD, low insight characterizes 33 percent to 45 percent of samples (Lewin et al., 2010; Storch, et al., 2008; Storch et al., 2014). Insight may vary with age: 80 percent of an older adolescent sample demonstrated higher insight compared to 50 percent in children ages 8–11 (Lewin et al., 2010). Children with low insight may struggle to engage with treatment and recognize that their concerns are unreasonable. As such, children with lower insight are often less likely to engage with ERP (Selles et al., 2020). Samples of adults often have higher proportions of individuals with absent insight, who retrospectively report experiencing their symptoms throughout childhood, suggesting that many individuals with lower insight may delay treatment seeking. Lower insight is also related to higher rates of family accommodation (Storch et al., 2014). Thus, clinicians should thoroughly assess for insight when evaluating pediatric patients and address poor insight in treatment planning.

Family Accommodation. Accommodation occurs when parents or caregivers intentionally or unintentionally encourage or participate in rituals or avoidance. It can take the form of a parent following the rules established by the child's anxiety; completing rituals or assisting a child to do rituals; or ignoring problem behaviors (e.g., "it's just a phase"; Storch et al., 2007; Watson et al., 2021). Accommodation often reduces anxiety in the short-term but begets more anxiety in the long-term. This arises from two behavioral cycles. From the perspective of the child, an obsession causes distress, eliciting compulsive behavior. When the child engages in compulsive behavior, such as reassurance-seeking, this temporarily decreases distress, and the reassurance is negatively reinforced, becoming more likely in the future (Abramowitz, 2006). From the caregivers' perspective, a distressed child causes their anxiety to increase, especially when compulsions are more severe (Flessner et al., 2011). By the same behavioral principles that strengthen the child's OCD, parents or caregivers negatively reinforce their own accommodation behaviors by decreasing their anxiousness about their child's anxiety when providing the reassurance that the child wants.

Because both parents and children are reinforced during accommodation cycles, treatment should focus on accommodation during ERP (Bertelsen et al., 2022). Therapists can work with parents to (a) provide psychoeducation, understand misconceptions about OCD, and learn how best to communicate with the family; followed by (b) concrete behaviors the family can do to reduce accommodative behaviors for the child through role-play and learning the principles of ERP (Demaria et al., 2021). In an uncontrolled study of 85 youth with OCD, a group ERP protocol (McKenney et al., 2020) was delivered separately to youth and parents. Parents learned how to decrease accommodation, create contingency management systems, and engage in self-care (Selles et al., 2018). A total of 56 percent of the sample were treatment responders and thirty-eight percent experienced remission. Although more research is needed to understand the causal role of accommodation in treating early onset ERP, its association with poorer therapy outcomes and OCD severity–coupled with the field's theoretical understanding of operant conditioning–suggest that addressing accommodation can improve ERP outcomes (Caporino, 2020; Lebowitz et al., 2020).

Pharmaceutical

Treatment considerations depend on clinical need. CBT is recommended for mild to moderate severity, and medications in combination with CBT are recommended for moderate to severe OCD (Geller & March, 2012). There is little information on how SRIs impact the developing brain (Mancuso et al., 2010). Mania has been reported as a heightened risk for children ages 10–14 taking antidepressants, including SSRIs (Martin et al., 2004). Therefore, current treatment algorithms recommend that mild to moderate cases include CBT-only treatment to limit potential medication side effects. For more severe cases, specifically in the presence of low insight or lack of motivation, treatment with medications is beneficial (Geller & March, 2012). Serotonin reuptake inhibitors (SRIs) are the typical first-line approaches, which include conventional SSRIs (i.e., fluo-voxamine, escitalopram) as well as clomipramine (Westwell-Roper & Stewart, 2019). A recent meta-analysis suggested that CBT with pharmacotherapy is more efficacious than either treatment alone, and escitalopram was found to be the most well tolerated and effective medication for early-onset OCD (Tao et al., 2022). However, the time frame included in these studies was short, and routine follow-up is often required in order to maximize treatment gains.

Tic-related OCD

Tics are characterized by sudden, rapid involuntary movements or sounds that may or may not be preceded by a premonitory urge (American Psychiatric Association, 2022). One-third of children with OCD are estimated to also be diagnosed with a tic disorder before age 18 (do Rosario-Campos et al., 2005), and 60 percent of children with OCD will present with tics but fail to meet diagnostic criteria for a tic disorder (Conelea et al., 2014). Although tic-related OCD is a diagnostic specifier, it has also been considered as a subtype of OCD, as these patients often have an earlier age of onset, male preponderance, higher rates of impulse control disorders, and higher rates of heritability (Conelea et al., 2014). OCD dimensional features also differ within this subgroup, as certain motor compulsions, intrusive violent/aggressive thoughts and imagery, and concerns with symmetry are more common than in non-tic-related OCD (Mansueto & Keuler, 2007). For these cases, it is important to consider which behaviors are tics and which behaviors are compulsions, and to take special care to delineate between a not-just-right experience and a premonitory urge.

Demographics

In a multicenter study with 813 patients, the mean age of onset for tic-related OCD in seven- to 13-year-olds was 11.97 years old (de Alvarenga et al., 2012; Katz et al., 2022). This may suggest a multimodal onset for OCD, with another pre-pubertal age of onset prior to puberty. Tic-related OCD has a male preponderance, with 53 percent of participants male (N = 124; Conelea et al., 2014). Owing to the propensity of children diagnosed with tic-related OCD, the condition is likely to affect the demographics of early-onset OCD, so future research should examine subgroup characteristics based on OCD specifier (i.e. tic-related, insight) rather than age of onset (Bloch, 2017b). There is a considerable dearth in research on racial and ethnic differences within tic-related OCD, as the few studies on early-onset OCD did not include comorbid tics (Kemp et al., 2021). Future studies should address this gap to maximize generalizability and inclusivity.

Clinical presentation

Clinically, tic-related OCD differs from early-onset OCD (more broadly) in several key ways. Many tic-related OCD cases present with broad sensory disturbances, sensations felt by the individual before performing a compulsion that can be mental or physical (Miguel et al., 2005). These differ from premonitory urges in tic disorders, as a premonitory urge is primarily a physical experience, such as an itch, localized energy within muscles, or hiccup-like pressure (Nam et al., 2019). By contrast, sensory disturbances are general feelings of discomfort, usually consisting of either urges, not-just-right experiences, or a sense of incompleteness (Miguel et al., 2005). These are more prevalent in comorbid tic disorders and OCD than either disorder alone, with a correlation between just-right feelings and comorbid OCD (Kwak et al., 2003). Premonitory urges and sensory experiences can both compel an individual to relieve the feeling with movement, either by engaging in a tic or doing a compulsion. These experiences are seen at a higher frequency in individuals with tic-related OCD. Of note, 72 percent of 813 OCD patients with comorbid Tourette's disorder reported sensory phenomena, including mental and physical sensations (de Alvarenga et al., 2012). For some individuals with tic-related OCD, tics can serve a compulsive function, in that tics are done repetitively or ritualistically to relieve obsessive distress or just-not-right experiences (e.g., repeating a shoulder shrug tic six times so it feels "just right," or to shake a "bad thought" off).

Across OCD symptom dimensions, some studies have found that individuals with tic-related OCD experienced higher severity within intrusive violent/sexual thoughts/images, religious, and hoarding domains compared to individuals with just OCD alone (de Alvarenga et al., 2012). Additionally, patients with tic-related OCD presented with higher severity than OCD alone on multiple other domains, namely miscellaneous and symmetry/ordering (Petter et al., 1998). However, subsequent studies have found no such elevation, with only counting compulsions, contamination obsessions, and sexual obsessions more common in OCD without tics (Storch, Stigge-Kaufman, et al., 2008). To reconcile the literature, less retrospective report, higher powered samples, and meta-analytic examinations are needed (Kloft et al., 2018).

Comorbidity

Tic-related OCD and non-tic related OCD differ in their comorbidities. ADHD is more common in tic-related OCD and may possibly contribute to the high comorbidity rates of ADHD also seen in early-onset OCD (de Alvarenga et al., 2012). Additionally, tic-related OCD has a higher comorbidity rate with impulse control disorders (i.e., oppositional defiant disorder, conduct disorder), anxiety disorders (i.e. separation anxiety, specific phobia, social anxiety disorder, generalized anxiety disorder), posttraumatic stress disorder, and excoriation disorder. Anxiety disorders and OCD are often comorbid, but the high rate of impulse control disorders within this sample suggests a potential relationship between impulsivity and motor disinhibition, commonly seen within ADHD, OCD, and Tourette's Disorder (TD; de Alvarenga et al., 2012). These symptoms contribute to a differing clinical profile than the symptoms in non-tic related OCD.

The most common comorbid tic-disorder with childhood OCD is TD. TD is characterized by the presence of multiple motor tics and at least one vocal tic for at least one year throughout the entire manifestation of the disorder, although not necessarily concomitantly (American Psychiatric Association, 2022). Anywhere between 18.7 percent (Nissen et al., 2017) and 46.2 percent (do Rosario-Campos et al., 2005) of individuals with early onset OCD will develop a tic disorder (including Tourette's) in their lifetime. TD seems strongly related to OCD: One-third of individuals with Tourette's will develop OCD, and the OCD that develops will be at its worst two years after tic-severity peaks (Bloch et al., 2006). OCD symptoms are also more likely than tics to persist into adulthood. This is important to note to patients and parents, as target symptoms may change over the course of treatment.

Genetics

Researchers have theorized that tic-related OCD carries a strong genetic load compared to typical OCD presentations. When comparing the two disorders separately, there seems to be no genome-wide significant variants that suggest a genetic linkage between these two disorders (Yu et al., 2015). However, when tic-related OCD cases were added to the overall OCD sample, the polygenic signal became significantly stronger, suggesting that tic-related OCD may have a differing genetic susceptibility. This was further demonstrated through examining a population from the National Patient Register in Sweden, which collected a sample of over 21,000 individuals with OCD. Estimated hazard ratios for the development of tic-related OCD ($n = 1,257$) in biological siblings sit at ten times more likely, compared to four times more likely in non-tic-related OCD ($n = 20,975$; Brander et al., 2021). To examine whether this was due to the high heritability of tic-disorders themselves, an analysis was conducted comparing OCD with comorbid ADHD to OCD without ADHD, as ADHD is also highly heritable. There was an increased risk for biological siblings of individuals with OCD and comorbid ADHD. However, when tic-related OCD cases were removed from this sample, the risk was no longer significantly elevated, indicating that tic disorders exclusively were not causing the high heritability effects. Overall, this suggests that there is distinct heritability for this subtype.

Treatment considerations

Psychoeducation

Current practice guidelines for treating chronic tics include psychoeducation as an integral component (Pringsheim et al., 2019), and psychoeducation has been similarly recommended in tic-related OCD for children, parents, and teachers (Bloch, 2017a). Psychoeducation includes information about the course, neurobiology, genetics, and treatment rationale for tic-disorders (Wilhelm et al., 2012). In a review of 22 studies, psychoeducation evidenced generally positive results on the knowledge and attitudes for adults and children, with mixed results when diagnostic labels were used (Nussey et al., 2013). Thus, some general points to convey to patients include the waxing/waning nature of tic severity, the worsening effects that stress/anxiety can have on tics, the peak period of tics in childhood (i.e., between 10–12 years old), and that OCD commonly co-occurs with tics (Bloch, 2017a).

Comprehensive Behavioral Intervention for Tics (CBIT) and CBT ERP

CBIT is a structured intervention that incorporates psychoeducation, habit reversal training, and a functional understanding of the antecedents and conditions that trigger tics to help mitigate their impairment (Woods et al., 2008). As CBIT is unlikely to assist with symptoms of impairing OCD (Zimmerman-Brenner et al., 2022), children and adolescents with comorbid OCD may require additional exposure and response prevention if the OCD worsens (Bloch et al., 2006). Evidence indicates that comorbid tic disorders do not adversely affect outcomes of CBT ERP (Himle et al., 2003; March et al., 2007). For example, 96 youth (aged 7–19) received 14 sessions of CBT ERP, with three-quarters of the sample meeting eligibility for a comorbid diagnosis (Storch, Merlo, et al., 2008). While comorbidity in general negatively impacted treatment outcome, the presence of Tourette's or chronic tic disorder did not.

Pharmaceutical

Pharmacological treatment of non-tic related OCD typically starts with SRIs (i.e. escitalopram, clomipramine etc). With no response, augmentation should occur (POTS, 2004). While past research has indicated that individuals with tic-related OCD responded worse to SSRIs than those without tics (McDougle, 1994; McDougle et al., 1993), research since then has found that SSRI response rates do not differ between individuals with tic-related and non-tic-related OCD (Husted et al., 2007; McGuire et al., 2015). Examining 11 SSRI trials utilizing a metanalytic approach, researchers found that comorbid Tourette's syndrome or tic disorders were not moderating factors on SSRI response (McGuire et al., 2015). For Tourette's syndrome alone, neuroleptics (both first and second generation) have been found to be the most efficacious (Budman, 2014), suggesting a viable augmentation strategy for tic-related OCD. In a naturalistic study, 68 percent of patients with tic-related OCD saw improvement in their tics when their SSRI was augmented with a neuroleptic (Masi et al., 2013). Given that neuroleptic monotherapy is not efficacious in treating OCD symptoms without an adjunctive anti-depressant, SSRIs should be utilized as a first-line approach for tic-related OCD as well, with pharmacological augmentation (i.e. neuroleptics) if the tics and OCD symptoms are not being properly addressed. Caution should be taken when prescribing a neuroleptic to a child, as they often cause side-effects (i.e. sedation, weight gain, extrapyramidal dysfunction) (Newcomer, 2004).

Summary

Early onset OCD is characterized broadly across the literature, primarily by its onset prior to age 18, as well as its comorbidity profile, symptom dimension attributes, and heightened genetic load. Tic-related OCD is also characterized by an earlier age of onset, typically in childhood. It remains an open question whether tic-related OCD is a special case of early-onset OCD, with differing dimensional attributes and treatment considerations. Although treatment is similar for both early and late onset OCD (CBT with ERP and/or SSRIs), providers must consider the unique functional role of the family in the maintenance of OCD symptoms. Psychoeducation is crucial for early-onset OCD, and particularly when tics are involved. Tic-related OCD also warrants targeting specific tic behaviors with additional CBT/ERP for OCD symptoms.

References

Abramovitch, A., Dar, R., Mittelman, A., & Wilhelm, S. (2015). Comorbidity between attention deficit/hyperactivity disorder and obsessive-compulsive disorder across the lifespan: A systematic and critical review. *Harvard Review of Psychiatry*, 23(4), 245–262. doi:10.1097/HRP.0000000000000050.

Abramowitz, J. S. (2006). The psychological treatment of obsessive-compulsive disorder. *The Canadian Journal of Psychiatry*, 51(7), 407–416.

American Psychiatric Association. (2022). *Diagnostic and statistical manual of mental disorders* (5th Ed., rev. text). doi:10.1176/appi.books.9780890425787.

Arnold, P. D., Askland, K. D., Barlassina, C., Bellodi, L., Bienvenu, O. J., & Black, D. (2018). Revealing the complex genetic architecture of obsessive–compulsive disorder using meta-analysis. *Molecular Psychiatry*, 23(5), 1181–1188. doi:10.1038/mp.2017.154.

Bertelsen, T. B., Himle, J. A., & Håland, Å. T. (2022). Bidirectional Relationship Between family accommodation and youth anxiety during cognitive-behavioral treatment. *Child Psychiatry & Human Development*, 1–8. doi:10.1007/s10578-021-01304-5.

Bloch, M. H. (2017a). Comorbidity in pediatric OCD: Tourette syndrome. In C. Pittenger (Ed.), *Obsessive-compulsive disorder: Phenomenology, pathophysiology, and treatment* (pp. 589–600). Oxford University Press.

Bloch, M. H. (2017b). Natural history and long-term outcome of OCD. In C. Pittenger (Ed.), *Natural history and long-term outcome of OCD* (pp. 47–56). Oxford University Press. doi:10.1093/med/9780190228163.003.0005.

Bloch, M. H., Landeros-Weisenberger, A., Rosario, M. C., Pittenger, C., & Leckman, J. F. (2008). Meta-Analysis of the symptom structure of obsessive-compulsive disorder. *American Journal of Psychiatry*, 165(12), 1532–1542. doi:10.1176/appi.ajp.2008.08020320.

Bloch, M. H., Peterson, B. S., Scahill, L., Otka, J., Katsovich, L., Zhang, H., & Leckman, J. F. (2006). Adulthood outcome of tic and obsessive-compulsive symptom severity in children with Tourette syndrome. *Archives of Pediatrics & Adolescent Medicine*, 160(1), 65–69. doi:10.1001/archpedi.160.1.65.

Brander, G., Kuja-Halkola, R., Rosenqvist, M. A., Rück, C., Serlachius, E., Fernández de la Cruz, L., Lichtenstein, P., Crowley, J. J., Larsson, H., & Mataix-Cols, D. (2021). A population-based family clustering study of tic-related obsessive-compulsive disorder. *Molecular Psychiatry*, 26(4), 1224–1233. doi:10.1038/s41380-019-0532-z.

Breslau, J., Aguilar-Gaxiola, S., Kendler, K. S., Su, M., Williams, D., & Kessler, R. C. (2006). Specifying race-ethnic differences in risk for psychiatric disorder in a USA national sample. *Psychological Medicine*, 36(1), 57–68. doi:10.1017/S0033291705006161.

Budman, C. L. (2014). The Role of atypical antipsychotics for treatment of Tourette's syndrome: An overview. *Drugs*, 74(11), 1177–1193. doi:10.1007/s40265-014-0254-0.

Caporino, N., E. (2020). Involving family members in exposure therapy for children and adolescents. In T. S. Peris, E. A. Storch, & J. F. McGuire (Eds), *Exposure therapy for children with anxiety and OCD: Clinician's guide to integrated treatment* (pp. 323–357). Academic Press.

Ching, T. H. W. & Williams, M. T. (2019). The role of ethnic identity in OC symptom dimensions among Asian Americans. *Journal of Obsessive-Compulsive and Related Disorders*, 21, 112–120. doi:10.1016/j.jocrd.2019.03.005.

Conelea, C. A., Walther, M. R., Freeman, J. B., Garcia, A. M., Sapyta, J., Khanna, M., & Franklin, M. (2014). Tic-related obsessive-compulsive disorder (OCD): Phenomenology and treatment outcome in the pediatric OCD treatment study II. *Journal of the American Academy of Child & Adolescent Psychiatry*, 53(12), 1308–1316. doi:10.1016/j.jaac.2014.09.014.

de Alvarenga, P. G., de Mathis, M. A., Dominguez Alves, A. C., do Rosário, M. C., Fossaluza, V., Hounie, A. G., Miguel, E. C., & Torres, A. R. (2012). Clinical features of tic-related obsessive-compulsive disorder: Results from a large multicenter study. *CNS Spectrums*, 17(2), 87–93. doi:10.1017/S1092852912000491.

Demaria, F., Pontillo, M., Tata, M. C., Gargiullo, P., Mancini, F., & Vicari, S. (2021). Psychoeducation focused on family accommodation: A practical intervention for parents of children and adolescents with obsessive-compulsive disorder. *Italian Journal of Pediatrics*, 47(1), 224. doi:10.1186/s13052-021-01177-3.

do Rosario-Campos, M. C., Leckman, J. F., Curi, M., Quatrano, S., Katsovitch, L., Miguel, E. C., & Pauls, D. L. (2005). A family study of early-onset obsessive-compulsive disorder. *American Journal of Medical Genetics Part B: Neuropsychiatric Genetics,* 136B(1), 92–97. doi:10.1002/ajmg.b.30149.

Farrell, L. & Barrett, P. (2006). Obsessive-compulsive disorder across developmental trajectory: Cognitive processing of threat in children, adolescents and adults. *British Journal of Psychology*, 97(1), 95–114. doi:10.1348/000712605X58592.

Farrell, L., Waters, A., Milliner, E., & Ollendick, T. (2012). Comorbidity and treatment response in pediatric obsessive-compulsive disorder: A pilot study of group cognitive-behavioral treatment. *Psychiatry Research*, 199(2), 115–123. doi:10.1016/j.psychres.2012.04.035.

Flament, M. F., Whitaker, A., Rapoport, J. L., Davies, M., Berg, C. Z., Kalikow, K., Sceery, W., & Shaffer, D. (1988). Obsessive Compulsive Disorder in Adolescence: An epidemiological study. *Journal of the American Academy of Child & Adolescent Psychiatry*, 27(6), 764–771. doi:10.1097/00004583-198811000-00018.

Flessner, C. A., Freeman, J. B., Sapyta, J., Garcia, A., Franklin, M. E., March, J. S., & Foa, E. (2011). Predictors of parental accommodation in pediatric obsessive-compulsive disorder: Findings from the pediatric obsessive-compulsive disorder treatment study (POTS) trial. *Journal of the American Academy of Child & Adolescent Psychiatry*, 50(7), 716–725. doi:10.1016/j.jaac.2011.03.019.

Garcia, A. M., Freeman, J. B., Himle, M. B., Berman, N. C., Ogata, A. K., Ng, J., Choate-Summers, M. L., & Leonard, H. (2009). Phenomenology of early childhood onset obsessive compulsive disorder. *Journal of Psychopathology and Behavioral Assessment*, 31(2), 104–111. doi:10.1007/s10862-008-9094-0.

Garcia, A. M., Sapyta, J. J., Moore, P. S., Freeman, J. B., Franklin, M. E., March, J. S., & Foa, E. B. (2010). Predictors and moderators of treatment outcome in the pediatric obsessive compulsive treatment study (POTS I). *Journal of the American Academy of Child & Adolescent Psychiatry*, 49(10), 1024–1033. doi:10.1016/j.jaac.2010.06.013.

Garcia-Delgar, B., Servera, M., Coffey, B. J., Lázaro, L., Openneer, T., Benaroya-Milshtein, N., Steinberg, T., Hoekstra, P. J., Dietrich, A., Morer, A., EMTICS collaborative group, Apter, A., Baglioni, V., Ball, J., Benaroya-Milshtein, N., Bognar, E., Burger, B., Buse, J., Cardona, F., ... Weidinger, E. (2022). Tic disorders in children and adolescents: Does the clinical presentation differ in males and females? A report by the EMTICS group. *European Child & Adolescent Psychiatry*, 31(10), 1539–1548. doi:10.1007/s00787-021-01751-4.

Geller, D. A. (2006). Obsessive-compulsive and spectrum disorders in children and adolescents. *Psychiatric Clinics of North America*, 29(2), 353–370. doi:10.1016/j.psc.2006.02.012.

Geller, D. A., & March, J. (2012). Practice parameter for the assessment and treatment of children and adolescents with obsessive-compulsive disorder. *Journal of the American Academy of Child & Adolescent Psychiatry*, 51(1), 98–113. doi:10.1016/j.jaac.2011.09.019.

Geller, D. A., Homayoun, S., & Johnson, G. (2021). Developmental considerations in obsessive compulsive disorder: Comparing pediatric and adult-onset cases. *Frontiers in Psychiatry*, 12, Article 678539. doi:10.3389/fpsyt.2021.678538.

Geller, D., Biederman, J., Faraone, S. V., Frazier, J., Coffey, B. J., Kim, G., & Bellordre, C. A. (2000). Clinical correlates of obsessive compulsive disorder in children and adolescents referred to specialized and non-specialized clinical settings. *Depression and Anxiety*, 11(4), 163–168. doi:10.1002/1520-6394.

Ginsburg, G. S., Kingery, J. N., Drake, K. L., & Grados, M. A. (2008). Predictors of treatment response in pediatric obsessive-compulsive disorder. *Journal of the*

American Academy of Child & Adolescent Psychiatry, 47(8), 868–878. doi:10.1097/CHI.0b013e3181799ebd.

Goodman, W. K., Price, L. H., Rasmussen, S. A., Riddle, M. A., & Rapoport, J. L. (1991). Children's Yale-Brown obsessive compulsive scale (CY-BOCS). *New Haven, Connecticut: Clinical Neuroscience Unit*, 29, 31–51.

Heyman, I., Fombonne, E., Simmons, H., Ford, T., Meltzer, H., & Goodman, R. (2001). Prevalence of obsessive–compulsive disorder in the British nationwide survey of child mental health. *British Journal of Psychiatry*, 179(4), 324–329. doi:10.1192/bjp.179.4.324.

Himle, J. A., Fischer, D. J., Van Etten, M. L., Janeck, A. S., & Hanna, G. L. (2003). Group behavioral therapy for adolescents with tic-related and non-tic–related obsessive–compulsive disorder. *Depression and Anxiety*, 17(2), 73–77. doi:10.1002/da.10088.

Hollingsworth, C. E., Tanguay, P. E., Grossman, L., & Pabst, P. (1980). Long-term outcome of obsessive-compulsive disorder in childhood. *Journal of the American Academy of Child Psychiatry*, 19(1), 134–144. doi:10.1016/s0002-7138(09)60658-0.

Husted, D. S., Shapira, N. A., Murphy, T. K., Mann, G. D., Ward, H. E., & Goodman, W. K. (2007). Effect of comorbid tics on a clinically meaningful response to 8-week open-label trial of fluoxetine in obsessive compulsive disorder. *Journal of Psychiatric Research*, 41(3–4),332–337. doi:10.1016/j.jpsychires.2006.05.007.

Katz, T. C., Bui, T. H., Worhach, J., Bogut, G., & Tomczak, K. K. (2022). Tourettic OCD: Current understanding and treatment challenges of a unique endophenotype. *Frontiers in Psychiatry*, 13, 929526. doi:10.3389/fpsyt.2022.929526.

Kemp, J., Barker, D., Benito, K., Herren, J., & Freeman, J. (2021). Moderators of psychosocial treatment for pediatric obsessive-compulsive disorder: Summary and recommendations for future directions. *Journal of Clinical Child & Adolescent Psychology*, 50(4), 478–485. doi:10.1080/15374416.2020.1790378.

Kessler, R. C., Petukhova, M., Sampson, N. A., Zaslavsky, A. M., & Wittchen, H.-U. (2012). Twelve-month and lifetime prevalence and lifetime morbid risk of anxiety and mood disorders in the United States. *International Journal of Methods in Psychiatric Research*, 21(3), 169–184. doi:10.1002/mpr.1359.

Kloft, L., Steinel, T., & Kathmann, N. (2018). Systematic review of co-occurring OCD and TD: Evidence for a tic-related OCD subtype? *Neuroscience & Biobehavioral Reviews*, 95, 280–314. doi:10.1016/j.neubiorev.2018.09.021.

Kwak, C., Dat Vuong, K., & Jankovic, J. (2003). Premonitory sensory phenomenon in Tourette's syndrome. *Movement Disorders*, 18(12), 1530–1533. doi:10.1002/mds.10618.

Lebowitz, E. R., Marin, C., Martino, A., Shimshoni, Y., & Silverman, W. K. (2020). Parent-Based Treatment as Efficacious as Cognitive-Behavioral Therapy for Childhood Anxiety: A Randomized Noninferiority Study of Supportive Parenting for Anxious Childhood Emotions. *Journal of the American Academy of Child & Adolescent Psychiatry*, 59(3), 362–372. doi:10.1016/j.jaac.2019.02.014.

Lewin, A. B., Bergman, R. L., Peris, T. S., Chang, S., McCracken, J. T., & Piacentini, J. (2010). Correlates of insight among youth with obsessive-compulsive disorder: Insight and Pediatric OCD. *Journal of Child Psychology and Psychiatry*, 51(5), 603–611. doi:10.1111/j.1469-7610.2009.02181.x.

Lochner, C., Fineberg, N. A., Zohar, J., van Ameringen, M., Juven-Wetzler, A., Altamura, A. C., Cuzen, N. L., Hollander, E., Denys, D., Nicolini, H., Dell'Osso, B., Pallanti, S., & Stein, D. J. (2014). Comorbidity in obsessive-compulsive disorder (OCD): A report from the International College of Obsessive–Compulsive Spectrum Disorders (ICOCS). *Comprehensive Psychiatry*, 55(7), 1513–1519. doi:10.1016/j.comppsych.2014.05.020.

Mancebo, M. C., Boisseau, C. L., Garnaat, S. L., Eisen, J. L., Greenberg, B. D., Sibrava, N. J., Stout, R. L., & Rasmussen, S. A. (2014). Long-term course of pediatric obsessive-compulsive disorder: 3 years of prospective follow-up. *Comprehensive Psychiatry*, 55(7), 1498–1504. doi:10.1016/j.comppsych.2014.04.010.

Mancuso, E., Faro, A., Joshi, G., & Geller, D. A. (2010). Treatment of pediatric obsessive-compulsive disorder: A review. *Journal of Child and Adolescent Psychopharmacology*, 20(4), 299–308. doi:10.1089/cap.2010.0040.

Mansueto, C. S. & Keuler, D. J. (2007). Tic or compulsion? It's Tourettic OCD. *FOCUS*, 5(3), 361–367. doi:10.1176/foc.5.3.foc361.

March, J. S., Franklin, M. E., Leonard, H., Garcia, A., Moore, P., Freeman, J., & Foa, E. (2007). Tics moderate treatment outcome with sertraline but not cognitive-behavior therapy in pediatric obsessive-compulsive disorder. *Biological Psychiatry*, 61(3), 344–347. doi:10.1016/j.biopsych.2006.09.035.

Martin, A., Young, C., Leckman, J. F., Mukonoweshuro, C., Rosenheck, R., & Leslie, D. (2004). Age effects on antidepressant-induced manic conversion. *Archives of Pediatrics & Adolescent Medicine*, 158(8), 773–780. doi:10.1001/archpedi.158.8.773.

Masi, G., Pfanner, C., & Brovedani, P. (2013). Antipsychotic augmentation of selective serotonin reuptake inhibitors in resistant tic-related obsessive-compulsive disorder in children and adolescents: A naturalistic comparative study. *Journal of Psychiatric Research*, 47(8), 1007–1012. doi:10.1016/j.jpsychires.2013.04.003.

McDougle, C. J. (1994). Haloperidol addition in fluvoxamine-refractory obsessive-compulsive disorder: A double-blind, placebo-controlled study in patients with and without tics. *Archives of General Psychiatry*, 51(4), 302–308. doi:10.1001/archpsyc.1994.03950040046006.

McDougle, C. J., Barr, L. C., Goodman, W. K., Pelton, G. H., Aronson, S. C., Anand, A., & Price, L. H. (1995). Lack of efficacy of clozapine monotherapy in refractory obsessive-compulsive disorder. *The American Journal of Psychiatry*, 152(12), 1812–1814. doi:10.1176/ajp.152.12.1812.

McDougle, C. J., Goodman, W. K., Leckman, J. F., Barr, L. C., Heninger, G. R., & Price, L. H. (1993). The efficacy of fluvoxamine in obsessive-compulsive disorder: Effects of comorbid chronic tic disorder. *Journal of Clinical Psychopharmacology*, 13(5), 354–358.

McGuire, J. F., Piacentini, J., Lewin, A. B., Brennan, E. A., Murphy, T. K., & Storch, E. A. (2015). A meta-analysis of cognitive behavior therapy and medication for child obsessive-compulsive disorder: Moderators of treatment efficacy, response, and remission. *Depression and Anxiety*, 32(8), 580–593. doi:10.1002/da.22389.

McKenney, K., Simpson, A., & Stewart, S. E. (2020). *OCD in Children and Adolescents: The "OCD is Not the Boss of Me" manual.* Guilford Press.

Miguel, E. C., Leckman, J. F., Rauch, S., do Rosario-Campos, M. C., Hounie, A. G., Mercadante, M. T., Chacon, P., & Pauls, D. L. (2005). Obsessive-compulsive disorder phenotypes: Implications for genetic studies. *Molecular Psychiatry*, 10 (3), 258–275. doi:10.1038/sj.mp.4001617.

Millet, B., Kochman, F., Gallarda, T., Krebs, M. O., Demonfaucon, F., Barrot, I., Bourdel, M. C., Olié, J. P., Loo, H., & Hantouche, E. G. (2004). Phenomenological and comorbid features associated in obsessive-compulsive disorder: Influence of age of onset. *Journal of Affective Disorders*, 79(1–3),241–246. doi:10.1016/S0165-0327(02)00351–00358.

Millet, N., Longworth, J., & Arcelus, J. (2017). Prevalence of anxiety symptoms and disorders in the transgender population: A systematic review of the literature. *International Journal of Transgenderism*, 18(1), 27–38. doi:10.1080/15532739.2016.1258353.

Murray, A. L., Booth, T., Eisner, M., Auyeung, B., Murray, G., & Ribeaud, D. (2019). Sex differences in ADHD trajectories across childhood and adolescence. *Developmental Science*, 22(1), e12721. doi:10.1111/desc.12721.

Nam, S. H., Park, J., & Park, T. W. (2019). Clinical aspects of premonitory urges in patients with Tourette's disorder. *Journal of the Korean Academy of Child and Adolescent Psychiatry*, 30(2), 50–56. doi:10.5765/jkacap.180025.

Nestadt, G., Samuels, J., Riddle, M., Bienvenu, O. J., Liang, K.-Y., LaBuda, M., Walkup, J., Grados, M., & Hoehn-Saric, R. (2000). A family study of obsessive-compulsive disorder. *Archives of General Psychiatry*, 57(4), 358. doi:10.1001/archpsyc.57.4.358.

Newcomer, J. W. (2004). Metabolic risk during antipsychotic treatment. *Clinical Therapeutics*, 26(12), 1936–1946. doi:10.1016/j.clinthera.2004.12.003.

Nissen, J., Powell, S., Koch, S. V., Crowley, J. J., Matthiesen, M., Grice, D. E., Thomsen, P. H., & Parner, E. (2017). Diagnostic validity of early-onset obsessive-compulsive disorder in the Danish Psychiatric Central Register: Findings from a cohort sample. *BMJ Open*, 7(9), e017172. doi:10.1136/bmjopen-2017-017172.

Nussey, C., Pistrang, N., & Murphy, T. (2013). How does psychoeducation help? A review of the effects of providing information about Tourette syndrome and attention-deficit/hyperactivity disorder. *Child: Care, Health and Development*, 39 (5), 617–627.

The Pediatric OCD Treatment Study (POTS) Team. (2004). Cognitive-behavior therapy, sertraline, and their combination for children and adolescents with obsessive-compulsive disorder: The pediatric OCD treatment study randomized controlled trial. *JAMA*, 292(16), 1969–1976. doi:10.1001/jama.292.16.1969.

Petter, T., Richter, M. A., & Sandor, P. (1998). Clinical features distinguishing patients with Tourette's syndrome and obsessive-compulsive disorder from patients with obsessive-compulsive disorder without tics. *The Journal of Clinical Psychiatry*, 59(9), 456–459. doi:10.4088/jcp.v59n0903.

Pringsheim, T., Okun, M. S., Müller-Vahl, K., Martino, D., Jankovic, J., Cavanna, A. E., Woods, D. W., Robinson, M., Jarvie, E., Roessner, V., Oskoui, M., Holler-Managan, Y., & Piacentini, J. (2019). Practice guideline recommendations summary: Treatment of tics in people with Tourette syndrome and chronic tic disorders. *Neurology*, 92(19), 896–906. doi:10.1212/WNL.0000000000007466.

Rasmussen, S. A. & Eisen, J. L. (1992). The epidemiology and clinical features of obsessive compulsive disorder. *The Psychiatric Clinics of North America*, 15(4), 743–758.

Ruscio, A. M., Stein, D. J., Chiu, W. T., & Kessler, R. C. (2010). The epidemiology of obsessive-compulsive disorder in the National Comorbidity Survey Replication. *Molecular Psychiatry*, 15(1), 53–63. doi:10.1038/mp.2008.94.

Selles, R. R., Belschner, L., Negreiros, J., Lin, S., Schuberth, D., McKenney, K., Gregorowski, N., Simpson, A., Bliss, A., & Stewart, S. E. (2018). Group family-based cognitive behavioral therapy for pediatric obsessive compulsive disorder: Global outcomes and predictors of improvement. *Psychiatry Research*, 260, 116–122. doi:10.1016/j.psychres.2017.11.041.

Selles, R. R., Højgaard, D. R. M. A., Ivarsson, T., Thomsen, P. H., McBride, N. M., Storch, E. A., Geller, D., Wilhelm, S., Farrell, L. J., Waters, A. M., Mathieu, S., & Stewart, S. E. (2020). Avoidance, insight, impairment recognition concordance, and cognitive-behavioral therapy outcomes in pediatric obsessive-compulsive disorder. *Journal of the American Academy of Child & Adolescent Psychiatry*, 59(5), 650–659.e2. doi:10.1016/j.jaac.2019.05.030.

Sobin, C., Blundell, M. L., & Karayiorgou, M. (2000). Phenotypic differences in early- and late-onset obsessive-compulsive disorder. *Comprehensive Psychiatry*, 41(5), 373–379. doi:10.1053/comp.2000.9009.

Storch, E. A., Geffken, G. R., Merlo, L. J., Jacob, M. L., Murphy, T. K., Goodman, W. K., ... & Grabill, K. (2007). Family accommodation in pediatric obsessive–compulsive disorder. *Journal of Clinical Child and Adolescent Psychology*, 36(2), 207–216. doi:10.1080/15374410701277929.

Storch, E. A., De Nadai, A. S., Jacob, M. L., Lewin, A. B., Muroff, J., Eisen, J., Abramowitz, J. S., Geller, D. A., & Murphy, T. K. (2014). Phenomenology and correlates of insight in pediatric obsessive–compulsive disorder. *Comprehensive Psychiatry*, 55(3), 613–620. doi:10.1016/j.comppsych.2013.09.014.

Storch, E. A., Merlo, L. J., Larson, M. J., Geffken, G. R., Lehmkuhl, H. D., Jacob, M. L., Murphy, T. K., & Goodman, W. K. (2008). Impact of comorbidity on cognitive-behavioral therapy response in pediatric obsessive-compulsive disorder. *Journal of the American Academy of Child & Adolescent Psychiatry*, 47 (5), 583–592. doi:10.1097/CHI.0b013e31816774b1.

Storch, E. A., Milsom, V. A., Merlo, L. J., Larson, M., Geffken, G. R., Jacob, M. L., Murphy, T. K., & Goodman, W. K. (2008). Insight in pediatric obsessive-compulsive disorder: Associations with clinical presentation. *Psychiatry Research*, 160(2), 212–220. doi:10.1016/j.psychres.2007.07.005.

Storch, E. A., Stigge-Kaufman, D., Marien, W. E., Sajid, M., Jacob, M. L., Geffken, G. R., Goodman, W. K., & Murphy, T. K. (2008). Obsessive-compulsive disorder in youth with and without a chronic tic disorder. *Depression and Anxiety*, 25(9), 761–767. doi:10.1002/da.20304.

Tanidir, C., Adaletli, H., Gunes, H., Kilicoglu, A. G., Mutlu, C., Bahali, M. K., Aytemiz, T., & Uneri, O. S. (2015). Impact of gender, age at onset, and lifetime tic disorders on the clinical presentation and comorbidity pattern of obsessive-compulsive disorder in children and adolescents. *Journal of Child and Adolescent Psychopharmacology*, 25(5), 425–431. doi:10.1089/cap.2014.0120.

Tao, Y., Li, H., Li, L., Zhang, H., Xu, H., Zhang, H., Zou, S., Deng, F., Huang, L., Wang, Y., Wang, X., Tang, X., Fu, X., & Yin, L. (2022). Comparing the efficacy of pharmacological and psychological treatment, alone and in combination, in children and adolescents with obsessive-compulsive disorder: A network meta-analysis. *Journal of Psychiatric Research*, 148, 95–102. doi:10.1016/j.jpsychires.2022.01.057.

Thomsen, P. H. (2013). Obsessive–compulsive disorders. *European Child & Adolescent Psychiatry*, 22(S1), 23–28. doi:10.1007/s00787-012-0357-7.

Tükel, R., Ertekin, E., Batmaz, S., Alyanak, F., Sözen, A., Aslantaş, B., Atli, H., & Ozyildirim, I. (2005). Influence of age of onset on clinical features in obsessive-compulsive disorder. *Depression and Anxiety*, 21(3), 112–117. doi:10.1002/da.20065.

van Grootheest, D. S., Cath, D. C., Beekman, A. T., & Boomsma, D. I. (2005). Twin studies on obsessive–compulsive disorder: A review. *Twin Research and Human Genetics*, 8(5), 450–458. doi:10.1375/twin.8.5.450.

Watson, P., Clarkin, J., & Lomax, C. (2021). What are the predictors of family accommodation of obsessive-compulsive behaviours in adults and youth with obsessive-compulsive disorder and their relatives? A systematic review. *Journal of Obsessive-Compulsive and Related Disorders*, 31, Article 100681.

Watson, H. J., & Rees, C. S. (2008). Meta-analysis of randomized, controlled treatment trials for pediatric obsessive-compulsive disorder. *Journal of Child Psychology and Psychiatry*, 49(5), 489–498. doi:10.1111/j.1469-7610.2007.01875.x.

Werling, D. M., & Geschwind, D. H. (2013). *Sex differences in autism spectrum disorders: Current Opinion in Neurology*, 26(2), 146–153. doi:10.1097/WCO.0b013e32835ee548.

Westwell-Roper, C., & Stewart, S. E. (2019). Challenges in the diagnosis and treatment of pediatric obsessive-compulsive disorder. *Indian Journal of Psychiatry*, 61(Suppl 1), S119–S130. doi:10.4103/psychiatry.IndianJPsychiatry_524_18.

Wilhelm, S., Peterson, A. L., Piacentini, J., Woods, D. W., Deckersbach, T., Sukhodolsky, D. G., Chang, S., Liu, H., Dziura, J., Walkup, J. T., & Scahill, L. (2012). Randomized trial of behavior therapy for adults with Tourette syndrome. *Archives of General Psychiatry*, 69(8), 795–803. doi:10.1001/archgenpsychiatry.2011.1528.

Williams, M. T., Elstein, J., Buckner, E., Abelson, J. M., & Himle, J. A. (2012). Symptom dimensions in two samples of African Americans with obsessive–compulsive disorder. *Journal of Obsessive-Compulsive and Related Disorders*, 1 (3), 145–152. doi:10.1016/j.jocrd.2012.03.004.

Woods, D. W., Piacentini, J., Chang, S., Deckersbach, T., Ginsburg, G., Peterson, A., Scahill, L. D., Walkup, J. T., & Wilhelm, S. (2008). *Managing Tourette syndrome: A behavioral intervention for children and adults therapist guide*. Oxford University Press.

Wu, Y., Lang, Z., & Zhang, H. (2016). Efficacy of cognitive-behavioral therapy in pediatric obsessive-compulsive disorder: A meta-analysis. *Medical Science Monitor*, 22, 1646–1653. doi:10.12659/MSM.895481.

Yu, D., Mathews, C. A., Scharf, J. M., Neale, B. M., Davis, L. K., Gamazon, E. R., Derks, E. M., Evans, P., Edlund, C. K., Crane, J., Fagerness, J. A., Osiecki, L., Gallagher, P., Gerber, G., Haddad, S., Illmann, C., McGrath, L. M., Mayerfeld, C., Arepalli, S., ... Pauls, D. L. (2015). Cross-disorder genome-wide analyses suggest a complex genetic relationship between Tourette's syndrome and OCD. *American Journal of Psychiatry*, 172(1), 82–93. doi:10.1176/appi. ajp.2014.13101306.

Zaboski, B. A., Gilbert, A., Hamblin, R., Andrews, J., Ramos, A., Nadeau, J. M., & Storch, E. A. (2019). Quality of life in children and adolescents with obsessive-compulsive disorder: The Pediatric Quality of Life Enjoyment and Satisfaction Questionnaire (PQ-LES-Q). *Bulletin of the Menninger Clinic*, 83(4), 377–397. doi:10.1521/bumc_2019_83_03.

Zimmerman-Brenner, S., Pilowsky-Peleg, T., Rachamim, L., Ben-Zvi, A., Gur, N., Murphy, T., Fattal-Valevski, A., & Rotstein, M. (2022). Group behavioral interventions for tics and comorbid symptoms in children with chronic tic disorders. *European Child & Adolescent Psychiatry*, 31(4), 637–648. doi:10.1007/s00787-020-01702-5.

Zohar, A. H. (1999). The epidemiology of obsessive-compulsive disorder in children and adolescents. *Child and Adolescent Psychiatric Clinics of North America*, 8(3), 445–460. doi:10.1016/S1056-4993(18)30163-30169.

15 Psychiatric Comorbidity of Pediatric OCRDs

Orri Smárason, Gudmundur Skarphedinsson and Davíð R. M. A. Højgaard

Historically, psychiatric comorbidity was not well understood and often viewed as a limitation of the diagnostic system rather than a reflection of the complexity of mental illness. As a result, individuals were often diagnosed with only one condition at a time (Krueger & Markon, 2006). In the 1980s, with the publication of the Diagnostic and statistical manual of mental disorders, third edition (DSM-III) (American Psychiatric Association, 1980), research began to show that comorbidity was common among individuals with mental health conditions. This led to a shift in the understanding of comorbidity as a reflection of the complexity of mental illness rather than a limitation of the diagnostic system (Lilienfeld, Waldman, & Israel, 1994). In the 1990s the appreciation of comorbidity led to the development of more comprehensive treatment approaches, such as integrated treatment, which addresses multiple conditions simultaneously. This approach recognizes that comorbid conditions can have a significant impact on treatment course and that addressing comorbidity is important for improving outcomes (Hirschfeld, 2001). In recent years, there has been a growing recognition of the importance of considering comorbidity when diagnosing and treating mental health conditions. The latest edition of the DSM (DSM-5) includes more information about comorbidity than earlier versions and encourages healthcare providers to consider comorbidity when making a diagnosis (American Psychiatric Association, 2013). In this chapter, the focus will be on the comorbidity of pediatric obsessive-compulsive and related disorders (OCRDs), tic disorders (TD), and health anxiety (HA). We will specifically discuss the nature and characteristics of these comorbid conditions, along with the theories and etiological factors that underlie their co-occurrence. Furthermore, we will address the developmental considerations related to assessment and treatment, highlighting the importance of age-appropriate and tailored approaches.

Obsessive Compulsive Disorder

A recent meta-analysis found that 64 percent of pediatric obsessive-compulsive disorder (OCD) patients met diagnostic criteria for at least

DOI: 10.4324/9781003517429-15

one other psychiatric disorder (Sharma et al., 2021). Comorbid disorders complicate the presentation of pediatric OCD in many ways, and their presence has consistently been associated with lower quality of life (Weidle, Ivarsson, Thomsen, Lydersen, & Jozefiak, 2015), attenuated treatment response (Geller, Biederman, et al., 2003), and greater functional impairment (Piacentini, Peris, Bergman, Chang, & Jaffer, 2007). Figure 15.1 provides an overview of comorbidity rates in pediatric OCD from a recent meta-analysis (Sharma et al., 2021). In addition to these comorbidities, rates of OCD are often elevated in other OCRD presentations, and those co-occurrences are discussed in the subsection pertaining to each OCRD.

Abbreviations: Major depressive disorder (MDD), Anxiety disorder (AD), Generalized anxiety disorder (GAD), Social anxiety disorder (SoAD), Panic disorder (PD), Specific phobia (SP), Tic disorders (TD), attention deficit hyperactivity disorder (ADHD).

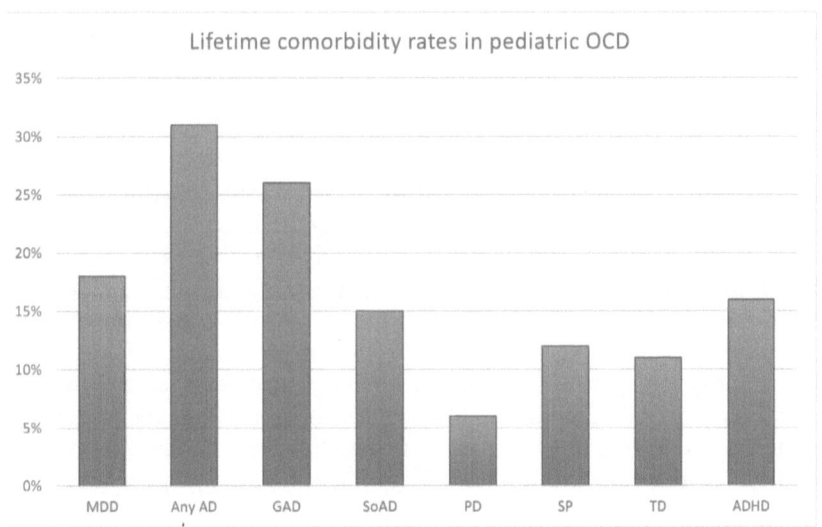

Abbreviations: Major depressive disorder (MDD), Anxiety disorder (AD), Generalized anxiety disorder (GAD), Social anxiety disorder (SoAD), Panic disorder (PD), Specific phobia (SP), Tic disorders (TD), attention deficit hyperactivity disorder (ADHD).

Figure 15.1 Rates of common comorbidities in pediatric OCD (Sharma et al., 2021).

OCD and anxiety disorders (AD)

Prevalence estimates for co-occurring AD with pediatric OCD range from 20–60 percent (Geller et al., 2001; Torp et al., 2015), with meta-analytic data suggesting a rate of just over 30 percent (Sharma et al., 2021). In adult OCD populations, ADs are the second most prevalent comorbid condition, only surpassed by mood disorders (Klein, Harris, Björgvinsson, & Kertz, 2020; Sharma et al., 2021). OCD was classified as an AD until DSM-5, owing to the central role of anxiety in OCD pathology. Obsessions generate anxiety/distress, and compulsions temporarily alleviate it. Avoidance behaviors, similar to those in AD, are also often seen in OCD (Tynes, White, & Steketee, 1990). However, anxiety and avoidance are non-specific symptoms associated with several other psychiatric disorders (e.g., depression, bipolar disorder, and schizophrenia). Further, many OCD presentations are driven by emotions distinct from anxiety (e.g., disgust, incompleteness and "not just right" experiences) (Storch, Abramowitz, & Goodman, 2008). Consequently, the DSM-5 reclassified OCD under the OCRD category (American Psychiatric Association, 2013; Sharma et al., 2021).

OCD and ADs share genetic, neurobiological, and psychological vulnerabilities (Pauls, Abramovitch, Rauch, & Geller, 2014; Storch, Abramowitz, et al., 2008). Family studies show that first-degree relatives of OCD patients are more likely to have OCD and ADs (Carter, Pollock, Suvak, & Pauls, 2004; Nestadt et al., 2001). Twin studies have also demonstrated overlapping genetic risk factors for OCD and ADs (López-Solà et al., 2016; Tambs et al., 2009). A large population register-based study in Sweden found moderate genetic correlations between OCD and ADs, strongest between OCD and generalized anxiety disorder (GAD), intermediate for OCD and social anxiety disorder, and weakest between OCD and panic disorder (Kendler, Abrahamsson, Ohlsson, Sundquist, & Sundquist, 2023). AD and OCD both involve chronic stress, amplified by cognitive misappraisals and distorted thinking patterns which lead to maladaptive, emotional responses such as avoidance and safety behaviors (Hellberg, Jacoby, & Wilhelm, 2020). These behaviors may be effective in reducing discomfort momentarily, but ultimately exacerbate symptoms by reinforcing inaccurate/unhelpful beliefs and preventing opportunities to extinguish fear and correct such beliefs (Hellberg et al., 2020; Rachman, 1997).

The co-occurrence of pediatric OCD and AD is associated with greater impairment, compared to when either condition occurs alone, likely leading to greater negative impact on child developmental trajectories (Angst et al., 2005; Grabe et al., 2000; Storch, Abramowitz, & Keeley, 2009). Parents have been found to rate younger children with OCD higher on measures of anxiety compared to adolescents, but this is mostly driven by higher scores for separation anxiety which is not found in youth self-reports or in clinician-administered diagnostic interviews (Smárason et al., 2021). Developmental level therefore does not significantly affect comorbid AD prevalence in pediatric OCD.

The significant overlap between AD and OCD can lead to challenges in differential diagnoses. Accurate conceptualization and tailored treatment approaches require comprehensive diagnostic and behavioral assessments when both conditions are present (Abramowitz & Jacoby, 2015). Intrusive thoughts occur frequently in both OCD and AD and can make distinguishing between the disorders challenging. However, in AD, intrusive thoughts are often focused on real-world problems, with overestimated catastrophic outcomes, while obsessions in OCD are usually ego-dystonic, and are often focused on irrational, highly improbable or impossible fears (Hellberg et al., 2020; Langlois, Freeston, & Ladouceur, 2000).

Comorbid AD does not seem to strongly impact treatment response to first-line OCD interventions (Storch, Larson, et al., 2008). This may be, in part, the result of high treatment overlap, as for both AD and OCD, cognitive behavioral therapy (CBT) is regarded as the first-line treatment option in children and adolescents, with serotonin reuptake inhibitors (SRI) as the first option for treatment augmentation for severe or complex cases (National Institute for Heath and Clinical Excellence, 2014). The guiding principles of CBT are the same for treatment of OCD and anxiety, although their application might be slightly different (Hellberg et al., 2020). For both disorders, a cognitive component is included where maladaptive beliefs, such as overestimation of personal responsibility or the need to control thoughts, are systematically challenged. The core component of treatment is behavioral and focused on exposure exercises. During exposures, patients test their fears through imagined or real-life experiences, while refraining from safety behaviors and compulsions. However, individual case conceptualizations, and empirically informed clinical judgment should be used to devise a treatment plan in conjunction with regular assessment of primary symptoms to modify treatment as needed.

OCD and depression

In children and adolescents with OCD, depression co-occurs in a about 15–20 percent of cases (Sharma et al., 2021; Storch et al., 2012) Comorbid depression in pediatric OCD is associated with greater OCD symptom severity, higher levels of functional impairment (Canavera, Ollendick, Ehrenreich May, & Pincus, 2010; Ivarsson, Melin, & Wallin, 2008; Peris et al., 2010), increased social problems, family conflict, and poorer family organization (Canavera et al., 2010). Additionally, it is associated with higher levels of suicidality (Angelakis, Gooding, Tarrier, & Panagioti, 2015), anxiety (Abramowitz, Storch, Keeley, & Cordell, 2007), and attenuated treatment response (Abramowitz, 2004; Meyer et al., 2014; Storch,

Larson, et al., 2008). However, when pre-treatment symptom severity is taken into account the impact comorbid depression has on treatment outcomes is less clear (Brown, Lester, Jassi, Heyman, & Krebs, 2015; Farrell, Waters, Milliner, & Ollendick, 2012; Leonard, Jacobi, Riemann, Lake, & Luhn, 2014).

Storch et al. (2012) found that functional impairment partially mediated the relationship between OCD and depressive symptom severity, suggesting that depression may arise from the impairment and avoidance caused by OCD. In such cases, depression may abate if interventions successfully target the primary OCD symptoms. Recent network analyses have explored links between OCD symptoms and depression in children and adolescents (Cervin et al., 2020; Jones, Mair, Riemann, Mugno, & McNally, 2018), indicating a strong link between obsessions and worry, a common symptom of depression (Cervin et al., 2020; Waszczuk, Brown, Eley, & Lester, 2015), and suggesting a complex reciprocal underlying mechanism linking OCD, anxiety and depression symptoms, which is also supported by their high levels of comorbidity (Cervin et al., 2020; Gentes & Ruscio, 2011).

Selective serotonin reuptake inhibitors (SSRI) and CBT are common and evidence-based treatment options for both OCD and depression (Bernaras, Jaureguizar, & Garaigordobil, 2019; Nazeer, Latif, Mondal, Azeem, & Greydanus, 2020). In some cases, targeting OCD symptoms and impairment, during CBT, should lead to improvements in depressive symptom severity as well. However, unlike when OCD and AD co-occur and exposure is the behavioral focus of treatment, depression treatment primarily emphasizes behavioral activation. In practice that may mean that therapists may need to concurrently treat depressive symptoms, potentially diluting treatment response. Other specific challenges of treating comorbid OCD and depression include that depression is often characterized by pervasive hopelessness which may lead to decreased motivation to engage in treatment. Similarly, reduced insight and low perceived self-competence in youth with depression may limit engagement with therapy (Brown et al., 2015; Peris et al., 2010). It is worth noting that many OCD treatment studies exclude depressed patients, particularly if depression is severe, limiting our understanding of treating these conditions concurrently. Current clinical practice guidelines advise that each comorbid disorder may require a separate treatment plan (Walter et al., 2022). When depression is particularly severe, it may merit acute and specific intervention prior to treating other OCD symptoms. However, transdiagnostic treatments that address the underlying vulnerabilities across these highly comorbid disorders, such as avoidance behavior or repetitive negative thinking, may be effective although they are understudied in youth with primary OCD (Ehrenreich-May et al., 2017; Weersing et al., 2012).

OCD, attention deficit hyperactivity disorder, and externalizing problems

The comorbidity rate of ADHD in children and adolescents with OCD is around 15–20 percent, with oppositional defiant disorder (ODD) around 12 percent (Sharma et al., 2021). Early childhood onset of OCD is particularly associated with comorbid ADHD (Brem, Grünblatt, Drechsler, Riederer, & Walitza, 2014). Studies show that children with comorbid ADHD and OCD experience more socialization and academic problems, and family dysfunction compared to those with OCD alone (Sukhodolsky, do Rosario-Campos, Scahill, Findley, & Leckman, 2005). Children with comorbid OCD and ADHD experience greater impairment and frequency of other comorbid diagnoses (Masi et al., 2006) and impaired educational functioning (Geller, Coffey, et al., 2003). Comorbid externalizing disorders are associated with lower family cohesion, greater OCD-specific functional impairment, and higher rates of comorbid tics (Langley, Lewin, Bergman, Lee, & Piacentini, 2010) and more behavioral, social, and attentional problems (Langley et al., 2010). While comorbid ADHD is associated with attenuated treatment response in children with OCD (Garcia et al., 2010; Storch, Merlo, et al., 2008), the evidence is mixed for other externalizing disorders (Garcia et al., 2010; Halldorsdottir & Ollendick, 2014; Storch et al., 2010). Further, those with both OCD and ADHD are more likely to experience relapse after successful inpatient treatment compared to patients without ADHD (Walitza et al., 2008).

Studies show independent familial risk factors for developing ADHD and OCD (Geller, Coffey, et al., 2003; Geller et al., 2007). First-degree relatives of children with comorbid ADHD and OCD are significantly more likely to have ADHD than relatives of healthy controls and children with OCD only, with no significant difference in the rate of ADHD between OCD only and healthy controls (Geller et al., 2007). ADHD and OCD are both associated with frontostriatal dysfunction, although ADHD is associated with frontostriatal hypoactivity (Konrad & Eickhoff, 2010) and OCD with frontostriatal hyperactivity (Norman et àl., 2017). Despite neurobiological differences (Norman et al., 2016), both disorders lead to overlapping neuropsychological deficits, suggesting that different neurological processes can lead to similar dysfunction (Cabarkapa, King, Dowling, & Ng, 2019). Specifically, both disorders are associated with impairments in executive function and particularly inhibition deficits (Abramovitch, Dar, Hermesh, & Schweiger, 2012; Norman et al., 2018). When assessing comorbid presentations and planning interventions, clinicians must be mindful of the potential interaction of symptoms. OCD symptoms and behavioral or attentional problems might affect each other in reciprocal ways. For instance, a child experiencing anxiety, owing to an OCD obsession may act out behaviorally (Peris et al., 2008). Similarly, attention difficulties can result from both obsessive preoccupation and

OCD-related worry (Langley et al., 2010). Abramowitz et al. (2015) suggest that ADHD-like symptoms resulting from OCD-specific symptomatology may commonly be misdiagnosed as ADHD.

Treating OCD with traditional first-line treatments (SSRI and/or CBT with ERP) can improve attentional deficits in cases with comorbid ADHD (Guzick et al., 2017). Untreated ADHD diminishes treatment response in pediatric OCD, so concurrent treatment is advised (Geller et al., 2002). The first line treatment for ADHD is stimulant medication, which may improve attention, and facilitate learning and retention of CBT skills for children with comorbid OCD, although this has only been demonstrated in case studies (King, Dowling, & Leow, 2017). However, limited evidence suggests that stimulant medication could exacerbate and provoke OCD symptoms (Jhanda, Singla, & Grover, 2016; Kouris, 1998; Woolley & Heyman, 2003). It is essential that clinicians closely monitor the severity of OCD symptoms when initiating stimulant treatment for comorbid ADHD.

OCD and autism

The rate of co-occurring autism in youth with OCD is around 6 percent (Sharma et al., 2021), while estimates of comorbid OCD rates in children with autism range from 2.6 percent to 37.2 percent (Leyfer et al., 2006; van Steensel, Bögels, & Perrin, 2011). Similar symptom topography between the two disorders may explain the wide range of prevalence rates between studies. Specifically, distinguishing between restricted, repetitive interests in autism and obsessions in OCD, and between repetitive or self-stimulatory behaviors in autism and compulsions in OCD can be challenging (Bedford, Hunsche, & Kerns, 2020). Clinicians should consider that in autism, repetitive behaviors tend to be calming, sensory seeking, ego-syntonic, and not linked to a specific purpose or thought, while in OCD they are ego-dystonic, cause distress, and are driven by anxiety or other uncomfortable emotional states associated with a specific obsessive thought (Bedford et al., 2020; Pazuniak & Pekrul, 2020).

OCD may present differently in individuals with autism, exhibiting more hoarding and ordering behaviors and fewer magical obsessions (Griffiths, Farrell, Waters, & White, 2017b; La Buissonnière-Ariza et al., 2018). It is unclear whether children and adolescents with OCD and comorbid autism experience more severe symptoms, However, youth with autism and OCD have increased functional impairment and a higher number of comorbid diagnoses (Griffiths, Farrell, Waters, & White, 2017a), poorer psychosocial functioning, use clinical services for longer and are prescribed medication more often and make lesser treatment gains (Martin et al., 2020). They also maintain less treatment gains six months after treatment termination (Griffiths et al., 2017b), relative to those with OCD only. In addition, it has been found that in children and adolescents with OCD, sub-clinical symptoms of autism are elevated (with reported rates ranging from 10–32.5 percent) (Arildskov et al., 2015; Griffiths et al., 2017a; Ivarsson & Melin, 2008).

Standard CBT programs for OCD are generally effective for those with autism diagnoses (Wolters, de Haan, Hogendoorn, Boer, & Prins, 2016), and autistic traits (Højgaard et al., 2023), although some studies have found that certain children with autism may benefit less than typically developing children (Murray, Jassi, Mataix-Cols, Barrow, & Krebs, 2015). Adapting CBT for autism yields comparable effect sizes to CBT for OCD in the general population (Flygare et al., 2020; Russell et al., 2013). Intensive CBT formats have also shown promise for adolescents with comorbid autism (Iniesta-Sepúlveda et al., 2018; Krebs, Murray, & Jassi, 2016). Another notable advancement is the development of function-based CBT (Fb-CBT), a novel treatment approach combining CBT principles and applied behavioral analysis (Bedford et al., 2020). SSRI medication appears to reduce OCD symptoms and repetitive behaviors in children and adolescents with comorbid OCD and autism (Reddihough et al., 2019). However adverse behavioral side effects may be common in young patients with autism, and caution should be used with initial dosing, and side effects must be closely monitored (Pazuniak & Pekrul, 2020; Reiersen & Handen, 2011).

OCD and other comorbidities

Sleep problems. Sleep related problems are common in pediatric OCD, with studies indicating that 27–84 percent of affected children and adolescents have significant sleep difficulties (Ivarsson & Skarphedinsson, 2015; Nabinger de Diaz, Farrell, Waters, Donovan, & McConnell, 2019; Sevilla-Cermeño et al., 2019; Storch, Murphy, et al., 2008). Children with OCD show reduced total sleep time and longer awake periods after sleep onset (Alfano & Kim, 2011). Adolescents with OCD have reduced total sleep time, reduced non-REM sleep time, and longer sleep onset latencies when compared to healthy controls (Insel et al., 1982; Rapoport, 1986). Sleep difficulties in pediatric OCD are associated with higher OCD symptom severity, more internalizing problems, more psychiatric comorbidity, more depressive symptoms, and more functional impairment (Nabinger de Diaz et al., 2019; Sevilla-Cermeño et al., 2019; Storch, Murphy, et al., 2008). Sleep problems tend to improve with CBT treatment (Ivarsson & Skarphedinsson, 2015; Storch, Murphy, et al., 2008), but the impact of sleep problems on OCD treatment outcomes is unclear. Some studies have found sleep problems to predict a less favorable CBT outcome (Ivarsson & Skarphedinsson, 2015), while others have found no such effect (Nabinger de Diaz et al., 2019; Sevilla-Cermeño et al., 2019).

Post-traumatic stress disorder and trauma exposure. Post-traumatic stress disorder (PTSD) rates have been found to be elevated in youth with

OCD compared to the general population and youth experiencing both OCD and PTSD may experience more severe OCD symptoms (Lafleur et al., 2011; Wislocki, Kratz, Martin, & Becker-Haimes, 2022). However, trauma exposure and subsequent PTSD symptoms are risk factors for many psychiatric problems, and there is very limited evidence to suggest a unique relationship between PTSD and OCD specifically (Wislocki et al., 2022). Whether exposure to a traumatic event may lead to the development or worsening of OCD is unclear. Some studies demonstrate a higher prevalence of traumatic events in youth with OCD while others find no relationship or even a lower prevalence of traumatic events in youth with OCD compared to youth with other psychiatric disorders (Ivarsson, Saavedra, Granqvist, & Broberg, 2016; Wislocki et al., 2022). One study has examined the impact of adverse childhood experiences (ACEs) on OCD treatment response. No significant associations between ACEs and CBT response were found, suggesting that CBT for pediatric OCD is effective regardless of ACE exposure (Vazquez et al., 2022).

Eating disorders. Eating disorders and OCD share numerous features as both are characterized by intrusive thoughts that are associated with negative affect and compulsive compensatory behaviors performed to reduce that negative affect (Coelho et al., 2019). Personality characteristics such a impulsivity, neuroticism, and perfectionism are also associated with both disorders (Altman & Shankman, 2009). A meta-analysis found a lifetime prevalence estimate of comorbid OCD in eating disorders of 13.9 percent (Drakes, Fawcett, Rose, Carter-Major, & Fawcett, 2021). In addition to the frequent co-occurrence of OCD and eating disorders, there is emerging data to support a genetic correlation with anorexia nervosa and OCD, suggesting a potential shared etiology (Aman et al., 2022; Cederlöf, Thornton, et al., 2015; Mas et al., 2013; Yilmaz et al., 2022). Whether the presence of a comorbid eating disorder attenuates OCD treatment response for children and adolescents remains unknown.

Schizophrenia and psychotic disorders

The prevalence of comorbid schizophrenia and psychotic disorders in OCD across the lifespan is estimated to be 4.5 percent, across all ages, and 3.5 percent in adults; however the prevalence in pediatric OCD is uncertain (Sharma et al., 2021). People first diagnosed with OCD were found to be three times more likely to later develop schizophrenia and five times more likely to later develop schizoaffective disorder in a large population-based study (Cederlöf, Lichtenstein, et al., 2015). The risk of later developing OCD if first diagnosed with schizophrenia or schizoaffective disorder was also increased. Although OCD and schizophrenia are well defined, it is important to assess insight, especially in pediatric OCD, to avoid a misdiagnosis of schizophrenia as bizarre behaviors and disorganized thoughts may well occur in pediatric OCD without psychosis (Rodowski, Cagande, & Riddle, 2008). When treating adolescents with concurrent OCD and schizophrenia, a higher dose of antipsychotic medicine may be needed than in the case of schizophrenia only (Baytunca et al., 2017), although the evidence for this is limited. Both positive and negative psychotic symptoms have been found to be higher when obsessive compulsive symptoms are present in schizophrenia (Cunill, Castells, & Simeon, 2009).

Tic disorders

Comorbidity in pediatric tic disorder (TD) is common (Hirschtritt, Lee, Pauls, & et al., 2015). In clinical samples children with TD will frequently meet criteria for two or more additional disorders (32.9 percent (Groth, Mol Debes, Rask, Lange, & Skov, 2017; Scahill, Sukhodolsky, Williams, & Leckman, 2005). Studies have also noted a high rate of comorbidity between TD, ADHD, and OCD, which suggests a shared neurobiological base (Grados, 2010), and shared genetic susceptibility (Abramovitch et al., 2015). TDs alone are very rarely the primary reason for psychiatric referral. Most children seek treatment, owing to their comorbid psychiatric conditions such as OCD, ADHD, or mood disorders (Khalifa & Knorring, 2007; Santangelo et al., 1994).

TD and ADHD

Attention-deficit/hyperactivity disorder (ADHD) is one of the most frequent comorbid conditions in pediatric TDs, with rates ranging from 40–80 percent in different studies (Coffey et al., 2000; Freeman et al., 2000; Hirschtritt et al., 2015). Usually, ADHD symptoms precede the tics onset. The co-occurrence of TD and ADHD is related to earlier tic onset (5.8 vs 6.2 years) (Roessner, Becker, Banaschewski, & Rothenberger, 2007). The etiologies of TD and ADHD include a combination of genetic and environmental factors (Homberg et al., 2016; Mathews & Grados, 2011). Studies have identified several genetic loci associated with tic disorders (Tsetsos et al., 2016), and there is evidence of strong heritability (Mathews & Grados, 2011). Prenatal exposure to toxins, infections, and stress are among environmental factors, also implicated in the development of both TD and ADHD (Bos-Veneman, Kuin, Minderaa, & Hoekstra, 2010; Homberg et al., 2016). The comorbidity of ADHD with TD in youth has also been associated with further psychopathology, such as OCD, ADs, mood disorders, sleep problems, social skills deficits, learning disorders and academic difficulties, ODD, CD, and anger control problems (Freeman et al., 2000; Hirschtritt et al., 2015; Roessner et al., 2007; Walkup et al., 1996). Developmental considerations for children and adolescents with TD and comorbid ADHD include the impact of these conditions on academic, social, and emotional functioning. Assessment of TD and

ADHD should include a thorough clinical evaluation, and it is important to note that TD and ADHD have can overlapping symptoms (e.g., rapid and recurrent motor movements) (Stewart et al., 2006). A comprehensive assessment, including a thorough medical, psychiatric, and psychological evaluation, is recommended to accurately diagnose both ADHD and TDs.

Treatment for both TD and ADHD typically includes a combination of pharmacotherapy and psychotherapy. Medications used to treat tic disorders include neuroleptics (e.g., haloperidol, pimozide) and alpha-2 agonists (e.g., clonidine, guanfacine; (Jankovic, 2020), while ADHD is most often treated with stimulants (e.g., methylphenidate, amphetamines), although non-stimulant medications are also used (e.g., atomoxetine, guanfacine; (Malmivaara, 2021). Treatment studies have specifically addressed the treatment of children with both disorders, including trials of psychostimulants and atomoxetine, in order to show effects for ADHD symptoms but without worsening tics symptoms (Pringsheim et al., 2019). Clonidine plus methylphenidate and methylphenidate are more likely than placebo to reduce tic severity and reduce ADHD symptoms (Kurlan, 2002), and atomoxetine has shown that it does not worsen tics in comparison to placebo, while reducing ADHD symptoms (Allen et al., 2005). Furthermore, the presence of ADHD does not seem to moderate response to behavioral treatment, such as Comprehensive Behavioral Intervention for Tics (Sukhodolsky et al., 2017), although one study has found a non-significant trend toward a reduced behavioral treatment response (Nissen et al., 2019).

TD and OCD

Comorbid OCD in individuals with TD is estimated to range from 20–50 percent (Coffey et al., 2000; Freeman, 2007; Freeman et al., 2000; Hirschtritt et al., 2015; Wanderer et al., 2012). TD usually occur before OCD and typically remit during adolescence or early adulthood (Pappert, Goetz, Louis, Blasucci, & Leurgans, 2003; Peterson, Pine, Cohen, & Brook, 2001). However, OCD tends to be more persistent (Leckman et al., 2010; Thomsen, 2000). OCD with comorbid TD has substantial evidence as a subtype, which is also reflected in the DSM-5's new tic-related specifier (Dell'Osso et al., 2017). TD with comorbid OCD is more common in males (Brander et al., 2021; Leckman et al., 1994; Nestadt et al., 2003) and is associated with earlier onset of OCD (Brander et al., 2021; Kloft, Steinel, & Kathmann, 2018), higher rates of symmetry, exactness, and sexual/aggressive obsessions, and touching, tapping, and rubbing compulsions (Darrow et al., 2017; de Vries et al., 2016; Hirschtritt et al., 2018), and sensory experiences before compulsions (Miguel, Baer, Coffey, & Rauch, 1997). Additionally, youth with TD and OCD tend to have higher rates of other comorbidities such as ADHD, ASD, epilepsy, and intellectual disability (Brander et al., 2021; Kloft et al., 2018). The exact causes of TDs with comorbid OCD are not known, but interactions between genetic, neurobiological, and environmental factors have been implicated (Mataix-Cols et al., 2013; Pauls, Alsobrook, Goodman, Rasmussen, & Leckman, 1995).

It is important to conduct a thorough clinical evaluation and to consider other potentially comorbid conditions, such as ADHD and AD (Szejko et al., 2022). Distinguishing between compulsions in OCD and complex tics can be challenging, particularly since they often occur together. The compulsions associated with OCD are intended to alleviate or reduce anxiety or discomfort and are typically carried out in response to an obsession (e.g., a fear of contamination). On the other hand, individuals with TDs have a compelling need to perform a specific action, such as carrying out certain movements the same number of times on both sides of the body, or until they experience a sense of "rightness" (American Psychiatric Association, 2013). Treatment for TD and OCD typically involves pharmacotherapy and psychotherapy. Neuroleptics and alpha-2 agonists are used to treat TDs (Jankovic, 2020), while SSRIs are used to treat OCD (Ivarsson et al., 2015). The response to SSRIs in this population is not clear as some studies report less response in TD with comorbid OCD (March et al., 2007; McDougle et al., 1993), while others show equal response as in non-tic-related OCD (Skarphedinsson et al., 2015). CBT with exposure and response prevention has been found effective in treating OCD with comorbid tic disorders or tic symptoms (Conelea et al., 2014; Højgaard et al., 2017), and comorbid OCD does not predict lesser response to behavior therapy for tics (Nissen, Parner, & Thomsen, 2019; Sukhodolsky et al., 2017). Further, there is some indication that children with TD and comorbid OCD symptoms might fare better in behavior therapy for tics compared to TD only (Nissen et al., 2019).

TD and comorbid anxiety or depression

Studies have shown that a significant proportion of children and adolescents with TD also experience anxiety and depression. The prevalence of ADs in individuals with TD ranges from 15–58 percent (Coffey et al., 2000; Freeman, 2007; Freeman et al., 2000; Hirschtritt et al., 2015; Wanderer et al., 2012). Previous studies suggest that the severity of tics is worse when children have a comorbid AD (Coffey et al., 2000; Johnco et al., 2016; Kurlan et al., 2002). The prevalence of depressive disorders ranges between 18–52 percent (Coffey et al., 2000; Hirschtritt et al., 2015; Kurlan, 2002). These rates are considerably higher than those observed in the general population (Merikangas et al., 2010), indicating an association between TD and these comorbid conditions.

The phenomenology of comorbid anxiety and depressive disorders in pediatric TD is complex, as symptoms may overlap and interact. The presence of comorbid anxiety and depressive disorders can exacerbate tic severity (Coffey et al., 2000), increase functional impairment, and lead to a lower quality of life for the affected individual (Coffey et al., 2000; Kurlan et al., 2002). TDs may have a shared etiology with internalizing disorders (Doering, Lichtenstein, Gillberg, Kuja-Halkola, & Lundström, 2021). Numerous situational elements may impact the manifestation and presentation of tics. A significant number of patients or their guardians observe heightened tic severity, owing to a combination of emotional conditions, such as arousal, excitement, frustration, stress, anxiety, fatigue, or boredom (Conelea & Woods, 2008). Neither anxiety nor depression appeared to moderate behavioral treatment outcomes in a recent meta-analysis (Sukhodolsky et al., 2017). However, a recent naturalistic study demonstrated that internalizing symptoms were associated with less reduction in functional impairment (Nissen et al., 2019).

Assessment of tic disorders and anxiety or depression should include a thorough clinical evaluation. It is also important to consider other comorbid conditions, such as OCD and ADHD, which are common in individuals with TD and ADs. Additionally, the presence of comorbid internalizing conditions may increase the risk of suicidal ideation later in life (Johnco et al., 2016). Clinicians should routinely screen for these comorbidities and tailor treatment plans accordingly to optimize outcomes.

TD and autism

Comorbidity rates of autism in TD are around 5–21 percent (Coffey et al., 2000; Freeman, 2007). The etiology of TDs and autism may involve shared genetic factors, pathogenic commonalities, and environmental influences. There is a significant overlap of genes associated with autism in TD patients compared to control subjects, suggesting key pathogenic similarities (Cukier et al., 2014). Common environmental factors like pre-natal stress (Fine, Zhang, & Stevens, 2014), as well as dysregulated inter-actions between the immune system (Frick & Pittenger, 2016), endocrine system, and the central nervous system, may contribute to the develop-mental abnormalities underlying both TD and autism (Hornig & Lipkin, 2013). Factor analyses of TD phenotypes suggest that autistic symptoms might signify a specific factor, potentially reflecting distinct causal factors for TD with significant comorbid autistic features (Huisman-van Dijk, van de Schoot, Rijkeboer, Mathews, & Cath, 2016).

Treatment for individuals with comorbid TD and autism should be tailored to address the specific needs of each patient, considering their unique combination of symptoms and challenges. Pharmacological inter-ventions, such as neuroleptics and alpha-2 agonists for TDs and psy-chostimulants for ADHD, may be helpful in managing symptoms (Pringsheim et al., 2019). Psychotherapeutic interventions, including CBT, social skills training, and specialized educational support, can also play a crucial role in addressing the unique challenges faced by these individuals (Andrén et al., 2022).

TD and ODD

Behavioral disturbances, such as ODD, CD, impulse control disorders, are frequently observed in individuals with TDs, with a prevalence rate of 12–30 percent (Freeman et al., 2000; Hirschtritt et al., 2015). Although the exact cause of the association between TD and ODD remains unclear, it has been proposed that both conditions could be linked to dysregulation within the brain's neurotransmitter systems, particularly involving dopamine (Roessner et al., 2022).

Treatment for youth with TD and ODD can be challenging, as interventions need to address the symptoms of both conditions. Comprehensive treatment plans may include behavioral therapies, such as CBT or Parent Management Training, as well as pharmacological interventions targeting the specific neurotransmitter imbalances involved. It is considered crucial to involve a multidisciplinary team of professionals, including psychiatrists and psychologists to effectively manage and treat these comorbid conditions (Kaur, Floyd, & Balta, 2022; Pringsheim et al., 2019; Roessner et al., 2022).

TD and sleep problems

Sleep disorders are prevalent in youth with TD, especially those with further comorbidities such as ADHD or OCD (Mol Debes, Hjalgrim, & Skov, 2008; Sambrani, Jakubovski, & Müller-Vahl, 2016), with rates ranging between 7–80 percent (Jiménez-Jiménez, Alonso-Navarro, García-Martín, & Agúndez, 2022). The most frequently reported sleep disorders include insomnia, excessive daytime sleepiness, persistent tics during sleep, arousal disorders, and periodic limb movement syndrome (Jiménez-Jiménez et al., 2022). However, the relationship between sleep disorders and the severity of TD remains unclear, with only a few studies addressing this aspect (Jiménez-Jiménez et al., 2022). Anxiety has been shown to contribute to sleep disorders in Tourette's, with a higher frequency of sleep-related problems in patients with comorbid anxiety. No specific guidelines currently exist for treating sleep disorders in TD, but effectively treating tics and comorbid conditions may improve sleep complaints.

TD and Anger problems

Rage attacks can be pronounced in youth with TD, with a range of 20–67 percent affected by rage attacks or aggressive behavior (Conte, Valente, Fioriello, & Cardona, 2020). Frequency of rage attacks is likely to rise with an increased comorbidity burden, particularly in cases involving ADHD and OCD (Conte et al., 2020).

Body-focused Repetitive Behaviors

Body focused repetitive behaviors (BFRB), like skin picking (excoriation), nail biting, and hair pulling (trichotillomania; Selles et al., 2015) are common in children, and tend to co-occur as around half of children diagnosed with a BFRB also have another form of the disorder simultaneously (Walther et al., 2014). Skin picking affects 10–40 percent of children (Achenbach & Rescorla, 2001), with onset often in childhood (Wilhelm et al., 1999) and higher prevalence in females. Adolescents who skin pick have significantly higher depression and anxiety scores, increased internalizing and externalizing problems, and significantly poorer quality of life, enjoyment, and satisfaction (Ricketts et al., 2022). Compulsive nail biting is the most prevalent BFRB, affecting 5–33 percent of children (Ghanizadeh, 2011) Nail biting is also possibly the most benign BFRB in terms of impairment and comorbid psychiatric symptoms (Selles et al., 2015). Nail biting has been found to commonly co-occur with Tourette Syndrome, ODD (Ghanizadeh & Mosallaei, 2009), attentional problems (Ghanizadeh, 2010), separation anxiety (Ghanizadeh, 2008) and to be associated with more internalizing symptoms (Selles et al., 2015). Hair pulling is associated with heightened social impairment and functional disability, anxiety disorders, disruptive behavior, attentional problems, and other body-focused repetitive behaviors (Duke, Keeley, Geffken, & Storch, 2010; Flessner, Woods, Franklin, Keuthen, & Piacentini, 2009; Santhanam, Fairley, & Rogers, 2008; Tolin, Franklin, Diefenbach, Anderson, & Meunier, 2007). Both compulsive hair pulling and nail biting have been associated with higher incidence of OCD in children and adolescents (Selles et al., 2018).

Body Dysmorphic Disorder

In a recent study using a large clinical sample of 172 children and adolescents with BDD, 72 percent presented with at least one additional mental disorder (Rautio et al., 2020). Some common comorbidities associated with BDD in this population included:

Depressive disorders (47 percent): Depressive disorders are common comorbidities with BDD. The negative self-image and persistent feelings of worthlessness associated with depressive disorders can intensify the distress caused by BDD.

Eating disorders (11 percent): BDD is sometimes linked with eating disorders like anorexia nervosa, bulimia nervosa, and binge-eating disorder. The preoccupation with body image and weight in individuals with eating disorders may overlap with the concerns related to BDD.

Social anxiety disorder (8 percent) and other anxiety disorders (11 percent): BDD frequently co-occurs with anxiety disorders, such as generalized anxiety disorder, social anxiety disorder, and panic disorder. The excessive worry and fear associated with anxiety disorders may exacerbate BDD symptoms and make it more difficult for children and adolescents to cope with their perceived flaws.

ADHD (10 percent): Some studies have suggested a possible link between BDD and ADHD in children and adolescents. The impulsivity and inattention associated with ADHD may contribute to the development or exacerbation of BDD symptoms.

OCD (6 percent): BDD and OCD share similarities in their symptomatology, such as intrusive thoughts and repetitive behaviors. In some cases, the two disorders may be difficult to distinguish from one another. It is not uncommon for children and adolescents with BDD to also have OCD, which can complicate treatment and management. Among people of all ages diagnosed with OCD, BDD has a lifetime prevalence of 2.8 percent (Sharma et al., 2021), but a recent study found an elevated prevalence of 9.4 percent in pediatric OCD, equal for males and females (Racz, Mathieu, McKenzie, & Farrell, 2022). Early identification and treatment of BDD and its comorbidities in children and adolescents are crucial for improving outcomes. Treatment typically involves a combination of psychotherapy, such as cognitive-behavioral therapy (CBT), and medication management. Family involvement in treatment may also be beneficial, as it helps to create a supportive environment for the child or adolescent.

Health Anxiety

In the DSM-5, hypochondriasis was replaced by somatic symptom disorder and illness anxiety disorder, collectively referred to here as health anxiety (HA). HA is understudied in child and adolescent populations, but evidence supports similar psychological distress and impairment as seen in adults (Rask, Elberling, Skovgaard, Thomsen, & Fink, 2012; Rask et al., 2016). In a study of 1886 Danish children aged 11–12 years, 161 children had high HA scores and of those, 20.5 percent were diagnosed with an emotional disorder, 6.2 percent with a neurodevelopmental disorder, and 74 percent had no comorbid disorder (Rask et al., 2016). HA is increased in children and adolescents with somatic illnesses, such as congenital heart disease (Oliver et al., 2020), and is associated with parental health concerns and depression (Wright, Reiser, & Delparte, 2017). The current diagnostic criteria may not match the manifestation of HA symptoms in children and adolescents, potentially leading to a misdiagnoses of OCD in some cases (Duholm, Højgaard, Skarphedinsson, Thomsen, & Rask, 2021). OCD can present with similar symptoms to HA, such as obsessions regarding health and somatic symptoms.

However, in the case of OCD, these symptoms will likely be accompanied by more compulsive behaviors to reduce distress, including but not limited to washing, cleaning, mental rituals, repeating behaviors and checking. The symptoms in OCD are also more likely to be ego-dystonic and unrealistic (Neziroglu, McKay, & Yaryura-Tobias, 2000). Around 30 percent of children and adolescents with OCD have been found to have symptoms of HA (Duholm et al., 2021; Villadsen et al., 2017), but it is unclear how many fulfill the diagnosis of somatic symptom disorder and illness anxiety disorder. Symptoms of illness anxiety disorder in adult OCD populations have been found to be associated with harm-related obsessions, checking compulsions and the overestimation of harm-related threat and responsibility (Reuman et al., 2017). In adults with health anxiety, the lifetime prevalence of OCD has been found to be 9.5 percent (Barsky, 1992), but the prevalence in younger populations is undetermined.

CBT and pharmacotherapy are effective for adult HA (Scarella, Boland, & Barsky, 2019). For children and adolescents with OCD, HA symptoms do not seem to affect CBT treatment outcomes, despite increased anxiety symptoms and a more heterogeneous OCD symptom profile (Duholm et al., 2021). There is also some evidence that mindfulness therapy, acceptance and commitment therapy, and stress management may be effective (Tyrer, 2018).

Hoarding Disorder

Hoarding can be classified as OCD-related hoarding or as hoarding disorder (HD) since the release of DSM-5 (American Psychiatric Association, 2013). Hoarding is considered OCD related when the hoarding behavior is direct consequence of obsessions or compulsions, such as difficulty discarding things to avoid harm or when discarding results in a feeling of incompleteness (American Psychiatric Association, 2013). A helpful sign to differentiate between HD and OCD-related hoarding is that OCD behaviors are mostly unwanted and do not provide pleasure. Excessive acquisition is also less common in OCD-related hoarding, and the items not discarded tend to have more of a bizarre nature, such as trash, nails, leftover food, or bodily discharge (Pertusa et al., 2008).

A review from 2019 found adult HD point prevalence at 2.6 percent, and pooled lifetime prevalence estimate at 1.7 percent (Postlethwaite, Kellett, & Mataix-Cols, 2019). The prevalence rate of HD in children is less clear but was 2 percent in an adolescent population study (Iervolino et al., 2009). The prevalence of HD in pediatric OCD is undetermined, but hoarding symptoms have been found in up to 30 percent of children and adolescents with OCD (Højgaard et al., 2019; Storch et al., 2007). The reason for the uncertain prevalence of hoarding disorder in children and adolescents is that the disorder is difficult to assess in these age groups as symptoms are often mild or masked by the interference of a parent or caregiver. However, since hoarding disorder is thought to usually begin before the age of 20 (Tolin, Meunier, Frost, & Steketee, 2010), it is important to improve assessment and diagnosis in the younger groups to allow early intervention. It is also worth considering that digital hoarding is becoming more recognized, especially among children and adolescents, and shares similarities with physical hoarding (Sweeten, Sillence, & Neave, 2018).

About 60 percent of children with hoarding have OCD symptoms (Burton et al., 2016). Other common psychological features commonly seen with hoarding disorder are indecisiveness, perfectionism, procrastination, avoidance, difficulties in planning, and being easily distracted (Frost & Hartl, 1996; Frost, Tolin, Steketee, & Oh, 2011; Steketee & Frost, 2003). Hoarding in youth with OCD has been found to be associated with executive functioning deficits, even when corrected for the impact of ADHD symptoms (Park et al., 2016). A strong association between ADHD and hoarding has been found in children and adolescents with OCD (Samuels et al., 2014). Hoarding symptoms in children and adolescents correlate uniquely with inattentive ADHD symptoms and fewer anxiety symptoms (Burton et al., 2016), as opposed to OCD-related hoarding, where a higher occurrence of comorbid anxiety is commonly found. Hoarding symptoms are common in children with autism spectrum disorders (ASD), with one study finding clinically significant hoarding symptoms in 25 percent of cases, correlating with anxiety and depressive symptoms, externalizing behavior, and attention problems (Storch et al., 2016).

CBT for adult HD (Tolin, Frost, Steketee, & Muroff, 2015) is effective, but few studies have examined its effectiveness in younger populations. Most existing studies have focused on OCD-related hoarding. When adapting the adult treatment manuals to younger populations, it is important to perform a thorough assessment of comorbid disorders before beginning treatment. This will help the clinician to distinguish pathological hoarding from normal saving and collecting behaviors, commonly seen in children (Plimpton, Frost, Abbey, & Dorer, 2009). In children and adolescents with OCD, hoarding has been effectively treated with CBT (Højgaard et al., 2019; Olino et al., 2011; Rozenman et al., 2019; Storch et al., 2011). Treatment for child and adolescent hoarding disorders should include parents and training of parents, exposure and response prevention, contingency management as well as cognitive training (Højgaard & Skarphedinsson, 2023).

Summary

OCRDs are frequently comorbid with each other and other psychiatric conditions. In general, comorbidity leads to greater symptom severity, significant developmental impact, greater functional impairment, and, in many cases, attenuated treatment response. Thus, it is crucial to comprehensively screen for potential comorbid conditions when assessing these disorders. Accurate conceptualization and tailored treatment approaches require comprehensive diagnostic and behavioral assessments in complex comorbid presentations.

References

Abramovitch, A., Dar, R., Hermesh, H., & Schweiger, A. (2012). Comparative neuropsychology of adult obsessive-compulsive disorder and attention deficit/ hyperactivity disorder: Implications for a novel executive overload model of OCD. *Journal of Neuropsychology*, 6(2), 161–191.

Abramovitch, A., Dar, R., Mittelman, A., & Wilhelm, S. (2015). Comorbidity between attention deficit/hyperactivity disorder and obsessive-compulsive disorder across the lifespan: A systematic and critical review. *Harvard Review of Psychiatry*.

Abramowitz, J. S. (2004). Treatment of obsessive-compulsive disorder in patients who have comorbid major depression. *Journal of Clinical Psychology*, 60(11), 1133–1141. doi:10.1002/jclp.20078.

Abramowitz, J. S. & Jacoby, R. J. (2015). Obsessive-compulsive and related disorders: A critical review of the new diagnostic class. *Annual Review of Clinical Psychology*, 11, 165–186.

Abramowitz, J. S., Storch, E. A., Keeley, M., & Cordell, E. (2007). Obsessive-compulsive disorder with comorbid major depression: what is the role of cognitive factors? *Behaviour Research and Therapy*, 45(10), 2257–2267.

Achenbach, T. M. & Rescorla, L. A. (2001). *Manual for the ASEBA School-Age Forms & Profiles*. Burlington, VT: University of Vermont, Research Center for Children, Youth, and Families.

Alfano, C. A. & Kim, K. L. (2011). Objective sleep patterns and severity of symptoms in pediatric obsessive compulsive disorder: a pilot investigation. *Journal of Anxiety Disorders*, 25(6), 835–839.

Allen, A., Kurlan, R., Gilbert, D., Coffey, B., Linder, S., Lewis, D., ... Sallee, F. (2005). Atomoxetine treatment in children and adolescents with ADHD and comorbid tic disorders. *Neurology*, 65(12), 1941–1949.

Altman, S. E. & Shankman, S. A. (2009). What is the association between obsessive–compulsive disorder and eating disorders? *Clinical Psychology Review*, 29 (7), 638–646.

Aman, M., Coelho, J. S., Lin, B., Lu, C., Westwell-Roper, C., Best, J. R., & Stewart, S. E. (2022). Prevalence of pediatric acute-onset neuropsychiatric syndrome (PANS) in children and adolescents with eating disorders. *Journal of Eating Disorders*, 10(1), 194. doi:10.1186/s40337-022-00707-6.

American Psychiatric Association. (1980). *Diagnostic and Statistical Manual of Mental Disorders (DSM-III)* (3rd Ed.). Arlington, VA: American Psychiatric Association.

American Psychiatric Association. (2013). *Diagnostic and Statistical Manual of Mental Disorders, Fifth Edition (DSM-5(TM))*. Arlington, VA: American Psychiatric Publishing.

Andrén, P., Jakubovski, E., Murphy, T. L., Woitecki, K., Tarnok, Z., Zimmerman-Brenner, S., ... Robinson, S. (2022). European clinical guidelines for Tourette syndrome and other tic disorders—Version 2.0. Part II: Psychological interventions. *European Child and Adolescent Psychiatry*, 31(3), 403–423.

Angelakis, I., Gooding, P., Tarrier, N., & Panagioti, M. (2015). Suicidality in obsessive compulsive disorder (OCD): a systematic review and meta-analysis. *Clinical Psychology Review*, 39, 1–15.

Angst, J., Gamma, A., Endrass, J., Hantouche, E., Goodwin, R., Ajdacic, V., ... Rossler, W. (2005). Obsessive-compulsive syndromes and disorders: significance of comorbidity with bipolar and anxiety syndromes. *European Archives of Psychiatry and Clinical Neuroscience*, 255(1), 65–71.

Arildskov, T. W., Hojgaard, D. R., Skarphedinsson, G., Thomsen, P. H., Ivarsson, T., Weidle, B., ... Hybel, K. A. (2015). Subclinical autism spectrum symptoms in pediatric obsessive-compulsive disorder. *European Child and Adolescent Psychiatry*, 25(7), 711–723. doi:10.1007/s00787-015-0782-5.

Barsky, A. J. (1992). Hypochondriasis and obsessive compulsive disorder. *Psychiatric Clinics of North America*.

Baytunca, B., Kalyoncu, T., Ozel, I., Erermiş, S., Kayahan, B., & Öngur, D. (2017). Early Onset Schizophrenia Associated With Obsessive-Compulsive Disorder: Clinical Features and Correlates. *Clinical Neuropharmacology*, 40(6), 243–245. doi:10.1097/wnf.0000000000000248.

Bedford, S. A., Hunsche, M. C., & Kerns, C. M. (2020). Co-occurrence, Assessment and Treatment of Obsessive Compulsive Disorder in Children and Adults With Autism Spectrum Disorder. *Current psychiatry reports*, 22(10), 53. doi:10.1007/s11920-020-01176-x.

Bernaras, E., Jaureguizar, J., & Garaigordobil, M. (2019). Child and adolescent depression: A review of theories, evaluation instruments, prevention programs, and treatments. *Frontiers in Psychology*, 10, 543.

Bos-Veneman, N. G., Kuin, A., Minderaa, R. B., & Hoekstra, P. J. (2010). Role of perinatal adversities on tic severity and symptoms of attention deficit/hyperactivity disorder in children and adolescents with a tic disorder. *Journal of Developmental and Behavioral Pediatrics*, 31(2), 100–106.

Brander, G., Kuja-Halkola, R., Rosenqvist, M. A., Rück, C., Serlachius, E., Fernández de la Cruz, L., ... Mataix-Cols, D. (2021). A population-based family clustering study of tic-related obsessive-compulsive disorder. *Molecular Psychiatry*, 26(4), 1224–1233.

Brem, S., Grünblatt, E., Drechsler, R., Riederer, P., & Walitza, S. (2014). The neurobiological link between OCD and ADHD. *Atten Defic Hyperact Disord*, 6 (3), 175–202. doi:10.1007/s12402-014-0146-x.

Brown, H. M., Lester, K. J., Jassi, A., Heyman, I., & Krebs, G. (2015). Paediatric Obsessive-Compulsive Disorder and Depressive Symptoms: Clinical Correlates and CBT Treatment Outcomes. *Journal of Abnormal Child Psychology*, 43(5), 933–942. doi:10.1007/s10802-014-9943-0.

Burton, C. L., Crosbie, J., Dupuis, A., Mathews, C. A., Soreni, N., Schachar, R., & Arnold, P. D. (2016). Clinical correlates of hoarding with and without comorbid obsessive-compulsive symptoms in a community pediatric sample. *Journal of the American Academy of Child and Adolescent Psychiatry*, 55(2), 114–121. e112.

Cabarkapa, S., King, J. A., Dowling, N., & Ng, C. H. (2019). Co-Morbid Obsessive–Compulsive Disorder and Attention Deficit Hyperactivity Disorder: Neurobiological Commonalities and Treatment Implications. *Frontiers in psychiatry*, 10. doi:10.3389/fpsyt.2019.00557.

Canavera, K. E., Ollendick, T. H., Ehrenreich May, J. T., & Pincus, D. B. (2010). Clinical correlates of comorbid obsessive–compulsive disorder and depression in youth. *Child Psychiatry and Human Development*, 41, 583–594.

Carter, A. S., Pollock, R. A., Suvak, M. K., & Pauls, D. L. (2004). Anxiety and major depression comorbidity in a family study of obsessive–compulsive disorder. *Depression and Anxiety*, 20(4), 165–174.

Cederlöf, M., Lichtenstein, P., Larsson, H., Boman, M., Rück, C., Landén, M., & Mataix-Cols, D. (2015). Obsessive-compulsive disorder, psychosis, and bipolarity: a longitudinal cohort and multigenerational family study. *Schizophrenia Bulletin*, 41(5), 1076–1083.

Cederlöf, M., Thornton, L. M., Baker, J., Lichtenstein, P., Larsson, H., Rück, C., ... Mataix-Cols, D. (2015). Etiological overlap between obsessive-compulsive disorder and anorexia nervosa: a longitudinal cohort, multigenerational family and twin study. *World Psychiatry*, 14(3), 333–338.

Cervin, M., Lázaro, L., Martínez-González, A. E., Piqueras, J. A., Rodríguez-Jiménez, T., Godoy, A., ... Storch, E. A. (2020). Obsessive-compulsive symptoms and their links to depression and anxiety in clinic- and community-based pediatric samples: A network analysis. *Journal of Affective Disorders*, 271, 9–18. doi:10.1016/j.jad.2020.03.090.

Coelho, J. S., Zaitsoff, S. L., Pullmer, R., Yamin, D. F., Anderson, S., Fernandes, A., & Stewart, S. E. (2019). Body checking in pediatric eating and obsessive-compulsive disorders. *Journal of Obsessive-Compulsive and Related Disorders*, 23, 100475. doi:10.1016/j.jocrd.2019.100475.

Coffey, B. J., Biederman, J., Smoller, J. W., Geller, D. A., Sarin, P., Schwartz, S., & Kim, G. S. (2000). Anxiety disorders and tic severity in juveniles with Tourette's disorder. *Journal of the American Academy of Child and Adolescent Psychiatry*, 39(5), 562–568.

Conelea, C. A., Walther, M. R., Freeman, J. B., Garcia, A. M., Sapyta, J., Khanna, M., & Franklin, M. (2014). Tic-Related Obsessive-Compulsive Disorder (OCD): Phenomenology and Treatment Outcome in the Pediatric OCD Treatment Study II. *Journal of the American Academy of Child and Adolescent Psychiatry*, 53(12), 1308–1316. doi:10.1016/j.jaac.2014.09.014.

Conelea, C. A. & Woods, D. W. (2008). The influence of contextual factors on tic expression in Tourette's syndrome: a review. *Journal of Psychosomatic Research*, 65(5), 487–496.

Conte, G., Valente, F., Fioriello, F., & Cardona, F. (2020). Rage attacks in Tourette syndrome and chronic tic disorder: a systematic review. *Neuroscience and Biobehavioral Reviews*, 119, 21–36.

Cukier, H. N., Dueker, N. D., Slifer, S. H., Lee, J. M., Whitehead, P. L., Lalanne, E., ... Hulme, W. F. (2014). Exome sequencing of extended families with autism reveals genes shared across neurodevelopmental and neuropsychiatric disorders. *Molecular Autism*, 5, 1–10.

Cunill, R., Castells, X., & Simeon, D. (2009). Relationships between obsessive-compulsive symptomatology and severity of psychosis in schizophrenia: a systematic review and meta-analysis. *Journal of Clinical Psychiatry*, 70(1), 70–82. doi:10.4088/jcp.07r03618.

Darrow, S. M., Hirschtritt, M. E., Davis, L. K., Illmann, C., Osiecki, L., Grados, M., ... Pauls, D. (2017). Identification of two heritable cross-disorder endophenotypes for Tourette syndrome. *American Journal of Psychiatry*, 174(4), 387–396.

de Vries, F. E., Cath, D. C., Hoogendoorn, A. W., van Oppen, P., Glas, G., Veltman, D. J., ... van Balkom, A. J. (2016). Tic-related versus tic-free obsessive-compulsive disorder: clinical picture and 2-year natural course. *The Journal of clinical psychiatry*, 77(10), 12464.

Dell'Osso, B., Marazziti, D., Albert, U., Pallanti, S., Gambini, O., Tundo, A., ... Scalone, L. (2017). Parsing the phenotype of obsessive-compulsive tic disorder (OCTD): a multidisciplinary consensus. *International Journal of Psychiatry in Clinical Practice*, 21(2), 156–159.

Doering, S., Lichtenstein, P., Gillberg, C., Kuja-Halkola, R., & Lundström, S. (2021). Internalizing and neurodevelopmental problems in young people: Educational outcomes in a large population-based cohort of twins. *Psychiatry Research*, 298, 113794.

Drakes, D. H., Fawcett, E. J., Rose, J. P., Carter-Major, J. C., & Fawcett, J. M. (2021). Comorbid obsessive-compulsive disorder in individuals with eating disorders: an epidemiological meta-analysis. *Journal of Psychiatric Research*, 141, 176–191.

Duholm, C. S., Højgaard, D. R., Skarphedinsson, G., Thomsen, P. H., & Rask, C. U. (2021). Health anxiety symptoms in pediatric obsessive–compulsive disorder: patient characteristics and effect on treatment outcome. *European Child and Adolescent Psychiatry*, 1–12.

Duke, D. C., Keeley, M. L., Geffken, G. R., & Storch, E. A. (2010). Trichotillomania: A current review. *Clinical Psychology Review*, 30(2), 181–193.

Farrell, L., Waters, A., Milliner, E., & Ollendick, T. (2012). Comorbidity and treatment response in pediatric obsessive-compulsive disorder: a pilot study of group cognitive-behavioral treatment. *Psychiatry Research*, 199(2), 115–123. doi:10.1016/j.psychres.2012.04.035.

Fine, R., Zhang, J., & Stevens, H. E. (2014). Prenatal stress and inhibitory neuron systems: implications for neuropsychiatric disorders. *Molecular Psychiatry*, 19 (6), 641–651.

Flessner, C. A., Woods, D. W., Franklin, M. E., Keuthen, N. J., & Piacentini, J. (2009). Cross-sectional study of women with trichotillomania: a preliminary examination of pulling styles, severity, phenomenology, and functional impact. *Child Psychiatry and Human Development*, 40, 153–167.

Flygare, O., Andersson, E., Ringberg, H., Hellstadius, A. C., Edbacken, J., Enander, J., ... Rück, C. (2020). Adapted cognitive behavior therapy for obsessive-compulsive disorder with co-occurring autism spectrum disorder: A clinical effectiveness study. *Autism*, 24(1), 190–199. doi:10.1177/1362361319856974.

Freeman, R. D. (2007). Tourette Syndrome International Database, C. (2007). Tic disorders and ADHD: answers from a world-wide clinical dataset on Tourette syndrome. *Eur. Child Adolesc Psychiatry*, 16, 15–23.

Freeman, R. D., Fast, D. K., Burd, L., Kerbeshian, J., Robertson, M. M., & Sandor, P. (2000). An international perspective on Tourette syndrome: selected findings from 3500 individuals in 22 countries. *Developmental Medicine and Child Neurology*, 42(7), 436–447.

Frick, L. & Pittenger, C. (2016). Microglial dysregulation in OCD, Tourette syndrome, and PANDAS. *Journal of immunology research*.

Frost, R. O. & Hartl, T. L. (1996). A cognitive-behavioral model of compulsive hoarding. *Behaviour Research and Therapy*, 34(4), 341–350.

Frost, R. O., Tolin, D. F., Steketee, G., & Oh, M. (2011). Indecisiveness and hoarding. *International Journal of Cognitive Therapy*, 4(3), 253–262.

Garcia, A. M., Sapyta, J. J., Moore, P. S., Freeman, J. B., Franklin, M. E., March, J. S., & Foa, E. B. (2010). Predictors and moderators of treatment outcome in the Pediatric Obsessive Compulsive Treatment Study (POTS I). *Journal of the American Academy of Child and Adolescent Psychiatry*, 49(10), 1024–1033; quiz 1086. doi:10.1016/j.jaac.2010.06.013.

Geller, D. A., Biederman, J., Faraone, S., Agranat, A., Cradock, K., Hagermoser, L., ... Coffey, B. J. (2001). Developmental aspects of obsessive compulsive disorder: findings in children, adolescents, and adults. *Journal of Nervous and Mental Disease*, 189(7), 471–477.

Geller, D. A., Biederman, J., Faraone, S. V., Cradock, K., Hagermoser, L., Zaman, N., ... Spencer, T. J. (2002). Attention-deficit/hyperactivity disorder in children and adolescents with obsessive-compulsive disorder: fact or artifact? *Journal of the American Academy of Child and Adolescent Psychiatry*, 41(1), 52–58. doi: S0890-8567(09)60588-60588 [pii] 10. 1097/00004583-200201000-00011.

Geller, D. A., Biederman, J., Stewart, S. E., Mullin, B., Farrell, C., Wagner, K. D., ... Carpenter, D. (2003). Impact of comorbidity on treatment response to paroxetine in pediatric obsessive-compulsive disorder: is the use of exclusion criteria empirically supported in randomized clinical trials? *Journal of Child and Adolescent Psychopharmacology, 13 Suppl* 1, S19–29.

Geller, D. A., Coffey, B., Faraone, S., Hagermoser, L., Zaman, N. K., Farrell, C. L., ... Biederman, J. (2003). Does comorbid attention-deficit/hyperactivity disorder impact the clinical expression of pediatric obsessive-compulsive disorder? *CNS Spectr*, 8(4), 259–264. Retrieved from www.ncbi.nlm.nih.gov/pubmed/12679741.

Geller, D. A., Petty, C., Vivas, F., Johnson, J., Pauls, D., & Biederman, J. (2007). Further Evidence for Co-Segregation between Pediatric Obsessive Compulsive Disorder and Attention Deficit Hyperactivity Disorder: A Familial Risk Analysis. *Biological Psychiatry*, 61(12), 1388–1394. doi:10.1016/j.biopsych.2006.09.026.

Gentes, E. L. & Ruscio, A. M. (2011). A meta-analysis of the relation of intolerance of uncertainty to symptoms of generalized anxiety disorder, major depressive disorder, and obsessive–compulsive disorder. *Clinical Psychology Review*, 31 (6), 923–933.

Ghanizadeh, A. (2008). Association of nail biting and psychiatric disorders in children and their parents in a psychiatrically referred sample of children. *Child and adolescent psychiatry and mental health*, 2, 1–7.

Ghanizadeh, A. (2010). Comorbidity of enuresis in children with attention-deficit/hyperactivity disorder. *Journal of Attention Disorders*, 13(5), 464–467.

Ghanizadeh, A. (2011). Nail biting; etiology, consequences and management. *Iranian journal of medical sciences*, 36(2), 73.

Ghanizadeh, A. & Mosallaei, S. (2009). Psychiatric disorders and behavioral problems in children and adolescents with Tourette syndrome. *Brain and Development*, 31(1), 15–19.

Grabe, H., Meyer, C., Hapke, U., Rumpf, H., Freyberger, H., Dilling, H., & John, U. (2000). Prevalence, quality of life and psychosocial function in obsessive-compulsive disorder and subclinical obsessive-compulsive disorder in northern Germany. *European Archives of Psychiatry and Clinical Neuroscience*, 250(5), 262–268.

Grados, M. A. (2010). The genetics of obsessive-compulsive disorder and Tourette syndrome: an epidemiological and pathway-based approach for gene discovery. *Journal of the American Academy of Child and Adolescent Psychiatry*, 49(8), 810–819, 819.e811–812. doi:10.1016/j.jaac.2010.04.009.

Griffiths, D. L., Farrell, L. J., Waters, A. M., & White, S. W. (2017a). ASD Traits Among Youth with Obsessive–Compulsive Disorder. *Child Psychiatry and Human Development*, 48(6), 911–921. doi:10.1007/s10578-017-0714-3.

Griffiths, D. L., Farrell, L. J., Waters, A. M., & White, S. W. (2017b). Clinical correlates of obsessive compulsive disorder and comorbid autism spectrum disorder in youth. *Journal of Obsessive-Compulsive and Related Disorders*, 14, 90–98. doi:10.1016/j.jocrd.2017.06.006.

Groth, C., Mol Debes, N., Rask, C. U., Lange, T., & Skov, L. (2017). Course of Tourette Syndrome and Comorbidities in a Large Prospective Clinical Study. *Journal of the American Academy of Child and Adolescent Psychiatry*, 56(4), 304–312. doi:10.1016/j.jaac.2017.01.010.

Guzick, A. G., McNamara, J. P., Reid, A. M., Balkhi, A. M., Storch, E. A., Murphy, T. K., ... Geffken, G. R. (2017). The link between ADHD-like inattention and obsessions and compulsions during treatment of youth with OCD. *Journal of Obsessive-Compulsive and Related Disorders*, 12, 1–8.

Halldorsdottir, T., & Ollendick, T. H. (2014). Comorbid ADHD: Implications for the treatment of anxiety disorders in children and adolescents. *Cognitive and Behavioral Practice*, 21(3), 310–322.

Hellberg, S. N., Jacoby, R. J., & Wilhelm, S. (2020). From OC Spectrum to Anxiety Disorders. In E. Bui, M. E. Charney, & A. W. Baker (Eds), *Clinical Handbook of Anxiety Disorders: From Theory to Practice* (pp. 105–140). Cham: Springer International Publishing.

Hirschfeld, R. M. (2001). The comorbidity of major depression and anxiety disorders: recognition and management in primary care. *Primary Care Companion to the Journal of Clinical Psychiatry*, 3(6), 244.

Hirschtritt, M. E., Darrow, S. M., Illmann, C., Osiecki, L., Grados, M., Sandor, P., ... Budman, C. L. (2018). Genetic and phenotypic overlap of specific obsessive-compulsive and attention-deficit/hyperactive subtypes with Tourette syndrome. *Psychological Medicine*, 48(2), 279–293.

Hirschtritt, M. E., Lee, P. C., Pauls, D. L., & et al. (2015). Lifetime prevalence, age of risk, and genetic relationships of comorbid psychiatric disorders in tourette syndrome. *JAMA psychiatry*, 72(4), 325–333. doi:10.1001/jamapsychiatry.2014.2650.

Højgaard, D. R. M. A., Arildskov, T. W., Skarphedinsson, G., Hybel, K. A., Ivarsson, T., Weidle, B., ... Thomsen, P. H. (2023). Do Autistic Traits Predict Outcome of Cognitive Behavioral Therapy in Pediatric Obsessive-Compulsive

Disorder? *Research on Child and Adolescent Psychopathology*, 51(8), 1083–1095. doi:10.1007/s10802-023-01078-5.

Højgaard, D. R. M. A. & Skarphedinsson, G. (2023). Cognitive behavioral therapy for child and adolescent hoarding disorder. In *Handbook of Lifespan Cognitive Behavioral Therapy* (pp. 109–121): Elsevier.

Højgaard, D. R. M. A., Skarphedinsson, G., Ivarsson, T., Weidle, B., Nissen, J. B., Hybel, K. A., … Thomsen, P. H. (2019). Hoarding in children and adolescents with obsessive–compulsive disorder: prevalence, clinical correlates, and cognitive behavioral therapy outcome. *European Child and Adolescent Psychiatry*, 28(8), 1097–1106. doi:10.1007/s00787-019-01276-x.

Højgaard, D. R. M. A., Skarphedinsson, G., Nissen, J. B., Hybel, K., Ivarsson, T., & Thomsen, P. (2017). Pediatric Obsessive-Compulsive Disorder with Tic symptoms: Clinical Presentation and Treatment Outcome. *European Child and Adolescent Psychiatry*, 26(6), 681–689. doi:10.1007/s00787-016-0936-0.

Homberg, J. R., Kyzar, E. J., Scattoni, M. L., Norton, W. H., Pittman, J., Gaikwad, S., … Diamond, D. M. (2016). Genetic and environmental modulation of neurodevelopmental disorders: translational insights from labs to beds. *Brain Research Bulletin*, 125, 79–91.

Hornig, M., & Lipkin, W. I. (2013). Immune-mediated animal models of Tourette syndrome. *Neuroscience and Biobehavioral Reviews*, 37(6), 1120–1138.

Huisman-van Dijk, H. M., van de Schoot, R., Rijkeboer, M. M., Mathews, C. A., & Cath, D. C. (2016). The relationship between tics, OC, ADHD and autism symptoms: A cross-disorder symptom analysis in Gilles de la Tourette syndrome patients and family-members. *Psychiatry Research*, 237, 138–146.

Iervolino, A. C., Perroud, N., Fullana, M. A., Guipponi, M., Cherkas, L., Collier, D. A., & Mataix-Cols, D. (2009). Prevalence and heritability of compulsive hoarding: a twin study. *American Journal of Psychiatry*, 166(10), 1156–1161.

Iniesta-Sepúlveda, M., Nadeau, J. M., Ramos, A., Kay, B., Riemann, B. C., & Storch, E. A. (2018). An Initial Case Series of Intensive Cognitive–Behavioral Therapy for Obsessive–Compulsive Disorder in Adolescents with Autism Spectrum Disorder. *Child Psychiatry and Human Development*, 49(1), 9–19. doi:10.1007/s10578-017-0724-1.

Insel, T. R., Gillin, J. C., Moore, A., Mendelson, W. B., Loewenstein, R. J., & Murphy, D. L. (1982). The sleep of patients with obsessive-compulsive disorder. *Archives of General Psychiatry*, 39(12), 1372–1377.

Ivarsson, T. & Melin, K. (2008). Autism spectrum traits in children and adolescents with obsessive-compulsive disorder (OCD). *Journal of Anxiety Disorders*, 22(6), 969–978. Retrieved from http://ovidsp.ovid.com/ovidweb.cgi?T=JS&CSC=Y&NEWS=N&PAGE=fulltext&D=medl&AN=18053683.

Ivarsson, T., Melin, K., & Wallin, L. (2008). Categorical and dimensional aspects of co-morbidity in obsessive-compulsive disorder (OCD). *European Child and Adolescent Psychiatry*, 17(1), 20–31. doi:10.1007/s00787-007-0626-z.

Ivarsson, T., Saavedra, F., Granqvist, P., & Broberg, A. G. (2016). Traumatic and adverse attachment childhood experiences are not characteristic of OCD but of depression in adolescents. *Child Psychiatry and Human Development*, 47, 270–280.

Ivarsson, T. & Skarphedinsson, G. (2015). Sleep problems and cognitive behavior therapy in pediatric obsessive-compulsive disorder have bidirectional effects. *Journal of Anxiety Disorders*, 30, 28–33.

Ivarsson, T., Skarphedinsson, G., Kornor, H., Axelsdottir, B., Biedilae, S., Heyman, I., ... March, J. (2015). The place of and evidence for serotonin reuptake inhibitors (SRIs) for obsessive compulsive disorder (OCD) in children and adolescents: Views based on a systematic review and meta-analysis. *Psychiatry Research*, 227(1), 93–103. doi:10.1016/j.psychres.2015.01.015.

Jankovic, J. (2020). Treatment of tics associated with Tourette syndrome. *Journal of Neural Transmission*, 127(5), 843–850.

Jhanda, S., Singla, N., & Grover, S. (2016). Methylphenidate-induced obsessive-compulsive symptoms: A case report and review of literature. *Journal of Pediatric Neurosciences*, 11(4), 316.

Jiménez-Jiménez, F. J., Alonso-Navarro, H., García-Martín, E., & Agúndez, J. A. (2022). Sleep Disorders and Sleep Problems in Patients With Tourette Syndrome and Other Tic Disorders: Current Perspectives. *Nature and Science of Sleep*, 1313–1331.

Johnco, C., McGuire, J. F., McBride, N. M., Murphy, T. K., Lewin, A. B., & Storch, E. A. (2016). Suicidal ideation in youth with tic disorders. *Journal of Affective Disorders*, 200, 204–211.

Jones, P. J., Mair, P., Riemann, B. C., Mugno, B. L., & McNally, R. J. (2018). A network perspective on comorbid depression in adolescents with obsessive-compulsive disorder. *Journal of Anxiety Disorders*, 53, 1–8. doi:10.1016/j.janxdis.2017.09.008.

Kaur, M., Floyd, A., & Balta, A.-M. (2022). Oppositional defiant disorder: Evidence-based review of behavioral treatment programs. *Annals of Clinical Psychiatry: Official Journal of the American Academy of Clinical Psychiatrists*, 34(1), 44–58.

Kendler, K. S., Abrahamsson, L., Ohlsson, H., Sundquist, J., & Sundquist, K. (2023). Obsessive-Compulsive Disorder and Its Cross-Generational Familial Association With Anxiety Disorders in a National Swedish Extended Adoption Study. *JAMA psychiatry*. doi:10.1001/jamapsychiatry.2022.4777.

Khalifa, N. & Knorring, A.-L. (2007). Tourette syndrome and other tic disorders in a total population of children: Clinical assessment and background. *Acta Paediatrica*, 94(11), 1608–1614. doi:10.1111/j.1651-2227.2005.tb01837.x.

King, J., Dowling, N., & Leow, F. (2017). Methylphenidate in the treatment of an adolescent female with obsessive-compulsive disorder and attention deficit hyperactivity disorder: a case report. *Australasian Psychiatry*, 25(2), 178–180.

Klein, K. P., Harris, E. K., Björgvinsson, T., & Kertz, S. J. (2020). A network analysis of symptoms of obsessive compulsive disorder and depression in a clinical sample. *Journal of Obsessive-Compulsive and Related Disorders*, 27, 100556. doi:10.1016/j.jocrd.2020.100556.

Kloft, L., Steinel, T., & Kathmann, N. (2018). Systematic review of co-occurring OCD and TD: Evidence for a tic-related OCD subtype? *Neuroscience and Biobehavioral Reviews*, 95, 280–314.

Konrad, K. & Eickhoff, S. B. (2010). Is the ADHD brain wired differently? A review on structural and functional connectivity in attention deficit hyperactivity disorder. *Human Brain Mapping*, 31(6), 904–916.

Kouris, S. (1998). Methylphenidate-induced obsessive-compulsiveness. *Journal of the American Academy of Child and Adolescent Psychiatry*, 37, 135–135.

Krebs, G., Murray, K., & Jassi, A. (2016). Modified Cognitive Behavior Therapy for Severe, Treatment-Resistant Obsessive-Compulsive Disorder in an

Adolescent With Autism Spectrum Disorder. *Journal of Clinical Psychology*, 72 (11), 1162–1173.

Krueger, R. F. & Markon, K. E. (2006). Understanding Psychopathology: Melding Behavior Genetics, Personality, and Quantitative Psychology to Develop an Empirically Based Model. *Current Directions in Psychological Science*, 15(3), 113–117. doi:10.1111/j.0963-7214.2006.00418.x.

Kurlan, R. (2002). Treatment of ADHD in children with tics: a randomized controlled trial. *Neurology*.

Kurlan, R., Como, P., Miller, B., Palumbo, D., Deeley, C., Andresen, E., ... McDermott, M. (2002). The behavioral spectrum of tic disorders: a community-based study. *Neurology*, 59(3), 414–420.

La Buissonnière-Ariza, V., Wood, J. J., Kendall, P. C., McBride, N. M., Cepeda, S. L., Small, B. J., ... Storch, E. A. (2018). Presentation and Correlates of Hoarding Behaviors in Children with Autism Spectrum Disorders and Comorbid Anxiety or Obsessive-Compulsive Symptoms. *Journal of Autism and Developmental Disorders*, 48(12), 4167–4178. doi:10.1007/s10803-018-3645-3.

Lafleur, D. L., Petty, C., Mancuso, E., McCarthy, K., Biederman, J., Faro, A., ... Geller, D. A. (2011). Traumatic events and obsessive compulsive disorder in children and adolescents: is there a link? *Journal of Anxiety Disorders*, 25(4), 513–519.

Langley, A. K., Lewin, A. B., Bergman, R., Lee, J. C., & Piacentini, J. (2010). Correlates of comorbid anxiety and externalizing disorders in childhood obsessive compulsive disorder. *European Child and Adolescent Psychiatry*, 19(8), 637–645.

Langlois, F., Freeston, M. H., & Ladouceur, R. (2000). Differences and similarities between obsessive intrusive thoughts and worry in a non-clinical population: Study 1. *Behaviour Research and Therapy*, 38(2), 157–173.

Leckman, J. F., Denys, D., Simpson, H. B., Mataix-Cols, D., Hollander, E., Saxena, S., ... Stein, D. J. (2010). Obsessive-compulsive disorder: a review of the diagnostic criteria and possible subtypes and dimensional specifiers for DSM-V. *Depression and Anxiety*, 27(6), 507–527.

Leckman, J. F., Grice, D. E., Barr, L. C., de Vries, A. L., Martin, C., Cohen, D. J., ... Rasmussen, S. A. (1994). Tic-related vs. non-tic-related obsessive compulsive disorder. *Anxiety*, 1(5), 208–215.

Leonard, R. C., Jacobi, D. M., Riemann, B. C., Lake, P. M., & Luhn, R. (2014). The effect of depression symptom severity on OCD treatment outcome in an adolescent residential sample. *Journal of Obsessive-Compulsive and Related Disorders*, 3(2), 95–101.

Leyfer, O. T., Folstein, S. E., Bacalman, S., Davis, N. O., Dinh, E., Morgan, J., ... Lainhart, J. E. (2006). Comorbid psychiatric disorders in children with autism: Interview development and rates of disorders. *Journal of Autism and Developmental Disorders*, 36, 849–861.

Lilienfeld, S. O., Waldman, I. D., & Israel, A. C. (1994). A critical examination of the use of the term and concept of comorbidity in psychopathology research. *Clinical Psychology: Science and Practice*, 1(1), 71.

López-Solà, C., Fontenelle, L. F., Bui, M., Hopper, J. L., Pantelis, C., Yücel, M., ... Harrison, B. J. (2016). Aetiological overlap between obsessive–compulsive related and anxiety disorder symptoms: Multivariate twin study. *The British Journal of Psychiatry*, 208(1), 26–33. doi:10.1192/bjp.bp.114.156281.

Malmivaara, A. (2021). What is the effect of pharmacological treatment for attention-deficit/hyperactivity disorder in children with comorbid tic disorders? A Cochrane Review summary with commentary. *Developmental Medicine and Child Neurology*, 63(1), 14–15. doi:10.1111/dmcn.14707.

March, J. S., Franklin, M. E., Leonard, H., Garcia, A., Moore, P., Freeman, J., & Foa, E. (2007). Tics moderate treatment outcome with sertraline but not cognitive-behavior therapy in pediatric obsessive-compulsive disorder. *Biological Psychiatry*, 61(3), 344–347.

Martin, A. F., Jassi, A., Cullen, A. E., Broadbent, M., Downs, J., & Krebs, G. (2020). Co-occurring obsessive–compulsive disorder and autism spectrum disorder in young people: prevalence, clinical characteristics and outcomes. *European Child and Adolescent Psychiatry*, 29(11), 1603–1611. doi:10.1007/s00787-020-01478-8.

Mas, S., Plana, M. T., Castro-Fornieles, J., Gassó, P., Lafuente, A., Moreno, E., … Lazaro, L. (2013). Common genetic background in anorexia nervosa and obsessive compulsive disorder: preliminary results from an association study. *Journal of Psychiatric Research*, 47(6), 747–754.

Masi, G., Millepiedi, S., Mucci, M., Bertini, N., Pfanner, C., & Arcangeli, F. (2006). Comorbidity of obsessive-compulsive disorder and attention-deficit/hyperactivity disorder in referred children and adolescents. *Comprehensive Psychiatry*, 47(1), 42–47. doi:10.1016/j.comppsych.2005.04.008.

Mataix-Cols, D., Boman, M., Monzani, B., Ruck, C., Serlachius, E., Langstrom, N., & Lichtenstein, P. (2013). Population-based, multigenerational family clustering study of obsessive-compulsive disorder. *JAMA psychiatry*, 70(7), 709–717. doi:10.1001/jamapsychiatry.2013.3.

Mathews, C. A. & Grados, M. A. (2011). Familiality of Tourette Syndrome, Obsessive-Compulsive Disorder, and Attention-Deficit/Hyperactivity Disorder: Heritability Analysis in a Large Sib-Pair Sample. *Journal of the American Academy of Child and Adolescent Psychiatry*, 50(1), 46–54. doi:10.1016/j.jaac.2010.10.004.

McDougle, C. J., Goodman, W. K., Leckman, J. F., Barr, L. C., Heninger, G. R., & Price, L. H. (1993). The efficacy of fluvoxamine in obsessive-compulsive disorder: effects of comorbid chronic tic disorder. *Journal of Clinical Psychopharmacology*, 13(5), 354–358.

Merikangas, K. R., He, J.-P., Brody, D., Fisher, P. W., Bourdon, K., & Koretz, D. S. (2010). Prevalence and treatment of mental disorders among US children in the 2001–2004 NHANES. *Pediatrics*, 125(1), 75–81.

Meyer, J. M., McNamara, J. P., Reid, A. M., Storch, E. A., Geffken, G. R., Mason, D. M., … Bussing, R. (2014). Prospective relationship between obsessive-compulsive and depressive symptoms during multimodal treatment in pediatric obsessive-compulsive disorder. *Child Psychiatry and Human Development*, 45(2), 163–172. doi:10.1007/s10578-013-0388-4.

Miguel, E. C., Baer, L., Coffey, B. J., & Rauch, S. L. (1997). Phenomenological differences appearing with repetitive behaviours in obsessive-compulsive disorder and Gilles de la Tourette's syndrome. *The British Journal of Psychiatry*, 170, 140.

Mol Debes, N. M., Hjalgrim, H., & Skov, L. (2008). Validation of the presence of comorbidities in a Danish clinical cohort of children with Tourette syndrome. *Journal of Child Neurology*, 23(9), 1017–1027.

Murray, K., Jassi, A., Mataix-Cols, D., Barrow, F., & Krebs, G. (2015). Outcomes of cognitive behaviour therapy for obsessive-compulsive disorder in young people with and without autism spectrum disorders: A case controlled study. *Psychiatry Research*, 228(1), 8–13. doi:10.1016/j.psychres.2015.03.012.

Nabinger de Diaz, N. A., Farrell, L. J., Waters, A. M., Donovan, C., & McConnell, H. W. (2019). Sleep-Related Problems in Pediatric Obsessive-Compulsive Disorder and Intensive Exposure Therapy. *Behavior Therapy*, 50(3), 608–620. doi:10.1016/j.beth.2018.09.008.

National Institute for Heath and Clinical Excellence. (2014). Anxiety disorders (pp. National Institute for Health and Clinical Excellence). Retrieved from www.nice.org.uk/guidance/qs53.

Nazeer, A., Latif, F., Mondal, A., Azeem, M. W., & Greydanus, D. E. (2020). Obsessive-compulsive disorder in children and adolescents: epidemiology, diagnosis and management. *Transl Pediatr*, 9(Suppl 1), S76–S93. doi:10.21037/tp.2019.10.02.

Nestadt, G., Addington, A., Samuels, J., Liang, K. Y., Bienvenu, O. J., Riddle, M., ... Cullen, B. (2003). The identification of OCD-related subgroups based on comorbidity. *Biological Psychiatry*, 53(10), 914–920. doi:10.1016/s0006-3223(02)01677-3.

Nestadt, G., Samuels, J., Riddle, M., Liang, K.-Y., Bienvenu, O., Hoehn-Saric, R., ... Cullen, B. (2001). The relationship between obsessive–compulsive disorder and anxiety and affective disorders: results from the Johns Hopkins OCD Family Study. *Psychological Medicine*, 31(3), 481–487.

Neziroglu, F., McKay, D., & Yaryura-Tobias, J. A. (2000). Overlapping and distinctive features of hypochondriasis and obsessive–compulsive disorder. *Journal of Anxiety Disorders*, 14(6), 603–614.

Nissen, J., Parner, E., & Thomsen, P. (2019). Predictors of therapeutic treatment outcome in adolescent chronic tic disorders. *BJPsych Open*, 5(5), e74.

Norman, L. J., Carlisi, C., Lukito, S., Hart, H., Mataix-Cols, D., Radua, J., & Rubia, K. (2016). Structural and functional brain abnormalities in attention-deficit/hyperactivity disorder and obsessive-compulsive disorder: a comparative meta-analysis. *JAMA psychiatry*, 73(8), 815–825.

Norman, L. J., Carlisi, C. O., Christakou, A., Chantiluke, K., Murphy, C., Simmons, A., ... Rubia, K. (2017). Neural dysfunction during temporal discounting in paediatric attention-deficit/hyperactivity disorder and obsessive-compulsive disorder. *Psychiatry Research: Neuroimaging*, 269, 97–105.

Norman, L. J., Carlisi, C. O., Christakou, A., Murphy, C. M., Chantiluke, K., Giampietro, V., ... Rubia, K. (2018). Frontostriatal Dysfunction During Decision Making in Attention-Deficit/Hyperactivity Disorder and Obsessive-Compulsive Disorder. *Biological Psychiatry: Cognitive Neuroscience and Neuroimaging*, 3(8), 694–703. doi:10.1016/j.bpsc.2018.03.009.

Olino, T. M., Gillo, S., Rowe, D., Palermo, S., Nuhfer, E. C., Birmaher, B., & Gilbert, A. R. (2011). Evidence for successful implementation of exposure and response prevention in a naturalistic group format for pediatric OCD. *Depression and Anxiety*, 28(4), 342–348. doi:10.1002/da.20789.

Oliver, A. M., Wright, K. D., Kakadekar, A., Pharis, S., Pockett, C., Bradley, T. J., ... Erlandson, M. C. (2020). Health anxiety and associated constructs in children and adolescents with congenital heart disease: A CHAMPS cohort study. *Journal of Health Psychology*, 25(10–11), 1355–1365.

Pappert, E. J., Goetz, C., Louis, E., Blasucci, L., & Leurgans, S. (2003). Objective assessments of longitudinal outcome in Gilles de la Tourette's syndrome. *Neurology*, 61(7), 936–940.

Park, J. M., Samuels, J. F., Grados, M. A., Riddle, M. A., Bienvenu, O. J., Goes, F. S., ... Geller, D. A. (2016). ADHD and executive functioning deficits in OCD youths who hoard. *Journal of Psychiatric Research*, 82, 141–148. doi:10.1016/j.jpsychires.2016.07.024.

Pauls, D. L., Abramovitch, A., Rauch, S. L., & Geller, D. A. (2014). Obsessive-compulsive disorder: an integrative genetic and neurobiological perspective. *Nature Reviews Neuroscience*, 15(6), 410–424. doi:http://dx.doi.org/10.1038/nrn3746.

Pauls, D. L., Alsobrook, J. P., 2nd, Goodman, W., Rasmussen, S., & Leckman, J. F. (1995). A family study of obsessive-compulsive disorder. *American Journal of Psychiatry*, 152(1), 76–84.

Pazuniak, M. & Pekrul, S. R. (2020). Obsessive–Compulsive Disorder in Autism Spectrum Disorder Across the Lifespan. *Child and Adolescent Psychiatric Clinics of North America*, 29(2), 419–432. doi:10.1016/j.chc.2019.12.003.

Peris, T. S., Bergman, R. L., Asarnow, J. R., Langley, A., McCracken, J. T., & Piacentini, J. (2010). Clinical and cognitive correlates of depressive symptoms among youth with obsessive compulsive disorder. *J.Clin.Child Adolesc.Psychol.*, 39(5), 616–626.

Peris, T. S., Bergman, R. L., Langley, A., Chang, S., McCracken, J. T., & Piacentini, J. (2008). Correlates of accommodation of pediatric obsessive-compulsive disorder: parent, child, and family characteristics. *Journal of the American Academy of Child and Adolescent Psychiatry*, 47(10), 1173–1181. doi:10.1097/CHI.0b013e3181825a91.

Pertusa, A., Fullana, M. A., Singh, S., Alonso, P., Menchón, J. M., & Mataix-Cols, D. (2008). Compulsive hoarding: OCD symptom, distinct clinical syndrome, or both? *American Journal of Psychiatry*, 165(10), 1289–1298.

Peterson, B. S., Pine, D. S., Cohen, P., & Brook, J. S. (2001). Prospective, longitudinal study of tic, obsessive-compulsive, and attention-deficit/hyperactivity disorders in an epidemiological sample. *Journal of the American Academy of Child and Adolescent Psychiatry*, 40(6), 685–695. doi:S0890–8567(09)60473–60471 [pii] 10. 1097/00004583–200106000–00014.

Piacentini, J., Peris, T. S., Bergman, R. L., Chang, S., & Jaffer, M. (2007). Functional impairment in childhood OCD: development and psychometrics properties of the Child Obsessive-Compulsive Impact Scale-Revised (COIS-R). *Journal of Clinical Child and Adolescent Psychology*, 36(4), 645–653. doi:10.1080/15374410701662790.

Plimpton, E. H., Frost, R. O., Abbey, B. C., & Dorer, W. (2009). Compulsive Hoarding in Children: Six Case Studies. *International Journal of Cognitive Therapy*, 2(1), 88–104. doi:10.1521/ijct.2009.2.1.88.

Postlethwaite, A., Kellett, S., & Mataix-Cols, D. (2019). Prevalence of hoarding disorder: A systematic review and meta-analysis. *Journal of Affective Disorders*, 256, 309–316.

Pringsheim, T., Holler-Managan, Y., Okun, M. S., Jankovic, J., Piacentini, J., Cavanna, A. E., ... Robinson, M. (2019). Comprehensive systematic review summary: treatment of tics in people with Tourette syndrome and chronic tic disorders. *Neurology*, 92(19), 907–915.

Rachman, S. (1997). A cognitive theory of obsessions. *Behaviour Research and Therapy*, 35(9), 793–802.

Racz, J. I., Mathieu, S. L., McKenzie, M. L., & Farrell, L. J. (2022). Paediatric Obsessive–Compulsive Disorder and Comorbid Body Dysmorphic Disorder: Clinical Expression and Treatment Response. *Child Psychiatry and Human Development*, 1–10.

Rapoport, J. L. (1986). Childhood obsessive compulsive disorder. *Journal of Child Psychology and Psychiatry and Allied Disciplines*, 27(3), 289–295.

Rask, C. U., Elberling, H., Skovgaard, A. M., Thomsen, P. H., & Fink, P. (2012). Parental-reported health anxiety symptoms in 5-to 7-year-old children: the Copenhagen Child Cohort CCC 2000. *Psychosomatics*, 53(1), 58–67.

Rask, C. U., Munkholm, A., Clemmensen, L., Rimvall, M. K., Ørnbøl, E., Jeppesen, P., & Skovgaard, A. M. (2016). Health anxiety in preadolescence-associated health problems, healthcare expenditure, and continuity in childhood. *Journal of Abnormal Child Psychology*, 44, 823–832.

Rautio, D., Jassi, A., Krebs, G., Andrén, P., Monzani, B., Gumpert, M., ... Jansson-Fröjmark, M. (2020). Clinical characteristics of 172 children and adolescents with body dysmorphic disorder. *European Child and Adolescent Psychiatry*, 1–12.

Reddihough, D. S., Marraffa, C., Mouti, A., O'Sullivan, M., Lee, K. J., Orsini, F., ... Kohn, M. (2019). Effect of Fluoxetine on Obsessive-Compulsive Behaviors in Children and Adolescents With Autism Spectrum Disorders: A Randomized Clinical Trial. *JAMA*, 322(16), 1561–1569. doi:10.1001/jama.2019.14685.

Reiersen, A. M., & Handen, B. (2011). Commentary on 'Selective serotonin reuptake inhibitors (SSRIs) for autism spectrum disorders (ASD)'. *Evid Based Child Health*, 6(4), 1082–1085. doi:10.1002/ebch.786.

Reuman, L., Jacoby, R. J., Blakey, S. M., Riemann, B. C., Leonard, R. C., & Abramowitz, J. S. (2017). Predictors of illness anxiety symptoms in patients with obsessive compulsive disorder. *Psychiatry Research*, 256, 417–422.

Ricketts, E. J., Peris, T. S., Grant, J. E., Valle, S., Cavic, E., Lerner, J. E., ... Piacentini, J. (2022). Clinical Characteristics of Youth with Trichotillomania (Hair-Pulling Disorder) and Excoriation (Skin-Picking) Disorder. *Child Psychiatry and Human Development*. doi:10.1007/s10578-022-01458-w.

Rodowski, M. F., Cagande, C. C., & Riddle, M. A. (2008). Childhood obsessive-compulsive disorder presenting as schizophrenia spectrum disorders. *Journal of Child and Adolescent Psychopharmacology*, 18(4), 395–401.

Roessner, V., Becker, A., Banaschewski, T., & Rothenberger, A. (2007). Psychopathological profile in children with chronic tic disorder and co-existing ADHD: additive effects. *Journal of Abnormal Child Psychology*, 35, 79–85.

Roessner, V., Eichele, H., Stern, J. S., Skov, L., Rizzo, R., Debes, N. M., ... Ganos, C. (2022). European clinical guidelines for Tourette syndrome and other tic disorders – version 2.0. Part III: pharmacological treatment. *European Child and Adolescent Psychiatry*, 1–17.

Rozenman, M., McGuire, J., Wu, M., Ricketts, E., Peris, T., O'Neill, J., ... Piacentini, J. (2019). Hoarding symptoms in children and adolescents with obsessive-compulsive disorder: Clinical features and response to cognitive-behavioral therapy. *Journal of the American Academy of Child and Adolescent Psychiatry*, 58(8), 799–805.

Russell, A. J., Jassi, A., Fullana, M. A., Mack, H., Johnston, K., Heyman, I., … Mataix-Cols, D. (2013). Cognitive behavior therapy for comorbid obsessive-compulsive disorder in high-functioning autism spectrum disorders: A randomized controlled trial. *Depression and Anxiety*, 30(8), 697–708. doi:10.1002/da.22053.

Sambrani, T., Jakubovski, E., & Müller-Vahl, K. R. (2016). New insights into clinical characteristics of Gilles de la Tourette syndrome: findings in 1032 patients from a single German center. *Frontiers in Neuroscience*, 10, 415.

Samuels, J., Grados, M. A., Riddle, M. A., Bienvenu, O. J., Goes, F. S., Cullen, B., … Nestadt, G. (2014). Hoarding in children and adolescents with obsessive-compulsive disorder. *Journal of Obsessive-Compulsive and Related Disorders*, 3 (4), 325–331. doi:10.1016/j.jocrd.2014.08.001.

Santangelo, S. L., Pauls, D. L., Goldstein, J. M., Faraone, S. V., Tsuang, M. T., & Leckman, J. F. (1994). Tourette's syndrome: what are the influences of gender and comorbid obsessive-compulsive disorder? *Journal of the American Academy of Child and Adolescent Psychiatry*, 33(6), 795–804.

Santhanam, R., Fairley, M., & Rogers, M. (2008). Is it trichotillomania? Hair pulling in childhood: A developmental perspective. *Clinical Child Psychology and Psychiatry*, 13(3), 409–418.

Scahill, L., Sukhodolsky, D. G., Williams, S. K., & Leckman, J. F. (2005). Public health significance of tic disorders in children and adolescents. *Advances in Neurology*, 96, 240–248.

Scarella, T. M., Boland, R. J., & Barsky, A. J. (2019). Illness anxiety disorder: psychopathology, epidemiology, clinical characteristics, and treatment. *Psychosomatic Medicine*, 81(5), 398–407.

Selles, R. R., Ariza, V. L. B., McBride, N. M., Dammann, J., Whiteside, S., & Storch, E. A. (2018). Initial psychometrics, outcomes, and correlates of the Repetitive Body Focused Behavior Scale: Examination in a sample of youth with anxiety and/or obsessive-compulsive disorder. *Comprehensive Psychiatry*, 81, 10–17.

Selles, R. R., Nelson, R., Zepeda, R., Dane, B. F., Wu, M. S., Carlos Novoa, J., … Storch, E. A. (2015). Body focused repetitive behaviors among Salvadorian youth: Incidence and clinical correlates. *Journal of Obsessive-Compulsive and Related Disorders*, 5, 49–54. doi:10.1016/j.jocrd.2015.01.008.

Sevilla-Cermeño, L., Andrén, P., Hillborg, M., Silverberg-Morse, M., Mataix-Cols, D., & Fernández de la Cruz, L. (2019). Insomnia in pediatric obsessive–compulsive disorder: prevalence and association with multimodal treatment outcomes in a naturalistic clinical setting. *Sleep Medicine*, 56, 104–110. doi:10.1016/j.sleep.2018.12.024.

Sharma, E., Sharma, L. P., Balachander, S., Lin, B., Manohar, H., Khanna, P., … Stewart, S. E. (2021). Comorbidities in Obsessive-Compulsive Disorder Across the Lifespan: A Systematic Review and Meta-Analysis. *Front Psychiatry*, 12, 703701. doi:10.3389/fpsyt.2021.703701.

Skarphedinsson, G., Compton, S., Thomsen, P. H., Weidle, B., Dahl, K., Nissen, J. B., … Ivarsson, T. (2015). Tics Moderate Sertraline, but Not Cognitive-Behavior Therapy Response in Pediatric Obsessive-Compulsive Disorder Patients Who Do Not Respond to Cognitive-Behavior Therapy. *Journal of Child and Adolescent Psychopharmacology*, 25(5), 432–439. doi:NLM. PMC4491151 10.1089/cap.2014.0167.

Smárason, O., Weidle, B., Hojgaard, D. R., Torp, N. C., Ivarsson, T., Nissen, J. B., ... Skarphedinsson, G. (2021). Younger versus older children with obsessive-compulsive disorder: Symptoms, severity and impairment. *Journal of Obsessive-Compulsive and Related Disorders*, 29, 100646.

Steketee, G. & Frost, R. (2003). Compulsive hoarding: current status of the research. *Clinical Psychology Review*, 23(7), 905–927.

Stewart, S. E., Illmann, C., Geller, D. A., Leckman, J. F., King, R., & Pauls, D. L. (2006). A controlled family study of attention-deficit/hyperactivity disorder and Tourette's disorder. *Journal of the American Academy of Child and Adolescent Psychiatry*, 45(11), 1354–1362.

Storch, E. A., Abramowitz, J., & Goodman, W. K. (2008). Where does obsessive-compulsive disorder belong in DSM-V? *Depression and Anxiety*, 25(4), 336–347. doi:10.1002/da.20488.

Storch, E. A., Abramowitz, J. S., & Keeley, M. (2009). Correlates and mediators of functional disability in obsessive-compulsive disorder. *Depression and Anxiety*, 26(9), 806–813. doi:10.1002/da.20481.

Storch, E. A., Lack, C. W., Merlo, L. J., Geffken, G. R., Jacob, M. L., Murphy, T. K., & Goodman, W. K. (2007). Clinical features of children and adolescents with obsessive-compulsive disorder and hoarding symptoms. *Comprehensive Psychiatry*, 48(4), 313–318. Retrieved from http://ovidsp.ovid.com/ovidweb.cgi?T=JS&CSC=Y&NEWS=N&PAGE=fulltext&D=medl&AN=17560950.

Storch, E. A., Larson, M., Merlo, L., Keeley, M., Jacob, M., Geffken, G., ... Goodman, W. (2008). Comorbidity of Pediatric Obsessive–Compulsive Disorder and Anxiety Disorders: Impact on Symptom Severity and Impairment. *Journal of Psychopathology and Behavioral Assessment*, 30(2), 111–120. doi:10.1007/s10862-007-9057-x.

Storch, E. A., Larson, M. J., Muroff, J., Caporino, N., Geller, D., Reid, J. M., ... Murphy, T. K. (2010). Predictors of functional impairment in pediatric obsessive-compulsive disorder. *Journal of Anxiety Disorders*, 24(2), 275–283. Retrieved from http://ovidsp.ovid.com/ovidweb.cgi?T=JS&CSC=Y&NEWS=N&PAGE=fulltext&D=medl&AN=20056376.

Storch, E. A., Lewin, A. B., Larson, M. J., Geffken, G. R., Murphy, T. K., & Geller, D. A. (2012). Depression in youth with obsessive-compulsive disorder: clinical phenomenology and correlates. *Psychiatry Research*, 196(1), 83–89.

Storch, E. A., Merlo, L. J., Larson, M. J., Geffken, G. R., Lehmkuhl, H. D., Jacob, M. L., ... Goodman, W. K. (2008). Impact of comorbidity on cognitive-behavioral therapy response in pediatric obsessive-compulsive disorder. *Journal of the American Academy of Child and Adolescent Psychiatry*, 47(5), 583–592.

Storch, E. A., Murphy, T. K., Lack, C. W., Geffken, G. R., Jacob, M. L., & Goodman, W. K. (2008). Sleep-related problems in pediatric obsessive-compulsive disorder. *Journal of Anxiety Disorders*, 22(5), 877–885. Retrieved from http://ovidsp.ovid.com/ovidweb.cgi?T=JS&CSC=Y&NEWS=N&PAGE=fulltext&D=medl&AN=17951025.

Storch, E. A., Nadeau, J. M., Johnco, C., Timpano, K., McBride, N., Jane Mutch, P., ... Murphy, T. K. (2016). Hoarding in Youth with Autism Spectrum Disorders and Anxiety: Incidence, Clinical Correlates, and Behavioral Treatment Response. *Journal of Autism and Developmental Disorders*, 46(5), 1602–1612. doi:10.1007/s10803-015-2687-z.

Storch, E. A., Rahman, O., Park, J. M., Reid, J., Murphy, T. K., & Lewin, A. B. (2011). Compulsive hoarding in children. *Journal of Clinical Psychology*, 67(5), 507–516. doi:https://doi.org/10.1002/jclp.20794.

Sukhodolsky, D. G., do Rosario-Campos, M. C., Scahill, L., Findley, D. B., & Leckman, J. F. (2005). Adaptive, Emotional, and Family Functioning of Children With Obsessive-Compulsive Disorder and Comorbid Attention Deficit Hyperactivity Disorder. *American Journal of Psychiatry*, 162(6), 1125–1132.

Sukhodolsky, D. G., Woods, D. W., Piacentini, J., Wilhelm, S., Peterson, A. L., Katsovich, L., ... Scahill, L. (2017). Moderators and predictors of response to behavior therapy for tics in Tourette syndrome. *Neurology*, 88(11), 1029–1036. Retrieved from www.ncbi.nlm.nih.gov/pmc/articles/PMC5384839/pdf/NEUROL OGY2016749267.pdf.

Sweeten, G., Sillence, E., & Neave, N. (2018). Digital hoarding behaviours: Underlying motivations and potential negative consequences. *Computers in Human Behavior*, 85, 54–60.

Szejko, N., Robinson, S., Hartmann, A., Ganos, C., Debes, N. M., Skov, L., ... Cath, D. C. (2022). European clinical guidelines for Tourette syndrome and other tic disorders-version 2.0. Part I: assessment. *European Child and Adolescent Psychiatry*, 31(3), 383–402. doi:10.1007/s00787-021-01842-2.

Tambs, K., Czajkowsky, N., Neale, M. C., Reichborn-Kjennerud, T., Aggen, S. H., Harris, J. R., & Kendler, K. S. (2009). Structure of genetic and environmental risk factors for dimensional representations of DSM–IV anxiety disorders. *The British Journal of Psychiatry*, 195(4), 301–307.

Thomsen, P. (2000). Obsessions: the impact and treatment of obsessive-compulsive disorder in children and adolescents. *Journal of Psychopharmacology*, 14 (2_suppl1), S31-S37.

Tolin, D. F., Franklin, M. E., Diefenbach, G. J., Anderson, E., & Meunier, S. A. (2007). Pediatric trichotillomania: descriptive psychopathology and an open trial of cognitive behavioral therapy. *Cognitive Behaviour Therapy*, 36(3), 129–144.

Tolin, D. F., Frost, R. O., Steketee, G., & Muroff, J. (2015). Cognitive behavioral therapy for hoarding disorder: a meta-analysis. *Depression and Anxiety*, 32(3), 158–166. doi:10.1002/da.22327.

Tolin, D. F., Meunier, S. A., Frost, R. O., & Steketee, G. (2010). Course of compulsive hoarding and its relationship to life events. *Depression and Anxiety*, 27 (9), 829–838.

Torp, N. C., Dahl, K., Skarphedinsson, G., Thomsen, P., Valderhaug, R., Weidle, B., ... Ivarsson, T. (2015). Effectiveness of cognitive behavior treatment for pediatric obsessive-compulsive disorder: Acute outcomes from The Nordic Long-term OCD Treatment Study (NordLOTS). *Behaviour Research and Therapy*, 64, 15–23. doi:10.1016/j.brat.2014.11.005.

Tsetsos, F., Padmanabhuni, S. S., Alexander, J., Karagiannidis, I., Tsifintaris, M., Topaloudi, A., ... Paschou, P. (2016). Meta-analysis of tourette syndrome and attention deficit hyperactivity disorder provides support for a shared genetic basis. *Frontiers in Neuroscience*, 10, 340.

Tynes, L. L., White, K., & Steketee, G. S. (1990). Toward a new nosology of obsessive compulsive disorder. *Comprehensive Psychiatry*, 31(5), 465–480.

Tyrer, P. (2018). Recent advances in the understanding and treatment of health anxiety. *Current psychiatry reports*, 20, 1–8.

van Steensel, F. J. A., Bögels, S. M., & Perrin, S. (2011). Anxiety Disorders in Children and Adolescents with Autistic Spectrum Disorders: A Meta-Analysis. *Clinical Child and Family Psychology Review*, 14(3), 302. doi:10.1007/s10567-011-0097-0.

Vazquez, M., Palo, A., Schuyler, M., Small, B. J., McGuire, J. F., Wilhelm, S., ... Storch, E. A. (2022). The Relationship Between Adverse Childhood Experiences, Symptom Severity, Negative Thinking, Comorbidity, and Treatment Response in Youth with Obsessive-Compulsive Disorder. *Child Psychiatry and Human Development*. doi:10.1007/s10578-022-01488-4.

Villadsen, A., Thorgaard, M. V., Hybel, K. A., Jensen, J. S., Thomsen, P. H., & Rask, C. U. (2017). Health anxiety symptoms in children and adolescents diagnosed with OCD. *European Child and Adolescent Psychiatry*, 26, 241–251. doi:10.1007/s00787-016-0884-8.

Walitza, S., Zellmann, H., Irblich, B., Lange, K. W., Tucha, O., Hemminger, U., ... Warnke, A. (2008). Children and adolescents with obsessive-compulsive disorder and comorbid attention-deficit/hyperactivity disorder: preliminary results of a prospective follow-up study. *J Neural Transm (Vienna)*, 115(2), 187–190. doi:10.1007/s00702-007-0841-2.

Walkup, J. T., Labuda, M. C., Singer, H. S., Brown, J., Riddle, M. A., & Hurko, O. (1996). Family study and segregation analysis of Tourette syndrome: evidence for a mixed model of inheritance. *American Journal of Human Genetics*, 59(3), 684.

Walther, M. R., Snorrason, I., Flessner, C. A., Franklin, M. E., Burkel, R., & Woods, D. W. (2014). The Trichotillomania Impact Project in Young Children (TIP-YC): Clinical Characteristics, Comorbidity, Functional Impairment and Treatment Utilization. *Child Psychiatry and Human Development*, 45(1), 24–31. doi:10.1007/s10578-013-0373-y.

Wanderer, S., Roessner, V., Freeman, R., Bock, N., Rothenberger, A., & Becker, A. (2012). Relationship of obsessive-compulsive disorder to age-related comorbidity in children and adolescents with Tourette syndrome. *Journal of Developmental and Behavioral Pediatrics*, 33(2), 124–133.

Waszczuk, M. A., Brown, H. M., Eley, T. C., & Lester, K. J. (2015). Attentional control theory in childhood: enhanced attentional capture by non-emotional and emotional distractors in anxiety and depression. *PloS One*, 10(11), e0141535.

Weidle, B., Ivarsson, T., Thomsen, P. H., Lydersen, S., & Jozefiak, T. (2015). Quality of life in children with OCD before and after treatment. *European Child and Adolescent Psychiatry*, 24(9), 1061–1074. doi:10.1007/s00787-014-0659-z.

Wilhelm, S., Keuthen, N. J., Deckersbach, T., Engelhard, I. M., Forker, A. E., Baer, L., ... Jenike, M. A. (1999). Self-injurious skin picking: clinical characteristics and comorbidity. *Journal of Clinical Psychiatry*, 60(7), 454–459.

Wislocki, K., Kratz, H. E., Martin, G., & Becker-Haimes, E. M. (2022). The Relationship Between Trauma Exposure and Obsessive–Compulsive Disorder in Youth: A Systematic Review. *Child Psychiatry and Human Development*. doi:10.1007/s10578-022-01352-5.

Wolters, L. H., de Haan, E., Hogendoorn, S. M., Boer, F., & Prins, P. J. M. (2016). Severe pediatric obsessive compulsive disorder and co-morbid autistic symptoms: Effectiveness of cognitive behavioral therapy. *Journal of Obsessive-Compulsive and Related Disorders*, 10, 69–77. doi:10.1016/j.jocrd.2016.06.002.

Woolley, J. B. & Heyman, I. (2003). Dexamphetamine for obsessive-compulsive disorder. *American Journal of Psychiatry*, 160(1), 183–183.

Wright, K. D., Reiser, S. J., & Delparte, C. A. (2017). The relationship between childhood health anxiety, parent health anxiety, and associated constructs. *Journal of Health Psychology*, 22(5), 617–626.

Yilmaz, Z., Schaumberg, K., Halvorsen, M., Goodman, E. L., Brosof, L. C., Crowley, J. J., ... Zerwas, S. C. (2022). Predicting eating disorder and anxiety symptoms using disorder-specific and transdiagnostic polygenic scores for anorexia nervosa and obsessive-compulsive disorder. *Psychological Medicine*, 1–15. doi:10.1017/s0033291721005079.

16 Neurobiology of Pediatric Obsessive-Compulsive Disorder

Augusto de las Casas, Shankar Nandakumar, Grace Pham, Yaman Kawamleh and Julia Ridgeway-Diaz

Introduction

This chapter pertains to the topic of the neurobiology of pediatric obsessive-compulsive disorder (OCD). It is divided into three subsections as follows:

1 The Neuroanatomy of Pediatric OCD: This section will review the circuitry of pediatric OCD. This section will discuss different functions of various brain regions and how they relate to pediatric OCD. It will also review neuroimaging studies and their findings related to this topic.
2 Neurotransmitter Systems and OCD: This section will review the serotonergic, dopaminergic, and glutamatergic neurotransmitter systems in the pathophysiology and management of OCD.
3 Current and Future Treatment Implications: This section will cover various treatments of OCD, including selective serotonin reuptake inhibitors (SSRIs) and Exposure Response Prevention (ERP) therapy, a type of Cognitive Behavioral Therapy (CBT). It will then conclude with future treatment possibilities, by looking at other receptor systems, emerging technologies, and other possible next steps.

The neuroanatomy of pediatric OCD

Understanding the neuroanatomy of OCD is crucial for gaining insights into the neural circuits and structures involved in its pathophysiology. This section delves into the intricate relationship between neuroanatomy and the neurobiology of pediatric OCD, as well as how it diverges from adult OCD. The greater availability of neuroimaging has provided additional insights into functional differences between children with OCD and their healthy counterparts.

At the heart of the neuroanatomy of pediatric OCD lies the Cortico-Striato-Thalamo-Cortical (CSTC) circuit, a complex network of brain

DOI: 10.4324/9781003517429-16

regions responsible for regulating thoughts, emotions, and behaviors. This circuitry is composed of the prefrontal cortex (PFC), the basal ganglia, and the thalamus. The PFC, particularly the orbitofrontal cortex (OFC) and anterior cingulate cortex (ACC), plays a pivotal role in OCD (van der Straten et al., 2018). The OFC is involved in evaluating the emotional significance of thoughts, while the ACC is responsible for error detection and cognitive control. The ACC is also involved in the assignment of salience, which is relevant to OCD, a disorder in which salience is abnormally assigned to and fixated on certain thoughts and behaviors with reduced ability to shift focus. Dysfunction within these regions contributes to the emergence of obsessions and compulsions (Fitzgerald et al., 1999). The basal ganglia, including the caudate nucleus and putamen (known jointly as the striatum), are central to the development of compulsions. They are responsible for motor control and habit formation. Dysregulation within the basal ganglia leads to the repetitive, ritualistic behaviors characteristic of OCD (Vattimo et al., 2019). The thalamus acts as a relay station within the CSTC circuitry, facilitating communication between different brain regions (Li & Mody, 2016). Dysregulation of thalamic function may amplify the intrusive nature of obsessions, as it contributes to the constant looping of distressing thoughts (Fitzgerald et al., 2000). There is no known primary locus of neuronal degeneration in OCD as there is in diseases such as Parkinson's disease; activity within the cortico-basal ganglia network is increased at rest relative to healthy individuals, is accentuated during provocation of symptoms, and is attenuated following successful treatment (Graybiel & Rauch, 2000). Interestingly, psychosurgical lesions of the anterior cingulum and thalamus can reduce OCD symptoms in treatment-resistant OCD (Rosenberg et al., 2001).

Research utilizing neuroimaging techniques, such as structural and functional magnetic resonance imaging (MRI), has revealed numerous neuroanatomical abnormalities in children and adolescents with OCD, including structural abnormalities, differences in cortical-thalamic connectivity, and striatal hyperactivity. Neuroimaging studies have shown alterations in gray matter volume, particularly within the PFC and basal ganglia (MacMaster et al., 2008). These structural changes correlate with the severity and duration of OCD symptoms. Functional MRI (fMRI) studies have demonstrated abnormal patterns of brain activation in pediatric OCD. Heightened activity in the OFC and ACC during symptom provocation tasks is indicative of their involvement in obsessions and compulsions (Huyser et al., 2011). The ACC was also found to be enlarged in children with OCD compared to healthy controls (Huyser et al., 2009). In general, pediatric OCD patients were found to have significantly more gray matter in the left and right putamen as well as the orbito-frontal cortex (Szeszko et al., 2008). Altered connectivity between the PFC and thalamus has been observed in pediatric OCD, which contributes to the faulty regulation of intrusive thoughts and compulsive behaviors (Bernstein et al., 2016). Excessive activity in the striatum, a key component of the basal ganglia, is associated with the repetitive nature of compulsions (Burguière et al., 2015). Overactivation of this region results in the stereotyped rituals seen in OCD.

Neuroimaging studies have shown that pediatric OCD is associated with abnormalities in brain regions like the PFC which continue to mature during adolescence (van der Straten et al., 2018). In contrast, adult OCD may involve different neural circuits that have reached a more stable developmental stage. Pediatric OCD is often associated with structural abnormalities in particular regions of the PFC, including the orbitofrontal cortex (OFC) and anterior cingulate cortex (ACC), as described above (van der Straten et al., 2018). These regions are critical for impulse control, emotion regulation, and decision-making. In contrast, adult OCD may exhibit less pronounced cortical abnormalities, suggesting a different neuroanatomical profile (Wang et al., 2022). While both pediatric and adult OCD involve the basal ganglia, the nature of their involvement may differ. Pediatric OCD often shows heightened basal ganglia activation, which correlates with the severity of compulsive behaviors (Maia et al., 2008). In contrast, adult OCD may exhibit different patterns of basal ganglia activity (Maia et al., 2008). Dysfunctional thalamic connectivity within the CSTC circuitry is a hallmark of both pediatric and adult OCD. However, the specific nature of these connectivity disruptions may vary, potentially contributing to differences in symptomatology and treatment response.

The CSTC circuitry, encompassing the PFC, basal ganglia, and thalamus, is central to the pathophysiology of OCD. Neuroimaging studies have provided critical insights into structural and functional abnormalities associated with the disorder. Integrating neuroanatomical findings with other aspects of the neurobiology of OCD, such as neurotransmitter systems and neurodevelopmental factors, yields a more comprehensive understanding of this complex condition.

Neurotransmitter systems and OCD

Introduction

Neurotransmitter systems, alongside genetic factors, environmental factors, structural factors, and many more, represent one dimension of the multifaceted development of OCD. While several neurotransmitters have been implicated in the pathophysiology of OCD, available data suggest that there are three predominant neurotransmitter systems involved: serotonin, dopamine, and glutamate; for each of these neurotransmitter systems, we will outline the relevant data.

It is important to frame the neurotransmitter data in the context of modern neuro-psychophysiological discourse. As stated earlier, OCD neuropathophysiology is thought to involve the cortico-striato-thalamo-cortical (CSTC) circuit which comprises both the direct and indirect pathways. The direct pathway disinhibits the circuit, leading to an increase in either motor movements, affective motivations, or cognitive associations, depending on the area of cerebral cortex involved. The indirect pathway inhibits the circuit, leading to a reduction in movement, affective motivation, or cognitive associations. Both pathways are active at any given time, creating a balance between hypokinesis and hyperkinesis, as well as a balance of cognitive and affective activity. In OCD, it is thought that the CSTC sub-circuit that involves the anterior cingulate and orbitofrontal cortices, the ventral striatum, the limbic territory of the substantia nigra pars reticulata, the globus pallidus interna, and certain thalamic nuclei is hyperactive. While patients with OCD have been found to have aberrancies in CSTC circuitry at several levels, among the most common is an impaired negative feedback loop involving reduced cortical inhibition of subcortical nodes. Complicating matters, however, is the fact that regulation of network activity is bidirectional, as can be seen with the high prevalence of OCD symptoms in patients with Huntington's disease, a condition marked by atophy of the caudate. It has been postulated that the pathophysiology of OCD involves functional changes to the CSTC circuit mediated by neurotransmitter imbalances. Serotonin, dopamine and glutamate are the most important neurotransmitters involved in these circuits and modulate the activity of both the direct and indirect circuits, thus modulating the frequency and severity of the cognitive, affective, and motor compulsions experienced by the patient.

Serotonin

The serotonergic neurotransmitter system, owing to the utility and widespread nature of its medications, is the neurotransmitter system most commonly associated with OCD. First line agents for OCD are the selective serotonin reuptake inhibitor (SSRI) class, followed by serotonin and norepinephrine reuptake inhibitors (SNRI). These medications reduce OCD symptoms through alterations in the serotonergic system, as their effectiveness is correlated with their degree of serotonin agonism (Derksen et al., 2020). In fact, a meta-analysis suggested clomipramine, a tricyclic antidepressant, shows superiority to SSRIs among individuals with OCD, with clomipramine being a stronger serotonergic drug than SSRIs (Ackerman & Greenland, 2002). This study was followed by a pediatric-focused meta-analysis which looked at 801 children with OCD through nine trials and found that clomipramine was associated with a greater benefit versus placebo than SSRIs versus placebo (Varigonda et al., 2016). The same study noted no evidence for a relationship between SSRI dosing and treatment effect and found that adults and children experienced a similar degree and time course of response. It is the side effect profile that largely places SSRIs as the first line treatment. However, it is important to note that about 30–40 percent of patients with OCD do not respond to serotonergic medications (Derksen et al., 2020). Having begun to establish its management-supported role, we will outline below additional studies that implicate the serotonergic system in OCD.

Clinical data

Among the strongest evidence in support of serotonin modulators in the treatment of OCD comes from clinical studies demonstrating their efficacy. Systematic reviews and meta-analysess have demonstrated that serotonergic antidepressants clomipramine, fluoxetine, fluvoxamine, behavioral therapy, and the combination of these medications with behavioral therapy were all superior to placebo in significantly reducing OCD symptoms in the short term. In particular, one meta-analysis of 20 randomized controlled trials found CBT to be more effective than SSRIs in terms of treatment efficacy, treatment response, and symptom/diagnostic remission (McGuire et al., 2015). A similar systematic review and meta-analysis in adult populations also found SSRIs to be superior to placebo for significant reduction of Yale-Brown Obsessive-Compulsive Scale (Y-BOCS) scores. The same study found CBT to be superior to antidepressants, and that the addition of SSRIs to the treatment of OCD patients already receiving CBT was not superior to patients receiving CBT and placebo (Öst et al., 2015). This meta-analysis was replicated similarly in children and produced similar findings with CBT yielding greater effect sizes, response rates, and remission rates compared to SSRIs and placebo, SSRIs yielding statistically significant effect sizes compared to placebo, but no potentiation effect from adding SSRIs to CBT (Öst et al., 2016). However, it has been postulated that CBT itself might also affect serotonergic systems: a 2018 positron emission tomography (PET) study demonstrated that independent of treatment modality (SSRIs or CBT), there are increases in global 5-HT synthesis capacity that correlates with reductions in OCD symptom severity (Lissemore et al., 2018). Thus, clinical evidence supports the implication of serotonin as a key neurotransmitter in the pathophysiology of OCD.

Receptors

Several serotonin receptors have been studied in the pathophysiology of OCD. The 5HT2A receptor is among the chief receptors implicated in this condition. A meta-analysis which examined the relationship between OCD and all previously identified polymorphisms in available studies for which there was significant enough evidence to calculate odds ratios found that OCD was associated with two serotonin-related polymorphisms–one in the 5HT2A receptor gene and another in the gene

5HTTLPR, a serotonin transporter (SERT) polymorphism encoded by gene *SLC6A4*–as well as two polymorphisms involved with catecholamine production (COMT and MAOA), discussed later (Taylor, 2013). OCD severity is generally associated with lower SERT binding, but in the thalamus and hypothalamus, this relationship appears to be inverted, and OCD symptom resolution correlates with increased SERT occupancy in these areas (Derksen et al., 2020). Directly pertaining to the pediatric OCD population, a 2002 association analysis demonstrated statistically significant differences in genotype and allele frequencies in a 5HT2A receptor polymorphism between individuals with OCD and controls (Walitza et al., 2002). Another 2017 meta-analysis, in which researchers sequenced coding and regulatory elements for several genes potentially involved in OCD, found the 5HT2A receptor, along with a synaptic functioning gene *NRXN1*, a synapse maintenance gene *CTTNBP2*, and a vesicle trafficking gene *REEP3*, all linked to compulsive behavior in OCD, glutamatergic and serotonergic signaling, and the cortico-striato-thalamic (CST) circuit (Noh et al., 2017). The 5HT2A receptor, in conjunction with 5-HT1A and 5-HT3A receptors to a lesser degree, are among the most abundant in the prefrontal cortex and can be exclusively found in certain populations of pyramidal neurons and inhibitory interneurons. Data suggests that serotonin functions in ameliorating OCD symptoms specifically by strengthening the prefrontal cortex's inhibitory signals in the CSTC circuit (Puig & Gulledge, 2011).

The hypothesis that serotonin activity improves OCD symptoms by strengthening inhibitory signals is one that was also arrived at incidentally through a 1992 study in which researchers reviewed data on patients with schizophrenia treated with clozapine, a D2, D4, 5-HT2A receptor blocker. Researchers observed the development and/or exacerbation of OCD symptoms (Baker, 1992). In that study, researchers postulated the involvement of the D4 receptor (discussed later) in their explanation for that phenomenon, but later studies illuminate that it may be antagonism of the 5HT2A receptor and its downstream effects on dopaminergic tone that caused these effects. In a 2014 literature review on the roles of second generation antipsychotics (SGAs) in the manifestation or exacerbation of OC symptoms in patients with schizophrenia, researchers found clozapine, followed by olanzapine (a D2, 5HT2A, and 5HT2C receptor blocker), were the SGAs with greatest propensity to create de novo OCD or exacerbate preexisting OCD symptoms, owing in part to the 5HT2A receptor antagonism of both drugs (Fonseka et al., 2014).

Studies have shown that administration of m-chlorophenylpiperazine (mCPP), a primary agonist at 5-HT1C with additional agonist properties at 5-HT1A, 5-HT1D, and 5-HT1C, induces OCD symptoms in animals and patients (Zohar et al., 1987; Gross-Isseroff et al., 2004). Similarly, administration of sumatriptan (5-HT1D agonist), exacerbated OCD symptoms in a double-blind randomized control trial (Koran et al., 2001).

However, while mCPP exacerbated OCD symptoms, administration of 6-chloro-2-[l-piperazinyl]-pyrazine (MK-212), a 5-HT1B, 5-HT1C, and 5-HT2 but not 5-HT1D agonist had no effect on OCD symptoms (Bastani et al., 1990). Thus, given mCPP's affinity and MK-212s non-affinity for the 5-HT1D receptor, there is evidence to suggest that it is this receptor that plays an integral role in the pathophysiology of OCD.

Genetics

In addition to the Taylor et al. (2013) meta-analysis (see above), additional literature shows mixed results in the association of 5HTTLPR and OCD. A 2003 family-based association study (FBAT) in which researchers used family-controlled transmission disequilibrium test (TDT) to family trios with OCD found that the *L* allele variant of the 5HTTPLR serotonin receptor gene may be a predictor of poor response to SSRI treatment in patients with OCD (Millet et al., 2003). A 2007 meta-analysis later found no association between any *L* or *S* polymorphisms of 5-HTTLPR and OCD (Lin, 2007). Additional studies on the 5HTTLPR polymorphism have also been done. A 2016 mega-analysis of a prospective cohort study in which researchers sought to replicate their prior findings of *S* allele (associated with decreased 5-HTT expression and serotonin reuptake) homozygotes of the 5HTTLPR polymorphism showing greater response to CBT in child anxiety disorders found no significant effect of 5HTTLPR genotype on CBT outcomes (Lester et al., 2016).

Other studies have been done looking into the association between OCD and the Stin2.12 allele of the VNTR polymorphism, a transcriptional regulator of 5-HTT whose function is affected by the number of tandem repeats. Baca-Garcia found such an association in her meta-analysis (Baca-Garcia et al., 2007). To further complicate the picture, a 2008 meta-analysis which looked at three genome-wide linkage studies and over 80 candidate gene studies (predominantly examining serotonergic and dopaminergic gene candidates) found no gene candidates achieve genome-wide significance, with only the glutamate transporter gene reliably replicated (Pauls, 2008). With this in mind, additional studies examining the replicability of some of this data are needed.

Dopamine

Dopamine is commonly known as the neurotransmitter associated with reward processing, including the anticipation of rewards. More relevant to OCD, the CSTC circuit, a primary pathway for OCD symptomatology, relies heavily on dopaminergic projections. Activation of D1 receptors in the striatum activates the direct pathway, and activation of D2 receptors exerts an inhibitory effect on the indirect pathway. Both of these actions result in an increase in activity of the CSTC circuits, which in the case of

OCD, is associated with an increase in symptoms (Hoffman, 2015). This formulation helps make clear the clinical and pathophysiological overlap between OCD and tic disorders. The motor and affective loops of the CSTC circuit are thought to be involved in tics, and it is well known that OCD and tics demonstrate a large amount of comorbidity, particularly in the pediatric population. The use of dopamine receptor blocking agents in the treatment of both OCD and tics is an intuitive choice given this understanding, although as a reminder that clinical practice is not always as straightforward as pathophysiological models, these medications are not first line treatments for either condition.

Clinical

Clinically, the use of some atypical antipsychotics has been seen to affect OCD symptoms, with sometimes conflicting findings. A 1999 case series found that risperidone, a D2 and 5HT2A antagonist, improved baseline OCD symptoms when used as augmentation of SSRI treatment (Fitzgerald et al., 1999). These data were later supported in a 2000 double-blind randomized controled trial in which thirty-six patients with a primary diagnosis of OCD refractory to 12 weeks of treatment with an SSRI were randomized in a double-blind manner to six weeks of risperidone or placebo. This study found that nine of 18 risperidone-treated subjects were responders whereas zero of 15 in the placebo addition group responded (McDougle et al., 2000). General clinical practice mirrors this, with risperidone used commonly as adjunctive treatment of OCD when SSRIs are insufficient. However, as discussed by Baker (1992) and Fonseka (2014), the use of second-generation antipsychotics may contribute to the exacerbation of OCD symptoms. This is seen clinically particularly with risperidone, olanzapine, and, most clearly, clozapine. This clinical experience is described in the literature, where a case study and case series found that risperidone use in patients with schizophrenia, while successful in treating psychotic symptoms, either produced de novo or exacerbated OC symptoms (Saini & Pande, 2018; Alevizos et al., 2002). This can be addressed by changing the antipsychotic dose, or in some instances, stopping and changing medications altogether, which typically results in resolution of symptoms (Naguy, 2017). Relative to adults, however, second generation antipsychotics have been much more rarely examined in youth.

The mechanism of the exacerbation of OCD symptoms by atypical antipsychotics is not totally understood, by it may be related to 5HT2A receptor affinity. Some researchers found that clozapine has a higher affinity for serotonin 5HT2A receptors than dopamine D2 receptors at low doses, and clozapine can exacerbate OCD symptoms upon initiation, with subsequent improvement of OCD symptoms at higher doses as D2 antagonism becomes more prominent (Ramasubbu et al., 2000). Cortical and subcortical 5HT2A receptors can act to reduce dopaminergic tone, and their antagonism can result in a release of inhibition on dopamine in the prefrontal cortex and nigrostriatal pathway. This increase in CSTC dopaminergic activity is postulated to drive the increase in OCD symptoms. As doses escalate, the increasing antagonistic occupancy of D2 receptors likely counterbalances this effect, leading eventually to a reduction in CSTC dopaminergic activity and thus a reduction in OCD symptoms. As doses escalate even further, the 5HT2A receptors can again become occupied, leading to a renewal of OCD symptom exacerbation. This exacerbation of OCD symptoms does not happen with all patients but can be seen in a significant minority of patients with preexisting OC tendencies. Researchers have also found that aripiprazole, with partial dopamine agonist properties, has been observed to induce OCD symptoms (Nafisa & Kakunje, 2022). These findings, taken together, suggest that dopamine agonism may worsen OCD, and antagonism may be therapeutic. Directly as its pertains to the pediatric population, de Nadai et al. (2011) in a literature review of the evidence base for pharmacotherapy of pediatric OCD and chronic tic disorders (CTDs) found that antipsychotics should only be used for the treatment of OCD and CTDs after failure of appropriate CBT and when symptoms are severely impairing functioning. This recommendation was given owing to the lack of randomized controlled trial (RCT) data supporting antipsychotic use and the risks of associated adverse effects including metabolic and cardiac effects. There continue to be minimal RCT data in children and adolescents testing atypical antipsychotics, and thus the extent to which clinical data would similarly implicate dopaminergic mechanisms of OCD in youth, although several open trials and case series suggest the effect would be similar in adults.

Receptors

As with the serotonergic system, much of the data on the role of dopamine receptors in OCD begin with animal studies. One mouse study investigated repetitive stereotyped behaviors, a corrolary to those seen in OCD, and found a link to aberrant dopamine signaling. Using selective D1 and D2 agonists, researchers found that the dopamine neurons in substantia nigra pars compacta (SNc) coordinate ventromedial striatum (VMS) and lateral orbitofrontal cortex (lOFC) microcircuits during self-grooming behavior. The SNc-VMS pathway promotes grooming via D1 receptors, whereas the SNc-lOFC pathway suppresses grooming via D2 receptors in a concept known as dual-gating (Xue et al., 2022). A pharmacological challenge study in rats supports this data; researchers found that the total amount of grooming behavior was increased by D1 agonism and decreased by D2 agonism (Berridge & Aldrige, 2000). In that same study, researchers also found that super-stereotypy, a term referring to "becoming trapped in sequential patterns or actions" (possibly analogous to OCD), was produced by dopamine D1 agonists in the basal ganglia (p. 1). Animal studies continue to support the idea of D1 receptor agonism in the pathophysiology of OCD: Cromwell et al. (1998) found D1A receptor-knockout mice exhibited a lower number, shorter duration, and more disrupted self-grooming bouts compared to healthy controls. Given the clinical data that supports the use of D2-blocking antipsychotics among adults with OCD, it is clear that both of these receptors play significant roles in mediating the symptomatology of OCD, although more research is needed to investigate whether this is the case in pediatric OCD, which has unique developmental considerations, such as asymmetry in sub-cortical structures (Kong, 2020).

There are human studies investigating the role of dopamine and dopamine receptors in OCD. A 2020 a systematic review of 11 neuroimaging studies found that striatal dopamine D2 receptor (D2R) density was decreased in OCD patients when compared to healthy controls, thought to be a result of downregulation as a response to execessive dopaminergic acvitity in those circuits (Dong et al., 2020). No significant correlation was found between striatal D2R density and disease severity in the study. The activity of the striatal dopamine transporter (DAT) was not found to be significantly different in OCD patients compared to control, although evidence was limited by small sample sizes (Dong et al., 2020).

Supporting the direct implication of dopamine receptors in antipsychotic contributions to OCD symptomatology, Baker also postulated the possibility of the D4 receptor antagonism in clozapine as a possible factor in the contribution to OCD symptom changes in patients with schizophrenia (1992). The D4 receptor has been found to be responsible for neuronal signaling in the mesolimbic system of the brain, implicated in OCD neurocircuitry. This is further supported by a genetic study in which researchers genotyped patients with OCD and matched controls for four loci previously identified as associated with OCD: a 40-base-pair repeat in the dopamine transporter gene, the TaqIA polymorphism and the serine/cysteine variation in the D2 dopamine receptor gene, an MscI polymorphism in the D3 dopamine receptor gene, and a 48-base-pair repeat in the D4 dopamine receptor gene. In this study, researchers found significant differences in allele frequencies between patients and controls for the D4 receptor gene (Billett et al., 1998). Given this data, the D4 receptor appears to be a promising receptor implicated in OCD pathophysiology.

Genetics

Studies have been done looking for associations between genetic factors related to dopamine and OCD. A 2003 meta-analysis using an FBAT to study genetic linkages between the D4 receptor and OCD found an absence of transmission of the allele 2 for the 48 bp repeat polymorphism of the *DRD4* gene, as well as significantly lower frequencies of the allele 2 in patients suffering from OCD compared to ethnically matched controls (Millet et al., 2003). Another study pursued investigation of candidate gene *SLC1A1*, which encodes excitatory amino acid transporters 1 and 3 (EAAT1 and EAAT3) which have glutamatergic activity. These investigators were able to produce EAAT3 ablation in mice via *SLC1A1* loss and found that this modification prevented expected increases in locomotor activity, stereotypy, and immediate early gene induction in the dorsal striatum following amphetamine administration compared to controls (Zike et al., 2017). In the same study, SLC1A1-STOP mice showed diminished grooming in response to a partial D1 agonist challenge, owing to reduced dopamine D1 receptor binding in the dorsal striatum and reduced extracellular dopamine concentrations in the dorsal striatum. Another meta-analysis found no association between the Met or Val polymorphisms of COMT and OCD (Azzam & Mathews, 2003). Taylor's 2013 meta-analysis, discussed above, found significant involvement of COMT and MAOA polymorphisms in OCD. As these are enzymes invovled in dopamine metabolism, this finding demonstrates another datapoint in support of dopaminergic associations in OCD.

These more focused studies can be assessed in the context of the Pauls (2008) meta-analysis which found no gene candidates achieve genome-wide significance with only the glutamate transporter gene with replicated findings. In the case of polygenic conditions like OCD, it can be difficult to clearly demonstrate the role of any one candidate gene in large analyses. Thus, despite Pauls' finding, it is clear that there is some evidence for the implication of both glutamate and dopamine-associated genetics in the pathophysiology of OCD. However, additional research must be done to clarify which genes and polymorphisms are significant contributors over others.

Glutamate

Not only is glutamate the primary excitatory neurotransmitter in the human brain, it is also a precursor to GABA, the primary inhibitory neurotransmitter. Glutamate receptors are either ionotropic (NMDA, AMPA, kainate) or metabotropic. The role of glutamate in the pathophysiology of OCD is already implicated through our current understanding that most dopaminergic and serotonergic studies involve direct modulation of glutamate (Hoffman, 2015; Karthik et al., 2020). Proton magnetic resonance spectroscopy (MRS) methods allow for the in vivo quantification of neurochemicals in localized brain regions including the CSTC network and are increasingly used in the research setting. A 2013 systematic review examined proton MRS methods to compare levels of various neurochemicals in OCD patients versus healthy individuals and examined structural and behavioral changes after treatment. The review found mixed results, implicating a necessity for additional research in total N-acetylaspartate (tNAA) levels in theACC and caudate, glutamate levels in the ACC and caudate, and total choline compounds (tCho) levels in the thalamus, parietal white matter, and hippocampus, all directly or closely related to glutamate. Better knowledge of these actions of these neurochemicals could lead to promising implications for OCD symptom modulation (Brennan et al., 2013). Below, we will outline additional studies that outline the discourse for this topic.

Clinical

Several clinical studies support significant glutamatergic involvement in OCD symptomatology. A randomized controlled trial in which 48 patients with SSRI-refractory OCD were randomized to 12 weeks of N-acetylcysteine, an NMDA modulator, versus placebo found significantly improved Y-BOCS scores and Clinical Global Impression-Severity of Illness scale scores when used as an add-on to SSRI treatment. The intervental group had 52.6 percent full responders compared to 15 percent of controls (Afshar et al., 2012). A double-blind placebo-controlled trial in which 60 treatment-resistant youth with moderate to severe childhood onset OCD were randomized to receive riluzole, a presynaptic glutamate-release inhibitor, versus placebo as adjunctive treatment to their existing regimen failed to demonstrate superiority of riluzole over placebo (Grant et al., 2014).

Receptors

Beginning again with an animal study, researchers who genetically engineered mice with a deletion of *SAPAP3*, a gene responsible for the effective functioning of NMDA and AMPA receptors, found that these mice displayed excessive self-grooming and anxiety-like behaviors, which subsided with repeated injections of fluoxetine (Welch et al., 2007). Similarly, mice deficient in neuron-specific transmembrane protein SLIT and NTRK-like protein-5 (SLITRK5) via genetically engineered SLITRK5-loss showed excessive self-grooming and increased anxiety-like behaviors with a lower number of glutamate receptors in the striatum compared to control mice, which improved with repeated administration of fluoxetine (Shmelkov et al., 2010). Arnold et al. (2004, 2006) and Sampaio et al. (2011) found the following genes associated with glutamate implicated in OCD: *SLC1A1* (codes for EAAC1, EAAT3), *GRIN2B* (codes for the 2B subunit of NMDA receptors), and *GRIK2/3* (codes for Kainate receptor subunits). Hence, the glutamatergic system appears to have an important role in mediating the pathophysiology of OCD.

Genetics

Studies examining the genetics associated with the glutamatergic role in OCD are overviewed in this subsection. A linkage study found modest evidence for linkage on chromosome 9p yielding the closest peak to *SLC1A1*, which encodes a glutamate transporter, and OCD (Willour et al., 2004). A genome-wide association study found a SNP near *BTBD3* (a regulator of transcription, ion channel assembly, ion channel gating, post-translational modification, and degradation of glutamate) which exceeded the genome-wide significance threshold (Stewart et al., 2013). The same study explains that this *BTBD3* SNP is additionally associated with *ISM1*, both associated with OCD and fear memory via their association with *ADCY8*; moreover, *ISM1* expression is associated with the expression of the glutamatergic genes *GRIK1, GRIK4, DLGAP3, SHANK3* and *ADARB2*. Another genetic study using FBAT testing for associations with OCD, along with additional analyses to test for familial genetic associations with the quantitative phenotype of lifetime OCD symptom severity found the 5072T/G variant of the NMDA receptor polymorphism *GRIN2B* to be significantly associated with OCD as well as a significant association with OCD diagnosis and the 5072G-5988T haplotype. And to state once more, Pauls (2008) found no gene candidates achieve genome-wide significance and only the glutamate transporter gene has replicated findings, lending some additional support to the involvement of glutamatergic genes in OCD, yet still highlighting the need for stronger, more robust data to establish this linkage.

Summary

In conclusion, there is ample evidence to suggest the role of the serotonergic, dopaminergic, and glutamatergic neurotransmitter systems in the pathophysiology and management of OCD. Generally speaking, despite the historical focus on serotonin and its related pharmacological use, glutamate has more recently been seen as the more central neurotransmitter related to OCD, with serotonin and dopamine acting as modulators of those glutamatergic systems. This is in alignment with the central role glutamate plays in the activation and regulation of the CSTC. There appears to be viability for medications that directly and indirectly alter each of these neurotransmitter systems in the sole or adjunct treatment of OCD, although several of the aforementioned medications are not without side effects.

Current and Future Treatments

Introduction

The treatment mainstay for pediatric OCD consists of therapy and medications, most importantly Exposure and Response Prevention Therapy (ERP) and SSRIs (McGuire et al., 2015; Öst et al., 2016). Before discussing how OCD treatments target specific neurobiological regions and mechanisms we must examine the most effective treatment options in pediatrics. SSRIs and CBT have both been found to be effective treatments. Per Varigonda et al. (2016) there is no evidence that suggests a relationship between dosing and treatment effect, and children and adults have demonstrated similar treatment times and courses with SSRIs. As noted, meta-analyses have found that the combination of SSRIs and ERP plus SSRIs tend to lead to improved outcomes relative to SSRIs alone or placebo alone, and that SSRIs lead to improved outcomes relative to placebo (McGuire et al., 2015; Öst et al., 2016). In addition to SSRIs, clomipramine has shown possibly even greater benefit for treatment of OCD (Varigonda et al., 2016). For patients that don't respond to these treatments, antipsychotics are the only treatments supported by empirical evidence. Alternative treatment options are being researched and will also be discussed below.

Multiple studies pinpoint genetic contribution to treatment response but specifying the exact abnormalities is a work in process (Grice, 2020). Our incomplete understanding of the neurobiology of OCD has limited efforts to target new treatments, but as we progress in our understanding new treatment modalities are emerging.

SSRIs

Multiple randomized clinical trials have established that SSRIs and clomipramine (a serotonergic tricyclic antidepressant) are the mainstay psychotropic treatments for OCD. The efficacy of SSRIs directed early research into serotonergic abnormalities in patients with OCD and into new serotonergic medications effective for treatment of OCD (Zohar et al., 1987; Goodman et al., 1995; Charney et al., 1988). The efficacy of SSRIs compared to other antidepressants in the treatment of OCD led to an early understanding that serotonin dysfunction plays a key role in the pathophysiology in OCD (Goodman et al., 1990). The most prominent hypotheses for SSRIs' efficacy is the drugs' presumed therapeutic action of decreasing the hyperactive orbitofrontal-subcortical circuits that drive OC behavior thereby balancing the direct and indirect CSTC pathways (Saxena et al., 1999).

Despite the efficacy of SSRIs, previous research has not uncovered any clear data that reduction of 5HT levels (via depleted tryptophan) specifically leads to worsening of OCD symptoms (Barr et al., 1994). PET studies that detect 5HT2A ligand levels also noted no significant difference between healthy patients and those with OCD (Simpson et al., 2011). Drug trials of other serotonin modulating agents such as ondansetron, buspirone, and tryptophan have not yielded clear results indicating efficacy, further clouding the identification of alternative treatment options (McDougle et al., 1993; Goodman et al., 1993; McDougle et al., 1991; Stern et al., 2019).

CBT (ERP)

Family-based exposure and ritual or response prevention therapy (ERP) has demonstrated considerable efficacy in the treatment of youth with OCD. ERP is a specific form of CBT that provides prolonged exposure to distressing situations or objects combined with prevention of rituals. Exposure to the feared stimulus occurs either in person or via imagination/ thoughts and resistance of rituals follows, in an effort to demonstrate that the failure to perform the ritual did not cause a feared disaster. The exercise also leads to desensitizaton to the provoked anxiety and distress and builds confidence that the distress can be tolerated without use of the ritual.

Studies have been performed to examine neural correlates of ERP in OCD in an attempt to better understand the neurobiology of the treatment. The findings have been inconsistent thus far but have led to proposed mechanisms that include the cingulo-opercular and orbito-striato-thalamic networks (Stern & Taylor, 2014). The cingulo-opercular network regulates attentional control with evidence from fMRI studies finding hyperactivity of this part of the brain during error processing tasks in people with OCD (Norman et al., 2019). The orbito-striato-thalamic network has been shown to normalize on fMRI studies after treatment with ERP (Saxena & Rauch, 2000). One study noted that increased pretreatment activation in these two aforementioned brain regions was associated with better treatment response to ERP (Norman et al., 2020).

Further research in children demonstrated decreased activity in the dorsolateral prefrontal cortex and left parietal cortex during executive functioning that improved after ERP treatment; this change also correlated with improved symptoms (Huyser et al., 2010). Moving forward, by demonstrating regions of the brain that are associated with OCD symptomatology or treatment we may find potential biomarkers that could direct new treatments (Norman et al., 2020).

Neurotropic genes are involved in synaptic plasticity, stress response, mood, and cognition. Some of their allelic variations have been studied to investigate possible associations with anxiety-related phenotypes. In children, a specific allele variation of Neurotrophic Growth Factor, a neurotropic gene, was associated with increased likelihood of being free of their primary anxiety disorder at follow-up (Lester et al., 2016). This early study demonstrated that genetic markers could possibly be used to inform clinical decisions regarding psychotherapeutic interventions and prognosis. *FAAH*, a gene in the endocannabinoid system that plays a role in anxiety and fear, has been studied to investigate whether particular variants are associated with stronger response to ERP. Results were conflicting and inconclusive (Mitjans et al., 2012).

While thus far it has been challenging to reliably identify specific gene variants that predict response to psychological treatment, further research is likely to provide insights into the relationship between genetics and psychological interventions. In time, this will lead to an expansion of the use of precision medicine in psychiatry (Lester et al., 2016).

NMDA receptor

The NMDA receptor is involved in fear extinction which underlies ERP's efficacy by playing a critical role in addressing aversion to conditioned stimuli (Mataix-Cols et al., 2017). Glycine is an allosteric agonist at the NMDA receptor in the central nervous system. Multiple drugs that modulate glycine function are available in practice and have been investigated in their use for patients with OCD (Greenberg et al., 2009). The findings thus far are inconclusive but there is potential in D-cyclo-serine, a partial agonist at the glycine/D-serine site of the NMDA receptor, in augmenting ERP by enhancement of extinction. A meta-analytic study showed that augmentation with the drug demonstrated a small but significant effect (Mataix-Cols et al., 2017). These studies have been inconclusive thus far.

The NMDA blocker memantine, commonly used for treatment of patients with Alzheimer's disease, has also been studied in OCD (Pittenger et al., 2015). Multiple studies have been performed on adult populations indicating positive response rates to the medication compared to placebo, but the strength of these studies has been questioned indicating need of further research on the efficacy of memantine for OCD (Ghaleiha, 2013; Haghighi, 2013; Modarresi et al., 2019; Andrade, 2019).

Glutamate is an amino acid that acts a primary excitatory neuro-transmitter in the adult brain and binds to the aforementioned NMDA receptor (Pittenger et al., 2011). GABA is an inhibitory neurotransmitter that coupled with glutamate modulates the cortico-striato-thalamo-cor-tical circuit that is implicated in the pathophysiology of OCD (Pittenger et al., 2011). Riluzole is a glutamate modulating agent approved by the FDA for treatment of amyotrophic lateral sclerosis and functions by both inhibiting presynaptic release of glutamate and attempting to increase clearance of the neurotransmitter (Pittenger, 2015; Sakurai et al., 2019). One RCT investigating riluzole was performed in children with OCD who had inadequate response to SSRIs. The study demon-strated no significant differences between the control group versus the group given riluzole (Grant et al., 2014). This was further complicated by reports of elevated transaminase levels and pancreatitis in two of the children given the medication. The drug troriluzole is a prodrug of rilu-zole that bypasses first pass metabolism and may offer promise in decreasing the risk of hepatotoxicity in children. However, there was an identified positive trend in the outpatient adult population in an RCT (Pittenger et al., 2015).

Cysteine

Cysteine is an amino acid that aids in glutamate modulation. The drug N-Acetylcysteine functions as a pro-drug of cysteine and has been used as an antidote for acetaminophen poisoning (Deepmala et al., 2015; Kupchik et al., 2012). A placebo controlled RCT in a pediatric OCD population aged 8–17 years found there may be initial improvement in OCD symptoms in this population. It may also help in alleviating symptoms of anxiety (Li, 2020).

Transcranial magnetic stimulation

Deep TMS (dTMS) has been approved by the FDA for the treatment of OCD based on recent paramount clinical trials (Carmi et al., 2019). The device stimulated deeper structures within the brain including the midline medial PFC and ACC, areas believed to be hyperactive in OCD (McCathern, 2020). The efficacy has further strengthened hypotheses that cortico-striatal hyperactivity may be one of the causes of OCD (Dunlop et al., 2016). Studies have shown significantly improved Y-BOCS scores in individuals treated with dTMS (Dunlop et al., 2016). Noninvasive neurostimulation has been minimally tested in youth with OCD and it remains to be seen whether these initial results translate.

Overall, the mainstay for OCD treatment in pediatric populations is CBT, SSRIs, and clomipramine. The exact mechanism of SSRIs' and clomipramine's success is not completely understood on a neurobiological level but is believed to be related to regulatory effects on the CSTC network. Other serotonergic drugs have not yielded the same positive results as SSRIs but this continues to be an area of exploration. More clearly, CBT has been shown to impact specific regions in the brain related to OCD including the cingulo-opercular network which regulates attentional control and the orbito-striato-thalamic network which plays a role in complex human behaviors such as evaluation, affect control, and reward-based decision-making. Much of the research used to look ahead at potential treatments stems from adult studies given the limited ability to study pediatric populations. Other potential neurobiological factors that could serve as potential targets for future treatments include glutamate, the NMDA receptor, cysteine, and glycine. For more severe cases, emerging research is examining the efficacy of interventional treatment options such as transcranial magnetic stimulation, deep brain stimulation, and neurosurgical options. All of these treatments are directly tied to areas of the brain believed to be relevant to OCD. Although OCD can be a debilitating disorder, it has also become one of the more treatable conditions in psychiatry, and there is great hope that our treatment options will only expand.

References

Ackerman, D. & Greenland, S. (2002). Multivariate Meta-Analysis of Controlled Drug Studies for Obsessive-Compulsive Disorder. *Journal of Clinical Psychopharmacology*, 22(3), 309–317.

Afshar, H., Roohafza, H., Mohammad-Beigi, H., Haghighi, M., Jahangard, L., Shokouh, P., Sadeghi, M., & Hafezian, H. (2012). N-acetylcysteine add-on treatment in refractory obsessive-compulsive disorder: a randomized, double-blind, placebo-controlled trial. *J Clin Psychopharmacol*, 32(6), 797–803.

Alevizos, B., Lykouras, L., Zervas, I. M., & Christodoulou, G. N. (2002). Risperidone-induced obsessive-compulsive symptoms: a series of six cases. *J Clin Psychopharmacol.* 22(5), 461–467.

American Psychiatric Association. *Diagnostic and Statistical Manual of Mental Disorders*, 5th Ed. (2013). American Psychiatric Association.

Andrade, C. (2019). Augmentation With Memantine in Obsessive-Compulsive Disorder. *The Journal of Clinical Psychiatry*, 80(6).

Arnold, P. D., Rosenberg, D. R., Mundo, E., Tharmalingam, S., Kennedy, J. L., & Richter, M. A. (2004). Association of a glutamate (NMDA) subunit receptor gene (GRIN2B) with obsessive-compulsive disorder: a preliminary study. *Psychopharmacology* (Berl), 174(4), 530–538.

Arnold, P. D., Sicard, T., Burroughs, E., Richter, M. A., & Kennedy, J. L. (2006). Glutamate Transporter Gene SLC1A1 Associated With Obsessive-compulsive Disorder. *Archives of General Psychiatry*, 63(7), 769–776.

Azzam, A. & Mathews, C. A. (2003). Meta-analysis of the association between the catecholamine-O-methyl-transferase gene and obsessive-compulsive disorder. *Am J Med Genet B Neuropsychiatr Genetics*, 123, 64–69.

Baca-Garcia, E., Vaquero-Lorenzo, C., Diaz-Hernandez, M., Rodriguez-Salgado, B., Dolengevich-Segal, H., Arrojo-Romero, M., Botillo-Martin, C., Ceverino, A., Piqueras, J. F., Perez-Rodriguez, M. M., & Saiz-Ruiz, J. (2007). Association between obsessive–compulsive disorder and a variable number of tandem repeats polymorphism in intron 2 of the serotonin transporter gene. *Progress in Neuro-Psychopharmacology & Biological Psychiatry*, 312), –420.

Baker, R. W., Chengappa, K. N., Baird, J. W., Steingard, S., Christ, M. A., & Schooler, N. R. (1992). Emergence of obsessive compulsive symptoms during treatment with clozapine. *J Clin Psychiatry*, 53(12), 439–442.

Barr L. C., Goodman W. K., McDougle C. J., et al. (1994). Tryptophan depletion in patients with obsessive-compulsive disorder who respond to serotonin reuptake inhibitors. *Arch Gen Psychiatry*, 51, 309–317.

Bastani, B., Nash, J. F., & Meltzer, H. Y. (1990). Prolactin and Cortisol Responses to MK-212, a Serotonin Agonist, in Obsessive-Compulsive Disorder. *Archives of General Psychiatry*, 47(9), 833–839. Cromwell, H. C., Berridge, K. C., Drago, J., & Levine, M. S. (1998). Action sequencing is impaired in D1A-deficient mutant mice. *Eur J Neurosci.* , 10(7), 2426–2432.

Bernstein, G. A., Mueller, B. A., Schreiner, M. W., Campbell, S. M., Regan, E. K., Nelson, P. M., Houri, A. K., Lee, S. S., Zagoloff, A. D., Lim, K. O., Yacoub, E. S., & Cullen, K. R. (2016). Abnormal striatal resting-state functional connectivity in adolescents with obsessive-compulsive disorder. *Psychiatry Research – Neuroimaging*, 247, 49–56.

Berridge K. C. & Aldridge J. W. (2000). Super-stereotypy II: enhancement of a complex movement sequence by intraventricular dopamine D1 agonists. *Synapse*, 37(3), 205–215.

Billett, E. A., Richter, M. A., Sam, F., Swinson, R. P., Dai, X. Y., King, N., Badri, F., Sasaki, T., Buchanan, J. A., Kennedy, J. L. (1998). Investigation of dopamine system genes in obsessive-compulsive disorder. *Psychiatr Genet*, 8(3), 163–169.

Brennan, B. P., Rauch, S. L., Jensen, J. E., & Pope, H. G.Jr. (2013). A critical review of magnetic resonance spectroscopy studies of obsessive-compulsive disorder. *Biol Psychiatry*, 73(1), 24–31.

Burguière, E., Monteiro, P., Mallet, L., Feng, G., & Graybiel, A. M. (2015). Striatal circuits, habits, and implications for obsessive-compulsive disorder. *Current Opinion in Neurobiology*, 30, 59–65.

Carmi, L., Tendler, A., Bystritsky, A., et al. (2019). Efficacy and safety of deep transcranial magnetic stimulation for obsessive-compulsive disorder: a prospective multicenter randomized double-blind placebo-controlled trial. *Am J Psychiatry*, 176, 931–938.

Charney, D. S., Goodman, W. K., & Price, L. H., et al. (1988). Serotonin function in obsessive-compulsive disorder. A comparison of the effects of tryptophan and m-chlorophenylpiperazine in patients and healthy subjects. *Arch Gen Psychiatry*, 45, 177–185.

Cromwell, H. C., Berridge, K. C., Drago, J., & Levine, M. S. (1998). Action sequencing is impaired in D1A-deficient mutant mice. *Eur J Neurosci.* , 10(7), 2426–2432.

Deepmala S. J., Slattery J., Kumar N., et al. (2015). Clinical trials of N-acetylcysteine in psychiatry and neurology: A systematic review. *Neurosci Biobehav Rev*, 55, 294–321.

De Nadai, A. S., Storch, E. A., McGuire, J. F., Lewin, A. B., & Murphy, T. K. (2011). Evidence-based pharmacotherapy for pediatric obsessive-compulsive disorder and chronic tic disorders. *J Cent Nerv Syst Dis*, 3, 125–142.

Derksen, M., Feenstra, M., Willuhn, I., & Denys, D. (2020). The serotonergic system in obsessive-compulsive disorder. *Handbook of Behavioral Neuroscience*, 31, 865–891.

Dong, M.-X., Chen, G.-H., & Hu, L. (2020). Dopaminergic System Alteration in Anxiety and Compulsive Disorders: A Systematic Review of Neuroimaging Studies. *Frontiers in Neuroscience*, 14, 608520–608520.

Dunlop, K., Woodside, B., Olmsted, M., et al. (2016). Reductions in cortico-striatal hyperconnectivity accompany successful treatment of obsessive-compulsive disorder with dorsomedial prefrontal rTMS. *Neuropsychopharmacology*, 41, 1395–1403.

Fitzgerald, K. D., MacMaster, F. P., Paulson, L. D., & Rosenberg, D. R. (1999). Neurobiology of childhood obsessive-compulsive disorder. *Child and Adolescent Psychiatric Clinics of North America*, 8(3), 533–575.

Fitzgerald, K. D., Moore, G. J., Paulson, L. A., Stewart, C. M., & Rosenberg, D. R. (2000). Proton Spectroscopic Imaging of the Thalamus in Treatment-Naive Pediatric Obsessive-Compulsive Disorder. *Biol Psychiatry*, 47, 174–182.

Fitzgerald, K. D., Stewart, C. M., Tawile, V., & Rosenberg, D. R. (1999). Risperidone augmentation of serotonin reuptake inhibitor treatment of pediatric obsessive compulsive disorder. *J Child Adolesc Psychopharmacol.* 9(2), 115–123.

Fonseka T. M., Richter M. A., & Müller D. J. (2014). Second generation anti-psychotic-induced obsessive-compulsive symptoms in schizophrenia: a review of the experimental literature. *Curr Psychiatry Rep*, 16(11), 510.

Ghaleiha, A., Entezari, N., Modabbernia, A., Najand, B., Askari, N., Tabrizi, M., Ashrafi, M., Hajiaghaee, R., & Akhondzadeh, S. (2013). Memantine add-on in moderate to severe obsessive-compulsive disorder: Randomized double-blind placebo-controlled study. *Journal of Psychiatric Research*, 47(2), 175–180.

Goodman, W. K., McDougle, C. J., & Barr, L. C., et al. (1993). Biological approaches to treatment-resistant obsessive compulsive disorder. *J Clin Psychiatry*, 54(Suppl), 16–26.

Goodman, W. K., McDougle, C. J., & Price, L. H., et al. (1995). m-Chlor-ophenylpiperazine in patients with obsessive-compulsive disorder: absence of symptom exacerbation. *Biol Psychiatry*, 38, 138–149.

Goodman, W. K, Price, L. H., & Delgado, P. L., et al. (1990). Specificity of serotonin reuptake inhibitors in the treatment of obsessive-compulsive disorder. Comparison of fluvoxamine and desipramine. *Arch Gen Psychiatry*, 47, 577–585.

Grant, P. J., Joseph, L. A., Farmer, C. A., Luckenbaugh, D. A., Lougee, L. C., Zarate, C. A.Jr, & Swedo, S. E. (2014). 12-week, placebo-controlled trial of add-on riluzole in the treatment of childhood-onset obsessive-compulsive disorder. *Neuropsychopharmacology*, 39(6), 1453–1459.

Graybiel, A. M. & Rauch, S. L. (2000). Toward a Neurobiology Review of Obsessive-Compulsive Disorder Dysfunction of the basal ganglia and associated cor. *Neuron*, 28.

Greenberg, W. M., Benedict, M. M., Doerfer, J., et al. (2009). Adjunctive glycine in the treatment of obsessive-compulsive disorder in adults. *J Psychiatr Res*, 43, 664–670.

Grice, D. E. (2020). Don't worry, the genetics of obsessive-compulsive disorder is finally catching up. *Biol Psychiatry*, 87, 1017–1018.

Gross-Isseroff, R., Cohen, R., Sasson, Y., Voet, H., & Zohar, J. (2004). Serotonergic Dissection of Obsessive Compulsive Symptoms: A Challenge Study with m-Chlorophenylpiperazine and Sumatriptan. *Neuropsychobiology*, 50(3), 200–205.

Haghighi, M., Jahangard, L., Mohammad-Beigi, H., Bajoghli, H., Hafezian, H., Rahimi, A., Afshar, H., Holsboer-Trachsler, E., & Brand, S. (2013). In a double-blind, randomized and placebo-controlled trial, adjuvant memantine improved symptoms in inpatients suffering from refractory obsessive-compulsive disorders (OCD). *Psychopharmacology*, 228(4), 633–640.

Hoffman, K. L. (2015). Obsessive Compulsive Disorder: Neurobiology and Treatment. *Reference Module in Biomedical Research*.

Huyser, C., Veltman, D. J., de Haan, E., & Boer, F. (2009). Paediatric obsessive-compulsive disorder, a neurodevelopmental disorder?. Evidence from neuroimaging. *Neuroscience and Biobehavioral Reviews*, 33(6), 818–830.

Huyser, C., Veltman, D. J., Wolters, L. H., et al. (2010). Functional magnetic resonance imaging during planning before and after cognitive-behavioral therapy in pediatric obsessive-compulsive disorder. *J Am Acad Child Adolesc Psychiatry*, 49, 1238–1248, 1248.e1–1248.e5.

Huyser, C., Veltman, D. J., Wolters, L. H., De Haan, E., & Boer, F. (2011). Developmental aspects of error and high-conflict-related brain activity in pediatric obsessive-compulsive disorder: A fMRI study with a Flanker task before and after CBT. *Journal of Child Psychology and Psychiatry and Allied Disciplines*, 52(12), 1251–1260.

Karthik, S., Sharma, L. P., & Narayanaswamy, J. C. (2020). Investigating the Role of Glutamate in Obsessive-Compulsive Disorder: Current Perspectives. *Neuropsychiatr Dis Treat*, 16, 1003–1013.

Kong, X. Z., Boedhoe, P. S. W., Abe, Y., et al. (2020). Mapping cortical and subcortical asymmetry in obsessive-compulsive disorder: findings from the ENIGMA consortium. *Biol Psychiatry*, 87, 1022–1034.

Koran, L. M., Pallanti, S., & Quercioli, L. (2001). Sumatriptan, 5-HT1D receptors and obsessive-compulsive disorder. *European Neuropsychopharmacology*, 11(2), 169–172.

Kupchik Y. M., Moussawi K., Tang X. C., et al. (2012). The effect of N-acetylcysteine in the nucleus accumbens on neurotransmission and relapse to cocaine. *Biol Psychiatry*, 71, 978–986.

Landeros-Weisenberger, A., & Bloch, M. H. (2020). *N-Acetylcysteine for Pediatric Obsessive-Compulsive Disorder: A Small Pilot Study. Journal of child and adolescent psychopharmacology*, 30(1), 32–37. Lester, K. J., Roberts, S., Keers, R., Coleman, J. R., Breen Gerome, W., Chloe C. Y., Xu, X., Arendt, K., Blatter-Meunier, J., Bögels, S., Cooper, P., Creswell, C., Heiervang, E. R., Herren Chantal, Hogendoorn, S. M., Hudson, J. L., Krause, K., Lyneham, H. J., McKinnon, A., ... Eley, T. C. (2016). Non-replication of the association between 5HTTLPR and response to psychological therapy for child anxiety disorders. *British Journal of Psychiatry*, 208(2), 182–188.

Li, B. & Mody, M. (2016). Cortico-striato-thalamo-cortical circuitry, working memory, and obsessive-compulsive disorder. *Frontiers in Psychiatry*, 7(May).

Li, F., Welling, M. C., Johnson, J. A., Coughlin, C., Mulqueen, J., Jakubovski, E., Coury, S.,

Lin, P. Y. (2007). Meta-analysis of the association of serotonin transporter gene polymorphism with obsessive–compulsive disorder. *Prog Neuropsychopharmacol Biol Psychiatry*, 31, 683–689.

Lissemore, J. I., Sookman, D., Gravel, P., Berney, A., Barsoum, A., Diksic, M., Nordahl, T. E., Pinard, G., Sibon, I., Cottraux, J., Leyton, M., & Benkelfat, C. (2018). Brain serotonin synthesis capacity in obsessive-compulsive disorder: effects of cognitive behavioral therapy and sertraline. *Transl Psychiatry*, 8(1), 82.

MacMaster, F. P., O'Neill, J., & Rosenberg, D. R. (2008). Brain imaging in pediatric obsessive-compulsive disorder. *Journal of the American Academy of Child and Adolescent Psychiatry*, 47(11), 1262–1272.

Maia, T. V., Cooney, R. E., & Peterson, B. S. (2008). The neural bases of obsessive – Compulsive disorder in children and adults. *Development and Psychopathology*, 20(4), 1251–1283.

Mataix-Cols, D., Fernández de la Cruz, L., Monzani, B, et al. (2017). D-Cycloserine augmentation of exposure-based cognitive behavior therapy for anxiety, obsessive-compulsive, and posttraumatic stress disorders: a systematic review and meta-analysis of individual participant data. *JAMA Psychiatry*, 74, 501–510.

McCathern, A.G. et al. (2020). Deep Transcranial Magnetic Stimulation for Obsessive Compulsive Disorder. *Expert review of neurotherapeutics*, 20(10), 1029–1036.

McDougle, C. J., Epperson, C. N., Pelton, G. H., Wasylink, S., & Price, L. H. (2000). A double-blind, placebo-controlled study of risperidone addition in serotonin reuptake inhibitor-refractory obsessive-compulsive disorder. *Arch Gen Psychiatry*, 57(8), 794–801.

McDougle, C. J., Goodman, W. K., Leckman, J. F., et al. (1993). Limited therapeutic effect of addition of buspirone in fluvoxamine-refractory obsessive-compulsive disorder. *Am J Psychiatry*, 150, 647–649.

McDougle, C. J., Price, L. H., Goodman, W. K., et al. (1991). A controlled trial of lithium augmentation in fluvoxamine-refractory obsessive-compulsive disorder: lack of efficacy. *J Clin Psychopharmacol*, 11, 175–184.

McGuire, J. F., Piacentini, J., Lewin, A. B., Brennan, E. A., Murphy, T. K., & Storch, E. A. (2015). A meta-analysis of cognitive behavior therpay and medication for child obsessive-compulsive disoder: Moderators of treatment efficacy, response, and remission. *Depression and Anxiety*, 32(8), 580–593.

Millet, B., Chabane, N., Delorme, R., Leboyer, M., Leroy, S., Poirier, M. F., Bourdel, M. C., Mouren-Simeoni, M. C., Rouillon, F., Loo, H., Krebs, M. O. (2003). Association between the dopamine receptor D4 (DRD4) gene and obsessive-compulsive disorder. *Am J Med Genet B Neuropsychiatr Genet*, 116B (1), 55–59.

Mitjans, M., Gastó, C., Catalán, R., Fañanás, L., & Arias, B. (2012). Genetic variability in the endocannabinoid system and 12-week clinical response to citalopram treatment: the role of the CNR1, CNR2 and FAAH genes. *Journal of Psychopharmacology* (Oxford), 26(10), 1391–1398.

Modarresi, A., Chaibakhsh, S., Koulaeinejad, N., & Koupaei SR. (2019). A systematic review and meta-analysis: Memantine augmentation in moderate to severe obsessive-compulsive disorder. *Psychiatry Res*, 282, 112602.

Nafisa, D. & Kakunje, A. (2022). Aripiprazole-induced obsessive-compulsive symptoms. *Ind Psychiatry J.*, 31(1), 158–161.

Naguy, A. (2017). Antipsychotics and OCD: Boon or Bane? *Indian Journal of Psychological Medicine*, 39(6), 830–831.

Noh H. J. et al. (2017). Integrating evolutionary and regulatory information with a multispecies approach implicates genes and pathways in obsessive-compulsive disorder. *Nat Commun*, 8(1), 774.

Norman L. J., Mannella, K. A., Yang, H., et al. (2020). Treatment-specific associations between brain activation and symptom reduction in OCD following CBT: a randomized fMRI trial. *Am J Psychiatry*, P202019080886.

Norman, L. J., Taylor, S. F., Liu, Y., et al. (2019). Error processing and inhibitory control in obsessive-compulsive disorder: a meta-analysis using statistical parametric maps. *Biol Psychiatry*, 85, 713–725.

Pauls, D. L. (2008). The genetics of obsessive compulsive disorder: A review of the evidence. *American Journal of Medical Genetics. Part C, Seminars in Medical Genetics*, 148C(2), 133–139.

Pediatric OCD Treatment Study (POTS) Team. (2004). Cognitive-behavior therapy, sertraline, and their combination for children and adolescents with obsessive-compulsive disorder: the Pediatric OCD Treatment Study (POTS) randomized controlled trial. *JAMA*, 292(16), 1969–1976.

Pittenger, C. (2015). Glutamatergic agents for OCD and related disorders. *Curr Treat Options Psychiatry*, 2, 271–283.

Pittenger, C., Bloch, M. H., Wasylink, S, et al. (2015). Riluzole augmentation in treatment-refractory obsessive-compulsive disorder: a pilot randomized placebo-controlled trial. *J Clin Psychiatry*, 76, 1075–1084.

Pittenger, C., Bloch, M. H., & Williams, K. (2011). Glutamate abnormalities in obsessive compulsive disorder: neurobiology, pathophysiology, and treatment. *Pharmacology & therapeutics*, 132(3), 314–332.

Puig, M. V. & Gulledge, A. T. (2011). Serotonin and prefrontal cortex function: neurons, networks, and circuits. *Mol Neurobiol*, 44(3), 449–464.

Ramasubbu, R., Ravindran, A., & Lapierre, Y. (2000). Serotonin and dopamine antagonism in obsessive-compulsive disorder: effect of atypical antipsychotic drugs. *Pharmacopsychiatry*, 33(6), 236–238.

Rosenberg, D. R., Macmillan, S. N., & Moore, G. J. (2001). Brain anatomy and chemistry may predict treatment response in paediatric obsessive-compulsive disorder. SPECIAL SECTION. *International Journal of Neuropsychopharmacology*, 4.

Saini, R. K. & Pande, V. (2018). Drug-Induced Obsessive Compulsive Disorder in Schizophrenia. *Med J Armed Forces India*. 64(2), 169–170.

Sakurai, H., Dording, C., Yeung, A., et al. (2019). Longer-term open-label study of adjunctive riluzole in treatment-resistant depression. *J Affect Disord*, 258, 102–108.

Sampaio, A. S., Fagerness, J., Crane, J., Leboyer, M., Delorme, R., Pauls, D. L., & Stewart, S. E. (2011). Association between polymorphisms in GRIK2 gene and obsessive-compulsive disorder: a family-based study. *CNS neuroscience & therapeutics*, 17(3), 141–147.

Saxena, S., Brody, A. L., Maidment, K. M., et al. (1999). Localized orbitofrontal and subcortical metabolic changes and predictors of response to paroxetine treatment in obsessive-compulsive disorder. *Neuropsychopharmacology*, 21, 683–693.

Saxena, S. & Rauch, S. L. (2000). Functional neuroimaging and the neuroanatomy of obsessive-compulsive disorder. *Psychiatr Clin North Am*, 23, 563–586.

Shmelkov, S. V., Hormigo, A., Jing, D., Proenca, C. C., Bath, K. G., Milde, T., Shmelkov, E., Kushner, J. S., Baljevic, M., Dincheva, I., Murphy, A. J., Valenzuela, D. M., Gale, N. W., Yancopoulos, G. D., Ninan, I, Lee F. S., Rafii, S. (2010). Slitrk5 deficiency impairs corticostriatal circuitry and leads to obsessive-compulsive-like behaviors in mice. *Nat Med*, 16(5), 598–602.

Simpson, H. B., Slifstein, M., Bender, J.Jr, et al. (2011). Serotonin 2A receptors in obsessive-compulsive disorder: a positron emission tomography study with [11C] MDL 100907. *Biol Psychiatry*, 70, 897–904.

Stern, E. R., Shahab, R., Grimaldi, S. J., et al. (2019). High-dose ondansetron reduces activation of interoceptive and sensorimotor brain regions. *Neuropsychopharmacology*, 44, 390–398.

Stern, E. R. & Taylor, S. F. (2014). Cognitive neuroscience of obsessive-compulsive disorder. *Psychiatr Clin North Am*, 37, 337–352.

Stewart, S. E., Yu, D., Scharf, J. M., Neale, B. M., Fagerness, J. A., Mathews, C. A., Arnold, P. D., Evans, P. D., Gamazon, E. R., Osiecki, L., McGrath, L., Haddad, S., Hezel, D., Illman, C., Konkashbaev, A., Pluzhnikov, A., Edlund, C.

K., Rauch, S. L., Moessner, R., ... Bellodi, L. (2013). Genome-wide association study of obsessive-compulsive disorder. *Molecular Psychiatry*, 18(7), 788–798.

Szeszko, P. R., Christian, C., Frank MacMaster, B., Lencz, T., Mirza, Y., Preeya Taormina, S., Easter, P., Michelle Rose, B., Michalopoulou, B. G., & Rosenberg, D. R. (2008). Gray Matter Structural Alterations in Psychotropic Drug-Naive Pediatric Obsessive-Compulsive Disorder: An Optimized Voxel-Based Morphometry Study. *Am J Psychiatry*, 165(10).

Taylor, S. (2013). Molecular genetics of obsessive–compulsive disorder: a comprehensive meta-analysis of genetic association studies. *Molecular Psychiatry*, 18(7), 799–805.

van Balkom, A. J. L. M., van Oppen, P., Vermeulen, A. W. A., van Dyck, R., Nauta, M. C. E., & Vorst, H. C. M. (1994). A meta-analysis on the treatment of obsessive compulsive disorder: A comparison of antidepressants, behavior, and cognitive therapy. *Clinical Psychology Review*, 14(5), 359–381.

van der Straten, A., Huyser, C., Wolters, L., Denys, D., & van Wingen, G. (2018). Long-Term Effects of Cognitive Behavioral Therapy on Planning and Prefrontal Cortex Function in Pediatric Obsessive-Compulsive Disorder. *Biological Psychiatry: Cognitive Neuroscience and Neuroimaging*, 3(4), 320–328.

Varigonda, A. L., Jakubovski, E., & Bloch, M. H. (2016). Systematic Review and Meta-Analysis: Early Treatment Responses of Selective Serotonin Reuptake Inhibitors and Clomipramine in Pediatric Obsessive-Compulsive Disorder. *Journal of the American Academy of Child and Adolescent Psychiatry*, 55(10), 851–859.

Vattimo, E. F. Q., Barros, V. B., Requena, G., Sato, J. R., Fatori, D., Miguel, E. C., Shavitt, R. G., Hoexter, M. Q., & Batistuzzo, M. C. (2019). Caudate volume differences among treatment responders, non-responders and controls in children with obsessive–compulsive disorder. *European Child and Adolescent Psychiatry*, 28(12), 1607–1617.

Walitza, S., Wewetzer, C., Warnke, A., Gerlach, M., Geller, F., Gerber, G., Görg, T., Herpertz-Dahlmann, B., Schulz, E., Remschmidt, H., Hebebrand, J., & Hinney A. (2002). 5-HT2A promoter polymorphism -1438G/A in children and adolescents with obsessive-compulsive disorders. *Mol Psychiatry*, 7(10), 1054–1057.

Wang, Z., Fontaine, M., Cyr, M., Rynn, M. A., Simpson, H. B., Marsh, R., & Pagliaccio, D. (2022). Subcortical shape in pediatric and adult obsessive-compulsive disorder. *Depression and Anxiety*, 39(6), 504–514.

Welch, J. M., Lu, J., Rodriguiz, R. M., Trotta, N. C., Peca, J., Ding, J. D., Feliciano, C., Chen, M., Adams, J. P., Luo, J., Dudek, S. M., Weinberg, R. J., Calakos, N., Wetsel, W. C., & Feng, G. (2007). Cortico-striatal synaptic defects and OCD-like behaviours in Sapap3-mutant mice. *Nature*, 448(7156), 894–900.

Willour, V. L., Yao Shugart, Y., Samuels, J., Grados, M., Cullen, B., Bienvenu, O. J., Wang, Y., Liang, K.-Y., Valle, D., Hoehn-Saric, R., Riddle, M., & Nestadt, G. (2004). Replication Study Supports Evidence for Linkage to 9p24 in Obsessive-Compulsive Disorder. *American Journal of Human Genetics*, 75(3), 508–513.

Xue, J., Qian, D., Zhang, B., Yang, J., Li, W., Bao, Y., Qiu, S., Fu, Y., Wang, S., Yuan, T. F., & Lu, W. (2022). Midbrain dopamine neurons arbiter OCD-like behavior. *Proc Natl Acad Sci U S A.*, 119(46), e2207545119.

Zike I. D., Chohan M. O., Kopelman J. M., Krasnow E. N., Flicker D., Nautiyal K. M., Bubser, M., Kellendonk, C., Jones, C. K., Stanwood, G., Tanaka, K. F., Moore, H., Ahmari, S. E., & Veenstra-VanderWeele, J. (2017). OCD candidate gene SLC1A1/EAAT3 impacts basal ganglia-mediated activity and stereotypic behavior. *Proc Natl Acad Sci U S A*. 114(22), 5719–5724.

Zohar, J., Mueller, E. A., Insel, T. R., Zohar-Kadouch, R. C., & Murphy, D. L. (1987). Serotonergic Responsivity in Obsessive-Compulsive Disorder: Comparison of Patients and Healthy Controls. *Archives of General Psychiatry*, 44(11), 946–951.

Öst, L.G., Havnen, A., Hansen, B., & Kvale, G. (2015). Cognitive behavioral treatments of obsessive–compulsive disorder. A systematic review and meta-analysis of studies published 1993–2014. *Clin. Psychol. Rev.* 40, 156–169.

Öst, L.-G., Riise, E. N., Wergeland, G. J., Hansen, B., & Kvale, G. (2016). Cognitive behavioral and pharmacological treatments of OCD in children: A systematic review and meta-analysis. *Journal of Anxiety Disorders*, 43, 58–69.

17 Assessment and Treatment Considerations for Sexual and Gender Minority Youth with OCD

Caitlin M. Pinciotti, Andreas Bezahler and Brian A. Feinstein

Characteristics and treatment of OCD among SGM individuals

Obsessive-compulsive disorder (OCD) is characterized by repetitive intrusive thoughts (i.e., obsessions) that cause marked anxiety accompanied by mental or physical actions (i.e., compulsions) that serve to reduce the anxiety (American Psychiatric Association, 2013). The content of obsessions is often theorized to be a manifestation of deeper "core fears," defined as the ultimate feared consequence that would occur if compulsions and avoidance behaviors were not used (Huppert & Zlotnick, 2012). Globally, OCD impacts 1–2percent of children, adolescents, and adults, with rates of pediatric OCD mirroring rates among adults (see Nazeer et al., 2020).

Despite increased empirical attention to pediatric OCD, a major gap exists with respect to OCD among sexual and gender minority (SGM) populations, especially youth. The available evidence indicates that SGM young adults are four to nine times more likely to be diagnosed with or treated for OCD compared to their cisgender and heterosexual peers (Oswalt & Lederer, 2017; Pelts & Albright, 2015). In contrast, two studies (one of undergraduate students with elevated OCD symptoms and one of adults with OCD) did not identify significant differences in OCD severity between SM and heterosexual adults (Pinciotti & Orcutt, 2021; Pinciotti et al., 2023). However, they did find that one symptom dimension – unacceptable thoughts (i.e., obsessions related to violence, sex, or religion) – was more severe among SM adults, especially those with "emerging identities" (e.g., asexual, queer, questioning; Pinciotti et al., 2023). Even less research has focused on OCD among GM populations, but one study of adults with OCD found that GM adults reported more severe OCD compared to cisgender adults in general and more severe contamination symptoms compared to cisgender men in particular (Pinciotti et al., 2022). Although this study did not identify significant gender differences in unacceptable thoughts, this symptom dimension was rated higher than all other symptom dimensions among GM adults, further

DOI: 10.4324/9781003517429-17

suggesting that unacceptable thoughts may be especially relevant to SGM individuals with OCD.

With respect to treatment, SM adults represent 16–38 percent of those in treatment for OCD, a proportion that is four to nine times greater than rates of SM identification in the US population (4–7 percent; Bezahler et al., 2023; Gates, 2011; Jones, 2021). Very few studies have examined OCD treatment outcomes among SGM populations, but one study found comparable outcomes between SM and heterosexual adults with OCD (Bezahler et al., 2022), while another study found that GM adults with OCD required significantly longer stays in intensive treatment to achieve comparable symptom reduction to their cisgender peers (Pinciotti et al., 2022). Given the dearth of research on clinical characteristics and treatment outcomes of SGM youth with OCD, it remains unclear whether these trends observed among adults would extend to youth.

Minority stress as a risk factor for OCD among SGM individuals

The predominant conceptual model used to explain the mental health disparities affecting SGM people is the minority stress model (Brooks, 1981; Meyer, 2003; Testa et al., 2015). The minority stress model posits that SGM people experience unique stressors related to their stigmatized identities and that these stressors contribute to their disproportionate rates of adverse mental health outcomes (e.g., depression, anxiety). Although it was initially developed to explain the mental health disparities affecting SM individuals, it was later extended to GM individuals (Testa et al., 2015). In the minority stress model, Meyer (2003) distinguishes between distal or external minority stressors (e.g., discrimination, victimization) and proximal or internal minority stressors (e.g., internalization of negative societal attitudes, expectations of future rejection, identity concealment). When the minority stress model was extended to GM individuals, non-affirmation of one's gender identity was added as a unique distal minority stressor experienced by transgender and nonbinary individuals (Testa et al., 2015).

Although the minority stress model has been used to explain the mental health disparities affecting SGM youth, it does not explicitly attend to developmental influences on minority stress processes. Adolescence is a critical developmental period for SGM youth. Not only are they still developing their identities (Kuper et al., 2018; Mustanski et al., 2013), but minority stress experienced during adolescence can have enduring effects on mental health into adulthood (Russell et al., 2011; Ryan et al., 2009). Goldbach and Gibbs (2017) explored the extent to which the minority stress model was relevant to the experiences of SM youth ages 13–19. They found that, similar to SM adults, SM youth reported experiencing both distal and proximal minority stressors.

However, they also found that SM youth's experiences were unique in certain ways.

SM youth were most likely to describe experiencing minority stress within their families and at school, two contexts in which youth generally lack autonomy (Goldbach & Gibbs, 2017). Given that adolescents typically rely on the financial support of their parents, family conflict related to an adolescent's sexual orientation or gender identity can have consequences ranging from psychological distress to homelessness (Keuroghlian et al., 2014; Puckett et al., 2015). In addition, adolescents are legally required to attend school, and SGM youth are more likely to be bullied at school (Centers for Disease Control, 2020; Johns et al., 2019), which has been implicated in absenteeism, lower educational attainment, and poorer mental health (Pearson et al., 2007; Russell et al., 2011). Of note, in a large survey of SGM youth, only 37 percent and 55 percent identified home and school, respectively, as SGM-affirming spaces (The Trevor Project, 2022). Goldbach and Gibbs (2017) also found that SM youth described the sexual identity development process itself as a stressor. Specifically, they described feeling different from their peers at an early age but not understanding the cause of this difference until later after developing an understanding of their sexual identity. Together, these findings suggest that the minority stress model is relevant to the experiences of SGM youth, but developmental considerations must be taken into account.

Meta-analyses have consistently demonstrated that minority stress is associated with adverse mental health outcomes among SGM youth (de Lange et al., 2022; Dürrbaum & Sattler, 2020). However, there has been a lack of empirical attention to the role of minority stress in OCD among SGM people, including youth. Although not directly related to OCD, one study found that sexual orientation-related rejection sensitivity and identity concealment were each associated with symptoms of body dysmorphic disorder (BDD), an obsessive-compulsive spectrum disorder, among SM adolescent and adult men (Oshana et al., 2020). In addition, there is evidence that discrimination related to other minoritized identities is associated with OCD symptom severity. For example, prior studies have demonstrated that more frequent racial discrimination is associated with greater endorsement of and higher distress from OCD symptoms among African American young adults and adults (Williams et al., 2017; Willis & Neblett, 2018). Therefore, although no prior studies have specifically examined minority stressors in relation to OCD among SGM people, related evidence provides indirect support for likely associations.

Based on the first author's clinical experiences, OCD presentations can, in some cases, intersect with SGM individuals' identity and minority stress experiences. These experiences can be explicitly associated with obsessional content (e.g., obsessive doubts about compatibility with a romantic partner of the same gender, i.e., relationship OCD), and/or implicitly associated with function of compulsions (e.g., perfecting appearance to reduce risk of being bullied) and underlying core fears (e.g., perceiving oneself as contaminated because of a core fear of being defective, as a result of one's identity, experiencing obsessions about making a mistake or unintentionally causing harm because of a core fear of being rejected owing to one's identity). Minority stress may lead to the development of core fears such as fears of being defective or unlovable, being negligent and responsible for harm, being forever plagued with distressing thoughts and feelings, living an inauthentic life, and being immoral or sinful, that manifest in a variety of different content themes.

Trauma and OCD among SGM individuals

In addition to experiencing minority stress, SGM youth are disproportionately exposed to potentially traumatic events relative to heterosexual and cisgender youth. For example, data from a US representative sample of high school students – the 2019 National Youth Risk Behavior Survey (YRBS) – revealed that SM youth were significantly more likely to experience multiple forms of victimization (e.g., sexually assaulted, being threatened or injured with a weapon at school) than were heterosexual youth (Centers for Disease Control, 2020). Similarly, using data from local versions of the 2017 YRBS, Johns et al. (2019) found that transgender youth were also significantly more likely to experience these same forms of victimization compared to cisgender youth. In addition, meta-analyses have found that SM adolescents are significantly more likely to experience sexual abuse, parental physical abuse, and victimization at school than are heterosexual adolescents (Friedman et al., 2011; Toomey & Russell, 2017). Together, these findings highlight the high rates of victimization among SGM youth and their disproportionate exposure relative to heterosexual and cisgender youth.

Given elevated rates of trauma exposure among SGM youth, it is important to consider its impact on OCD. Nearly one in seven adults with severe OCD attributed the onset of their OCD to trauma, often occurring during childhood (Pinciotti & Fisher, 2022). In general, childhood trauma, especially neglect and abuse, is associated with more severe OCD and co-occurring mental health problems as well as greater suicide risk (Barzilay et al., 2019; Çoban & Tan, 2020; Khosravani et al., 2017; Kilic et al., 2020). The effect of childhood trauma on OCD severity is particularly strong for youth assigned female at birth and when the trauma occurred prior to puberty (Barzilay et al., 2019).

Although no prior studies have directly examined the role of trauma exposure in OCD among SGM youth or adults, one study found that bisexual men with a history of childhood sexual abuse were two times more likely to be diagnosed with OCD compared to gay men with a history of childhood sexual abuse (Batchelder et al., 2021). In addition, prior research has demonstrated that sexual abuse and assault are more strongly associated with OCD compared to other types of trauma (Barzilay et al., 2018; Jaisoorya et al., 2015), and SGM youth are disproportionately affected by sexual violence relative to heterosexual and cisgender youth (Centers for Disease Control, 2020; Marshal et al., 2011; Johns et al., 2019). Although speculative, if SGM individuals perceive that they were victimized because of their identity, then the victimization may have a greater impact and be more strongly associated with OCD risk and severity (Gothelf et al., 2004; Steinberg et al., 2013). In sum, SGM youth are disproportionately affected by trauma, and trauma exposure is a well-documented risk factor for OCD. Although the association between trauma exposure and OCD has yet not been examined among SGM youth, the available evidence suggests a likely connection.

Case conceptualization for SGM youth with OCD

Case conceptualization should consider the whole person, not simply their OCD, to have the most complete picture of each unique person's experiences and responses that inform the presentation and maintenance of their OCD. An individual's SGM identity and experiences related to their identity may have no bearing at all on their OCD. When OCD symptoms appear to have manifested in response to minority stress, however, these external and internal experiences must be considered as part of the patient's case conceptualization.

The cognitive-behavioral model of OCD posits that symptoms develop because of cognitive and behavioral reactions to intrusive thoughts (Gibbs, 1996). While intrusive thoughts are overwhelmingly common in people with or without OCD (Purdon & Clark, 1993), what differentiates those with OCD is their tendency to appraise these thoughts as threatening, personally important, highly unacceptable, and/or immoral (Abramowitz et al., 2007). Because of these appraisals, compulsions and avoidance behaviors are used to neutralize or suppress the intrusive thought and to prevent feared outcomes. This results in temporary relief from anxiety, yet paradoxically intensifies the emotional valence and perceived importance of the intrusive thought, thereby making the thought more likely to reoccur (Abramowitz et al., 2009). Over time, the cycle of OCD is strengthened and maintained through repeated use of neutralizing, suppression, and avoidance strategies.

It is intuitive that the intrusive thoughts that are particularly relevant and meaningful for an individual are likely to be viewed as more threatening and personally important than those that are not, such as intrusive thoughts that threaten an individual's values, beliefs, and life roles (e.g., as a student, friend, or family member). Minority stress is an important facet of early life experiences and critical incidents that are theorized to shape the beliefs and assumptions individuals develop that ultimately inform the content of the intrusive thoughts that are most likely to "stick" (Salkovskis, 1999). This may be why unacceptable thoughts, such as those involving violence, sex, or religion, may be endorsed more strongly by SGM individuals compared to other OCD symptoms (Pinciotti et al., 2023; Pinciotti et al., 2022; Pinciotti & Orcutt, 2021). Unacceptable thoughts are the most stigmatized, including by professionals, and are associated with rejection and shame (Glazier et al., 2015; Wetterneck et al., 2014). SGM youth who are already sensitized to stigma and rejection, and perhaps have developed stigmatized core beliefs about themselves, owing to minority stress, may be more reactive to these intrusive thoughts out of concern that the thoughts will compound the experiences of rejection and stigmatization they are already experiencing (Pinciotti et al., 2023; Pinciotti et al., 2022; Pinciotti & Orcutt, 2021). This reactivity only increases the salience of such thoughts and inadvertently reinforces the OCD cycle. Irrespective of OCD, minority stress has the potential to contribute to the development of a system of beliefs in which SGM youth feel as though they are unwanted, unlovable, and defective because of their identity, and those with OCD may feel overly responsible for preventing harm in the form of further stigmatization and rejection.

Protective and avoidance behaviors may also be borne out of minority stress experiences but generalize and intensify to such a degree that they become compulsive. For example, a bisexual adolescent may have developed a core fear of being sinful and destined to hell stemming from minority stress experiences in which they were told by family members that their sexual orientation was a sin. In response, they may engage in excessive and ritualized praying to repent for their perceived sin of being bisexual, and over time this behavior may generalize to all perceived sins.

Assessment considerations for SGM youth

It is important to highlight that self-report assessment measures of OCD considered to be the "gold standard" have not been specifically examined in SGM populations. This represents a crucial gap in need of further research because commonly used measures for other mental health concerns (e.g., depression, anxiety) have shown to perform differently among SGM people compared to non-SGM people (Borgogna et al., 2021). Evidence of elevations on the intrusive thoughts subscale of the Dimensional Obsessive-Compulsive Scale (DOCS; Abramowitz et al., 2010) among SGM people (Pinciotti et al., 2023; Pinciotti et al., 2022; Pinciotti & Orcutt, 2021) suggests either that these symptoms are truly more common in this population, as described above, or that the subscale may tap into common cognitive and behavioral processes for SGM people that are unrelated to OCD symptoms (i.e., "intrusive thoughts" about sex or sexuality may not actually be obsessions). Until more is known about the extent to which these gold-standard assessments of OCD measure the intended constructs among SGM people, they should be used and interpreted with caution with SGM patients, and clinicians are encouraged to ask follow-up questions to ensure that self-reported symptoms are truly specific to OCD.

Assessing minority stress

Given that most SGM youth experience and are impacted by minority stress, it is important to assess these experiences and incorporate them into case conceptualization and treatment planning when working with SGM youth with OCD. During clinical intake, clinicians are advised to ask about experiences with distal and proximal minority stressors and their impact on mental health broadly, and on OCD specifically. Clinicians should use appropriate caution and sensitivity when asking about minority stress to avoid making assumptions about a given youth's experiences. For example, asking a leading, closed-ended question such as "Your parents must have really struggled with your identity. Did they reject you when you came out?" can communicate to the patient that the clinician believes parental rejection is inevitable for SGM youth. Instead, questions can be phrased in an open-ended manner (e.g., "Has anyone ever treated you differently or rejected you because of your identity? If so, how did that impact you?") Doing so creates space to discuss the possibility of having experienced rejection or mistreatment without, assuming that all SGM youth share this experience.

Similarly, given the role of trauma in OCD, it is important to assess exposure to potentially traumatic events and their possible impact on the youth's symptoms. When assessing trauma history, it can be pertinent to ask whether and how any endorsed traumatic events were related to anti-SGM stigma. Language is again important when assessing trauma to avoid implicitly communicating that the young person is to blame for the trauma because of their identity. Rather than asking "Do you think you were attacked you because of your identity?", consider instead "Do you think you were attacked because of their prejudice against transgender and nonbinary people?" If the patient perceives the experience to have occurred because of prejudice against them, then the clinician could go on to assess how the experience impacted the patient's beliefs (e.g., about their identity, other people, and safety).

Self-report measures are often used to collect baseline information about a patient's experience and to monitor progress throughout treatment. Unfortunately, most measures of minority stress assess one specific type (e.g., discrimination or internalized stigma), and few were specifically developed for SGM youth. In exceptions, the Sexual Minority Adolescent Stress Inventory (SMASI; Schrager et al., 2018) can be used to assess multiple types of sexual orientation-related minority stress (e.g., family rejection, internalized homonegativity, negative disclosure experiences, negative expectancies) and the adolescent extension of the Gender Minority Stress and Resilience Measure (GMSR-A; Hidalgo et al., 2019) can be used to assess multiple types of gender-related stress (e.g., discrimination, rejection, victimization, non-affirmation of one's gender identity, internalized transphobia, negative expectations for the future).

In addition to minority stress, it is also important to assess resilience factors related to one's SGM identity. Doing so not only provides valuable information to inform case conceptualization and treatment planning; it also communicates that there are strengths related to being a member of the SGM community. The GMSR-A assesses both minority stress (noted above) and resilience factors (pride in one's gender identity and community connectedness) for GM youth. Although the SMASI only assesses minority stress, other measures can be used to assess resilience factors for SM youth such as the Lesbian, Gay, and Bisexual Positive Identity Measure (Riggle et al., 2014), which was originally developed for adults. In addition to identity-specific forms of resilience, it is also advisable to assess general protective factors such as family and peer support (e.g., such as by using the Multidimensional Scale of Perceived Social Support; Zimet et al., 1990).

Assessing intersections of OCD symptoms and identity-related experiences

When working with SGM youth with OCD, it is important to consider and assess the extent to which OCD symptoms are connected to or maintained by minority stress-related beliefs and experiences. To be clear, OCD is not caused by a person's SGM identity. Instead, beliefs about one's identity (e.g., negative societal attitudes that have been internalized) and exposure to minority stress (e.g., discrimination) can serve as catalysts for the development and maintenance of OCD, such as through obsessions and compulsions that are rooted in core fears connected to internalized stigma and shame related to one's identity. These intersections of symptoms and experiences will not be relevant for all SGM youth with OCD, so clinicians should use caution when assessing this and avoid making assumptions or being forceful in one's questioning if the patient denies intersections between their symptoms and identity-related beliefs and experiences.

Clinicians should use clinical judgment in determining whether and when such questions should be asked. Given the sensitivity of assessing the extent to which a patient's symptoms intersect with beliefs or experiences related to their identity, establishment of rapport is critical. Rushing into assessing intersections of symptoms and experiences may damage rapport and cause the patient to discontinue the assessment or not want to engage in treatment. Youth should experience their provider as affirming (not simply tolerant) of their identity and understanding of the unique experiences – both positive and negative – of SGM youth. If a clinician decides to assess the intersections of symptoms and experiences, they can ask whether the youth believes that any of the thoughts, images, sensations, or urges (for obsessions) or behaviors or actions (for compulsions) that they endorsed are in any way connected to experiences they have had related to their sexual orientation or gender identity (e.g., discrimination). Clinicians can also normalize that some, but not all, SGM youth with OCD describe their symptoms as being connected to beliefs or experiences related to their identity, and that the patient is not alone if that is true for them as well.

Differentiating sexual orientation and gender-themed OCD from identity rumination

Given the threat of experiencing minority stress in everyday interactions and important relationships, as well as the developmentally appropriate identity exploration that occurs during adolescence, it is no surprise that OCD can latch onto themes related to sexual orientation and gender identity. Sexual orientation (SO) and gender-themed OCD are centered on doubts about one's sexual orientation or gender identity, fear of becoming another sexual orientation or gender identity, and/or fears that others will perceive one as another sexual orientation or gender identity (Williams, 2008). Individuals with SO- or gender-themed OCD may attempt to "figure out" their identity through compulsions involving body scanning and checking for arousal, reassurance seeking and self-assurance, searching online to read about SGM people's experiences and monitoring one's reactions, mentally reviewing one's interactions with people of the gender to which they obsess about potential attraction, testing one's response to dressing in a way that could lead to be perceived as a different gender, avoiding cues related to SGM populations (e.g., media content or peers), and/or testing and comparing physiological arousal to sexual content and activity involving people of different genders (Pinciotti et al., 2022; Safer et al., 2016; Williams & Wetterneck, 2019).

SO- and gender-themed OCD develop in response to over-interpretation of unwanted sexual- or gender identity-related thoughts, and these identity-related intrusive thoughts are characterized by significant doubt and result in attempts to quell this doubt using repetitive, compulsive behaviors. Several documented case examples have described SGM individuals who experienced obsessions about being heterosexual or cisgender (Goldberg, 1984; Williams & Ching, 2016; Williams & Wetterneck, 2019). The onset of SO- and gender-themed OCD may coincide with periods of sexual and gender identity development during adolescence, owing to a combination of experiencing minority stress at school, having less experience or knowledge about gender and sexuality, and increased physiological reactions associated with puberty (Williams & Wetterneck, 2019). The lifetime prevalence of SO-OCD is approximately 12 percent (Williams &

Farris, 2011), and sexual obsessions are present in 18–27 percent of youth with OCD, with 30–33 percent of these sexual obsessions involving themes related to sexual orientation (Fernández de la Cruz et al., 2013; Weidle et al., 2022). Gender-themed OCD is less well studied so the prevalence is currently unknown, however its prevalence is likely to increase in tandem with increases in anti-transgender policies in the US and globally.

SO- and gender-themed OCD may present similarly to non-OCD-related identity rumination, referred to as typical identity rumination, which can be challenging for clinicians to discern. Identity rumination develops in reaction to internalized stigma and may be conceptualized as a means of coming to accept one's identity and coping with minority stress (Galupo & Bauerband, 2016). Regardless of sexual orientation, exploration of sexual identity is a normative developmental process during adolescence (Savin-Williams, 2011), and rumination about one's sexual orientation or gender identity is common among SGM people, especially those who experience uncertainty about their identity (Borders et al., 2014). Therefore, it is crucial to be able to differentiate OCD from developmentally appropriate identity exploration, uncertainty, and rumination to ensure appropriate treatment. A critical distinguishing factor is that SO- and gender-themed obsessions are ego-dystonic in that they are inconsistent with historical patterns of the individual's felt identity, attractions, and behaviors, whereas identity rumination is ego-syntonic and consistent with these patterns, even if they evoke distress (Luxon et al., 2021; Pinciotti et al., 2022; Williams, 2008). For example, an adolescent who is lesbian or gay with typical identity rumination may feel sexually aroused by thoughts of and experiences with people of the same gender but may ruminate on these experiences because of fear of stigma and rejection from peers and family members. In contrast, an adolescent with SO-OCD centered on being lesbian or gay may feel more sexually aroused by thoughts of and experiences with people of a different gender but feel anxious about the possibility that they may find same-gender sexual experiences enjoyable or arousing and are concerned about the consequences of being lesbian or gay (e.g., losing one's current romantic partner). The adolescent with SO-OCD will likely have difficulty disengaging from other-gender thoughts and engage in compulsive checking and reassurance behaviors to assuage their doubt about their identity. Williams (2008) and Luxon et al. (2021) provide detailed guidelines for differential diagnosis of SO- and gender-themed OCD and identity-based rumination.

Treatment considerations for SGM youth

Cognitive behavioral therapy with exposure and response prevention (ERP) is an evidence-based, gold-standard treatment for pediatric OCD

(Storch & Merlo, 2006). The focus of this section is on unique considerations for the application of this treatment with SGM youth.

Providing identity-affirming treatment

It is expected that, at a minimum, all clinicians can provide competent and affirming care to SGM patients, including but not limited to: ensuring intake paperwork has inclusive demographic options, introducing oneself with pronouns, asking patients what name and pronouns they use, reflecting on and challenging one's own potential biases, being aware of and addressing mistreatment in the home, maintaining a basic understanding of different sexual and gender identities, remaining up-to-date on currently accepted language related to sexual orientation and gender identity, remaining up-to-date on sociopolitical conditions affecting SGM people (e.g., recent legislation restricting the rights of SGM people in the US), and being mindful of not contributing – whether unintentional or otherwise – to patients' minority stress within sessions (see Boroughs et al., 2015 for a discussion of minimum standards of developing SGM-specific cultural competence).

Some ERP clinicians become fixated on using exposures to target all situations which evoke anxiety and/or avoidance without consideration of the unique experiences of SGM youth. SGM individuals may expect rejection and discrimination, and subsequently feel anxious, when meeting new people, in situations that have the potential for being outed, or in situations that center the gender binary and/or involve gender markers (e. g., public restrooms, clothing stores, healthcare settings; Rood et al., 2016). With the rise of anti-SGM rhetoric, political and school policies, and hate crimes in the US and globally, it is critical that clinicians understand that avoidance can be adaptive and protective, and does not need to be targeted with ERP, particularly if doing so could expose patients to actual risk (e.g., asking a GM youth to use a public restroom could carry actual risk for violence).

Clinicians should also refrain from incorporating minority stress into exposure work. For example, a GM patient who avoids correcting individuals who misgender them (i.e., uses the wrong pronouns) does not need to be encouraged to use ERP in session to challenge their anxiety by correcting the clinician's incorrect use of pronouns. This exposure exercise not only intentionally subjects the patient to a microaggression perpetrated by a trusted authority figure, it also perpetuates the belief that it is the responsibility of GM youth to educate and empathize with cisgender people regardless of the emotional toll (Pinciotti et al., 2022). Intentionally creating minority stress is harmful, unnecessary, and damaging to therapeutic rapport; patients who wish to practice coping with minority stress can do so outside of session when these situations naturally occur or can use imaginal exposure to past minority stress experiences if they are requesting to approach and habituate to these painful emotions without artificially adding to their history of minority stress (Burton et al., 2019).

When treating adolescents with SO- and gender-themed OCD, clinicians should ensure that treatment is justice-based so that exposure exercises do not further marginalize, tokenize, out, or otherwise harm the SGM community (see Pinciotti et al., 2022). Justice-based treatment is defined as "an equitable, thorough, and compassionate lens through which to conceptualize and implement mental health treatment so that all impacted persons – client, provider, and society – are respected" (Pinciotti et al., 2022). Using this lens, any exposure that capitalizes on and reinforces stereotypes about SGM people (e.g., a masculine person dressing femininely), reinforces misinformation (e.g., a worry script about suddenly becoming SGM), tokenizes and/or outs SGM people (e.g., shaking hands with a person who "looks" SGM), normalizes disgust (e. g., looking at a photo that invokes disgust of two same-gender people kissing), normalizes the use of slurs (e.g., writing a transphobic slur), or perpetuates the hyper-sexualization of SGM people (e.g., describing sexual acts between people of the same-gender to someone else) should be avoided. These exposures should be replaced with exposures that target the core fear underlying the surface level SO- or gender themed obsession (e.g., describing other lived experiences involving deception or inauthenticity), encourage tolerating uncertainty about SGM-related fears (e.g., socializing with people who may or may not be SGM), and that provide corrective information about SGM people (e.g., read about definitions of different identity labels).

On occasion, a clinician may recommend a change in the patient's level of care (i.e., standard outpatient, intensive outpatient, partial hospitalization, or residential treatment programs), either through "stepping up" to higher levels of care when symptoms or comorbid presentation are too severe and/or functionality is too impaired, or "stepping down" to lower levels of care when symptom severity and functionality has improved. Referrals should only be made to treatment programs and clinicians who provide justice-based treatment and SGM-affirming care. If unsure, clinicians should consider inquiring as to these practices such as by asking about policies related to use of patient's chosen name and pronouns, inclusive patient identification and data collection, non-discrimination, mandated staff training in SGM-affirming care, support for SGM employees, engagement with local SGM communities, promotion of SGM-affirming information and resources, implementation of justice-based OCD treatment, and gender-inclusive restrooms and rooming (if residential). To assist with this decision making, the Human Rights Campaign has developed a healthcare equality index score that is publicly available that represents the extent to which a healthcare facility provides equitable and inclusive care to SGM patients and their families based on a number of detailed criteria (Human Rights Campaign, 2022).

Addressing intersections of OCD symptoms and identity-related experiences

The extent to which any OCD symptoms are connected to beliefs or experiences related to one's SGM identity should be considered as a relevant treatment target and strategies other than exposure-based techniques will be more sensitive and affirming to use because they can address the internalized beliefs associated with these symptoms. Obsessions or compulsions tied to identity and minority stress should not be challenged through exposure therapy which can contribute to minority stress within the therapy room, thereby damaging rapport and reinforcing patients' internalized stigma and shame. Consider a transgender adolescent with contamination concerns who feels that they themselves are contaminated or disgusting because of their gender identity and feels particularly contaminated when using public restrooms in which the possibility of being identified as transgender and experiencing violence could occur. It would be harmful to emphasize the possibility that the adolescent is, in fact, contaminated and disgusting because of their gender identity, with phrases such as: "Maybe you are contaminated, maybe not. You must sit with this possibility." Rather, the clinician can approach the internalized transphobia and shame driving this personal attribution with positive identity-based affirmation and compassion-based strategies.

Modeling for the adolescent that their identity should be celebrated, such as through affirming statements and content and opportunities to connect with the transgender community, can help the adolescent identify and process their shame, understand how their internalized transphobia has developed through external messaging, and learn how to love and celebrate themselves. Self-compassion exercises (e.g., Neff & Germer, 2018), including ones that are specific to transgender identities (e.g., Lorenz, 2020), may be helpful to integrate. Exposure practices, then, can be used to target those aspects of OCD that are unrelated to the patient's identity. In the above example, perhaps the adolescent also feels contamination related to sticky substances and residues and this concern has no relation to their identity, in which case the clinician could use traditional ERP to target these fears.

Working with families

Families of youth with OCD tend to be characterized by disrupted family functioning and high distress, and respond to this distress and upheaval with hostility and blame (Peris et al., 2008; Piacentini et al., 2003). Family functioning impacts treatment outcomes for youth, such that greater conflict and parental blame as well as lower family cohesion are associated with worse treatment outcomes (Peris et al., 2012). Although many SGM youth have supportive families, others experience rejection, abuse and neglect, and increased arguments, conflict, and discrimination following identity disclosure (DeChants et al., 2022).

In such instances, these home experiences are not only likely to worsen mental health for SGM youth as described above, but present as significant barriers to treatment. Namely, effective treatment for youth with OCD is largely contingent upon supportive family involvement. The aforementioned OCD-related familial conflict may be further compounded by SGM-related conflict and create a home environment that is untenable. As a result, clinicians should also strongly consider regular family sessions in which they can serve as a protective moderator for the youth, and work collaboratively with families to reframe problematic beliefs and behaviors. This may involve meeting privately with caregivers to have these conversations so that the youth is not further impacted by hearing and internalizing these anti-SGM messages. Clinicians should also be clear about when families should redirect or challenge behaviors that may present as compulsions and when they should support them. For example, youth may change identity labels and pronouns during periods of identity exploration; these behaviors should not be treated as compulsions to be resisted when gender-themed OCD is not present. In situations where anti-SGM behaviors in the home do not improve, or are intensifying over the course of treatment, clinicians may consider alternative treatment settings such as "stepping up" to SGM-affirming higher levels of care that would provide the youth with space away from unsupportive family where they can focus more specifically on their OCD treatment without fear of mistreatment or abuse.

Clinicians should engage in conversations with the caregivers and the youth patient to discuss what information will be kept private and in what cases information may be shared. Clinicians should be mindful of the potential that patients may not be "out" to caregivers about their sexual orientation or gender identity, owing to several potential factors, including knowledge of caregivers' prejudicial attitudes, expectations of rejection, and concerns about potential mistreatment or abuse. Although research has found some positive benefits to being "out" (Beals et al., 2009), this is not the case for all youth and in all contexts. For example, being more open about one's identity is associated with better mental health for gay and lesbian youth, but worse mental health for those who are questioning their sexual orientation (Rentería et al., 2022). Clinicians should never disclose a patient's sexual orientation or gender identity to others without the patient's consent, and they should never coerce patients to disclose their identity as this could create highly unsafe situations and cause potentially irreparable damage to the therapeutic relationship. If a transgender or nonbinary patient is not "out" to family, the clinician should discuss with the patient their preferences regarding the clinicians' conversations with family members and be prepared to use a different name and/or different pronouns with family members to protect the patient's privacy regarding their identity.

Conclusion

Increasing rates of SGM-identification among youth coupled with higher rates of OCD among SGM individuals likely resulting from minority stress requires that clinicians who treat youth with OCD develop and maintain competence in providing identity-affirming assessment and treatment to SGM youth. Conceptualization, assessment, and treatment must consider and thoughtfully address the impact of minority stress on the presentation, severity, and maintenance of OCD.

References

Abramowitz, J. S., Deacon, B. J., Olatunji, B. O., Wheaton, M. G., Berman, N. C., Losardo, D., ... Hale, L. R. (2010). Assessment of obsessive-compulsive symptom dimensions: Development and evaluation of the Dimensional Obsessive-Compulsive Scale. *Psychological Assessment*, 22(1), 180–198. doi:10.1037/a0018260.

Abramowitz, J. S., Nelson, C. A., Rygwall, R., & Khandker, M. (2007). The cognitive mediation of obsessive-compulsive symptoms: a longitudinal study. *Journal of Anxiety Disorders*, 21(1), 91–104. doi:10.1016/j.janxdis.2006.05.003.

Abramowitz, J. S., Taylor, S., & McKay, D. (2009). Obsessive-compulsive disorder. *The Lancet*, 374(9688), 491–499. doi:10.1016/S0140-6736(09)60240–60243.

American Psychiatric Association. (2013). *Diagnostic and statistical manual of mental disorders* (5th ed.). https://doi.org/10.1176/appi.books.9780890425596.

Barzilay, R., Patrick, A., Calkins, M. E., Moore, T. M., Gur, R. C., & Gur, R. E. (2019). Association between early-life trauma and obsessive compulsive symptoms in community youth. *Depression and Anxiety*, 36(7), 586–595. doi:10.1002/da.22907.

Batchelder, A. W., Fitch, C., Feinstein, B. A., Thiim, A., & O'Cleirigh, C. (2021). Psychiatric, substance use, and structural disparities between gay and bisexual men with histories of childhood sexual abuse and recent sexual risk behavior. *Archives of Sexual Behavior*, 50(7), 2861–2873. doi:10.1007/s10508-021-02037-1.

Beals, K. P., Peplau, L. A., & Gable, S. L. (2009). Stigma management and well-being: The role of perceived social support, emotional processing, and suppression. *Personality and Social Psychology Bulletin*, 35(7), 867–879. doi:10.1177/0146167209334783.

Bezahler, A., Feinstein, B. A., Falkenstein, M. J., & Kuckertz, J. M. (2023). Emerging trends in sexual minority identification and clinical implications for treating OCD and related disorders. *The Behavior Therapist, 46(5)*, 194–199.

Bezahler, A., Kuckertz, J. M., Schreck, M., Narine, K., Dattolico, D., & Falkenstein, M. J. (2022). Examination of outcomes among sexual minorities in treatment for obsessive-compulsive and related disorders. *Journal of Obsessive-Compulsive and Related Disorders*, 33, 100724. doi:10.1016/j.jocrd.2022.100724.

Borders, A., Guillén, L. A., & Meyer, I. H. (2014). Rumination, sexual orientation uncertainty, and psychological distress in sexual minority university students. *The Counseling Psychologist*, 42(4), 497–523. doi:10.1177/001100001452700.

Borgogna, N. C., Brenner, R. E., & McDermott, R. C. (2021). Sexuality and gender invariance of the PHQ-9 and GAD-7: Implications for 16 identity groups. *Journal of Affective Disorders*, 278, 122–130. doi:10.1016/j.jad.2020.09.069.

Boroughs, M. S., Bedoya, C. A., O'Cleirigh, C., & Safren, S. A. (2015). Toward defining, measuring, and evaluating LGBT cultural competence for psychologists. *Clinical Psychology: Science and Practice*, 22(2), 151–171. doi:10.1111/cpsp.12098.

Brooks, V. R. (1981). *Minority stress and lesbian women*. Lexington, MA: Lexington Books.

Burton, C. L., Wang, K., & Pachankis, J. E. (2019). Psychotherapy for the spectrum of sexual minority stress: Application and technique of the ESTEEM treatment model. *Cognitive and Behavioral Practice*, 26(2), 285–299. doi:10.1016/j.cbpra.2017.05.001.

Centers for Disease Control. (2020). *Youth Risk Behavior Surveillance System – United States and selected sites, 2019*. www.cdc.gov/healthyyouth/data/yrbs/2019_tables/pdf/2019_MMWR-SS_Tables.pdf.

Çoban, A. & Tan, O. (2020). Attention deficit hyperactivity disorder, impulsivity, anxiety, and depression symptoms mediating the relationship between childhood trauma and symptoms severity of obsessive-compulsive disorder. *Archives of Neuropsychiatry*, 57(1), 37–43. doi:10.29399/npa.23654.

DeChants, J. P., Shelton, J., Anyon, Y., & Bender, K. (2022). "It kinda breaks my heart": LGBTQ young adults' responses to family rejection. *Family Relations*, 71(3), 968–986. doi:10.1111/fare.12638.

de Lange, J., Baams, L., van Bergen, D. D., Bos, H. M. W., & Bosker, R. J. (2022). Minority stress and suicidal ideation and suicide attempts among LGBT adolescents and young adults: A meta-analysis. *LGBT Health*, 9(4), 222–237. doi:10.1089/lgbt.2021.0106.

Dürrbaum, T. & Sattler, F. A. (2020). Minority stress and mental health in lesbian, gay male, and bisexual youths: A meta-analysis. *Journal of LGBT Youth*, 17(3), 298–314. doi:10.1080/19361653.2019.1586615.

Fernández de la Cruz, L., Barrow, F., Bolhuis, K., Krebs, G., Volz, C., Nakatani, E., Heyman, I., & Mataix-Cols, D. (2013). Sexual obsessions in pediatric obsessive-compulsive disorder: Clinical characteristics and treatment outcomes. *Depression and Anxiety*, 30(8), 732–740. doi:10.1002/da.22097.

Galupo, M. P. & Bauerband, L. A. (2016). Sexual Orientation Reflection and Rumination Scale: Development and psychometric evaluation. *Stigma and Health*, 1(1), 44–58.

Gates, G. J. (2011). *How many people are lesbian, gay, bisexual, and transgender?* UCLA School of Law Williams Institute. Retrieved from: https://williamsinstitute.law.ucla.edu/publications/how-many-people-lgbt.

Gibbs, N. A. (1996). Nonclinical populations in research on obsessive-compulsive disorder: A critical review. *Clinical Psychology Review*, 16(8), 729–773. doi:10.1016/S0272-7358(96)00043-8.

Glazier, K., Wetterneck, C., Singh, S., Williams, M. (2015) Stigma and shame as barriers to treatment for obsessive-compulsive and related disorders. *Journal of Depression and Anxiety*, 4, 191. doi:10.4191/2167-1044.1000191.

Goldbach, J. T. & Gibbs, J. J. (2017). A developmentally informed adaptation of minority stress for sexual minority adolescents. *Journal of Adolescence*, 55, 36–50. doi:10.1016/j.adolescence.2016.12.007.

Goldberg, R. L. (1984). Heterosexual panic. *American Journal of Psychoanalysis*, 44, 209–211. doi:10.1007/bf01248300.

Gothelf, D., Aharonovsky, O., Horesh, N., Carty, T., & Apter, A. (2004). Life events and personality factors in children and adolescents with obsessive-compulsive disorder and other anxiety disorders. *Comprehensive Psychiatry*, 45(3), 192–198. doi:10.1016/j.comppsych.2004.02.010.

Hidalgo, M. A., Petras, H., Chen, D., & Chodzen, G. (2019). *The Gender Minority Stress and Resilience Measure: Psychometric validity of an adolescent extension. Clinical Practice in Pediatric Psychology*, 7(3), 278–290. doi:10.1037/cpp0000297.

Human Rights Campaign. (2022). *Healthcare equality index 2022*. Retrieved from www.hrc.org/resources/healthcare-equality-index.

Huppert, J. D. & Zlotnick, E. (2012). Core fears, values, and obsessive-compulsive disorder: A preliminary clinical-theoretical outlook. *Psicoterapia Cognitiva e Comportamentale*, 18(1), 91–102.

Jaisoorya, T. S., Janardhan Reddy, Y. C., Thennarasu, K., Beena, K. V., Beena, M., & Jose, D. C. (2015). An epidemological study of obsessive compulsive disorder in adolescents from India. *Comprehensive Psychiatry*, 61, 106–114. doi:10.1016/j.comppsych.2015.05.003.

Johns, M. M., Lowry, R., Andrzejewski, J., Barrios, L. C., Demissie, Z., McManus, T., Rasberry, C. N., Robin, L., & Underwood, J. M. (2019). Transgender identity and experiences of violence victimization, substance use, suicide risk, and sexual risk behaviors among high school students – 19 states and large urban school districts, 2017. *Morbidity and Mortality Weekly Report*, 68(3), 67–71. doi:10.15585/mmwr.mm6803a3.

Jones, J. M. (February 24, 2021). LGBT identification rises to 5.6 percent in latest U.S. estimate. *Gallup*. Retrieved from https://news.gallup.com/poll/329708/lgbt-identification-rises-latest-estimate.aspx.

Keuroghlian, A. S., Shtasel, D., & Bassuk, E. L. (2014). Out on the street: A public health and policy agenda for lesbian, gay, bisexual, and transgender youth who are homeless. *American Journal of Orthopsychiatry*, 84(1), 66–72. doi:10.1037/h0098852.

Khosravani, V., Kamali, Z., Ardakani, R. J., & Ardestani, M. S. (2017). The relation of childhood trauma to suicide ideation in patients suffering from obsessive-compulsive disorder with lifetime suicide attempts. *Psychiatry Research*, 255, 139–145. doi:10.1016/j.psychres.2017.05.032.

Kilic, F., Karakoc, A. A., Isik, U., Donmez, F., & Demirdas, A. (2020). Childhood traumas and suicide probability in obsessive-compulsive disorder patients with and without suicide attempts. *The Journal of Psychiatry and Neurological Sciences*, 33(4), 402–409. doi:10.14744/DAJPNS.2020.00108.

Kuper, L. E., Wright, L., & Mustanski, B. (2018). Gender identity development among transgender and gender nonconforming emerging adults: An intersectional approach. *International Journal of Transgenderism*, 19(4), 436–455. doi:10.1080/15532739.2018.1443869.

Lorenz, T. N. (2020). *The trans self-care workbook*. Philadelphia, PA: Jessica Kingsley.

Lucassen, M. F. G., Stasiak, K., Samra, R., Frampton, C. M. A., & Merry, S. N. (2017). Sexual minority youth and depressive symptoms or depressive disorder: A systematic review and meta-analysis of population-based studies. *Australian and New Zealand Journal of Psychiatry*, 51(8), 774–787.

Luxon, A. M., Chasson, G. S., Williams, M. T., Skinta, M., & Galupo, M. P. (2021). Brooding over the closet: Differentiating sexual orientation rumination and sexual orientation obsessions. *Journal of Cognitive Psychotherapy*, 35(3), 167–182. doi:10.1891/JCPSY-D-20-00013.

Marshal, M. P., Dietz, L. J., Friedman, M. S., Stall, R., Smith, H. A., McGinley, J., Thoma, B. C., Murray, P. J., D'Augelli, A. R., & Brent, D. A. (2011). Suicidality and depression disparities between sexual minority and heterosexual youth: A meta-analytic review. *Journal of Adolescent Health*, 49(2), 115–123.

Meyer I. H. (2003). Prejudice, social stress, and mental health in lesbian, gay, and bisexual populations: Conceptual issues and research evidence. *Psychological Bulletin*, 129(5), 674–697. doi:10.1037/0033-2909.129.5.674.

Mustanski, B., Kuper, K., & Greene, G. J. (2013). Development of sexual orientation and identity. In D. L. Tolman & L. M. Diamond (Eds), *Handbook of Sexuality and Psychology* (Vol. 1, pp. 597–628). Washington, DC: American Psychological Association.

Nazeer, A., Latif, F., Mondal, A., Azeem, M. W., & Greydanus, D. E. (2020). Obsessive-compulsive disorder in children and adolescents: epidemiology, diagnosis and management. *Translational Pediatrics*, 9(Suppl 1), S76–S93. doi:10.21037/tp.2019.10.02.

Neff, K. & Germer, C. (2018). *The mindful self-compassion workbook: A proven way to accept yourself, build inner strength, and thrive*. New York: Guilford Press.

Oshana, A., Klimek, P., & Blashill, A. J. (2020). Minority stress and body dysmorphic disorder symptoms among sexual minority adolescents and adult men. *Body Image*, 34, 167–174. doi:10.1016/j.bodyim.2020.06.001.

Oswalt, S. & Lederer, A. (2017). Beyond depression and suicide: The mental health of transgender college students. *Social Sciences*, 6(1), 20. doi:10.3390/socsci6010020.

Pearson, J., Muller, C., & Wilkinson, L. (2007). Adolescent same-sex attraction and academic outcomes: the role of school attachment and engagement. *Social Problems*, 54, 523–542. doi:10.1525/sp.2007.54.4.523.

Pelts, M. D. & Albright, D. L. (2015). An exploratory study of student service members/veterans' mental health characteristics by sexual orientation. *Journal of American College Health*, 63(7), 508–512. doi:10.1080/07448481.2014.947992.

Peris, T. S., Bergman, R. L., Langley, A., Chang, S., McCracken, J. T., & Piacentini, J. (2008). Correlates of accommodation of pediatric obsessive-compulsive disorder: Parent, child, and family characteristics. *Journal of the American Academy of Child & Adolescent Psychiatry*, 47(10), 1173–1181. doi:10.1097/CHI.0b013e3181825a91.

Peris, T. S., Roblek, T., Langley, A., Benazon, N., & Piacentini, J. (2008). Parental responses to obsessive compulsive disorder: development and validation of the parental attitudes and behaviors scale (PABS). *Child and Family Behavior Therapy*, 30, 199–214.

Peris, T. S., Sugar, C. A., Bergman, R. L., Chang, S., Langley, A., & Piacentini, J. (2012). Family factors predict treatment outcome for pediatric obsessive-compulsive disorder. *Journal of Consulting and Clinical Psychology*, 80(2), 255–263. doi:10.1037/a0027084.

Piacentini, J., Bergman, R. L., Keller, M., & McCracken, J. (2003). Functional impairment in children and adolescents with obsessive-compulsive disorder. *Journal of Child and Adolescent Psychopharmacology*, 13(2, Supplement 1), 61–69. doi:10.1089/104454603322126359.

Pinciotti, C. M., Feinstein, B. A., & Williams, M. T. (2023). *Sexual orientation differences in OCD symptom profiles in a clinical sample.* Manuscript under review.

Pinciotti, C. M. & Fisher, E. K. (2022). Perceived traumatic and stressful etiology of obsessive-compulsive disorder. *Psychiatry Research Communications*, 2(2), 100044. doi:10.1016/j.psycom.2022.100044.

Pinciotti, C. M. & Orcutt, H. K. (2021). Obsessive-compulsive symptoms in sexual minorities. *Psychology of Sexual Orientation and Gender Diversity*, 8(4), 487–495. doi:10.1037/sgd0000437.

Pinciotti, C. M., Nuñez, M., Riemann, B. C., & Bailey, B. E. (2022). Clinical presentation and treatment trajectory of gender minority patients with obsessive-compulsive disorder. *Journal of Cognitive Psychotherapy*, 36(1), 42–59. doi:10.1891/jcpsy-d-20-00022.

Pinciotti, C. M., Smith, Z., Singh, S., Wetterneck, C. T., & Williams, M. T. (2022). Call to action: Recommendations for justice-based treatment of obsessive-compulsive disorder with sexual orientation and gender themes. *Behavior Therapy*, 53(2), 153–169. doi:10.1016/j.beth.2021.11.001.

Puckett, J. A., Woodward, E. N., Mereish, E. H., & Pantalone, D. W. (2015). Parental rejection following sexual orientation disclosure: Impact on internalized homophobia, social support, and mental health. *LGBT Health*, 2(3), 265–269. doi:10.1089/lgbt.2013.0024.

Purdon, C. & Clark, D. A. (1993). Obsessive intrusive thoughts in nonclinical subjects. Part I. Content and relation with depressive, anxious and obsessional symptoms. *Behaviour Research and Therapy*, 31(8), 713–720. doi:10.1016/0005-7967(93)90001-B.

Rentería, R., Feinstein, B. A., Dyar, C., & Watson, R. J. (2022). Does outness function the same for all sexual minority youth? Testing its associations with different aspects of well-being in a sample of youth with diverse sexual identities. *Psychology of Sexual Orientation and Gender Diversity.* doi:10.1037/sgd0000547.

Riggle, E. D. B., Mohr, J. J., Rostosky, S. S., Fingerhut, A. W., & Balsam, K. F. (2014). A multifactor Lesbian, Gay, and Bisexual Positive Identity Measure (LGB-PIM). *Psychology of Sexual Orientation and Gender Diversity*, 1(4), 398–411. doi:10.1037/t37069-000.

Rood, B. A., Reisner, S. L., Surace, F. I., Puckett, J. A., Maroney, M. R., & Pantalone, D. W. (2016). Expecting rejection: Understanding the minority stress experiences of transgender and gender-nonconforming individuals. *Transgender Health*, 1(1), 151–164. doi:10.1089/trgh.2016.0012.

Russell, S. T., Ryan, C., Toomey, R. B., Diaz, R. M., & Sanchez, J. (2011). Lesbian, gay, bisexual, and transgender adolescent school victimization: implications for young adult health and adjustment. *Journal of School Health*, 81(5), 223–230. doi:10.1111/j.1746-1561.2011.00583.x.

Ryan, C., Huebner, D., Diaz, R. M., & Sanchez, J. (2009). Family rejection as a predictor of negative health outcomes in white and Latino lesbian, gay, and bisexual young adults. *Pediatrics*, 123(1), 346–352. doi:10.1542/peds.2007-3524.

Safer, D. L., Bullock, K. D., & Safer, J. D. (2016). Obsessive-compulsive disorder presenting as gender dysphoria/gender incongruence: A case report and literature review. *AACE Clinical Case Reports*, 2(3), e268–e271. doi:10.4158/EP161223.CR.

Salkovskis, P. M. (1999). Understanding and treating obsessive – compulsive disorder. *Behaviour Research and Therapy*, 37, S29–S52.

Savin-Williams, R. C. (2011). Identity development among sexual-minority youth. In *Handbook of identity theory and research* (pp. 671–689). New York: Springer.

Schrager, S. M., Goldbach, J. T., & Mamey, M. R. (2018). Development of the Sexual Minority Adolescent Stress Inventory. *Frontiers in Psychology*, 9, 319. doi:10.3389/fpsyg.2018.00319.

Steinberg, T., Shmuel-Baruch, S., Horesh, N., & Apter, A. (2013). Life events and Tourette syndrome. *Comprehensive Psychiatry*, 54(5), 467–473. doi:10.1016/j.comppsych.2012.10.015.

Storch, E. A. & Merlo, L. J. (2006). Obsessive-compulsive disorder: Strategies for using CBT and pharmacotherapy. *Journal of Family Practice*, 55(4), 329–334.

Testa, R. J., Habarth, J., Peta, J., Balsam, K., & Bockting, W. (2015). Development of the gender minority stress and resilience measure. *Psychology of Sexual Orientation and Gender Diversity*, 2(1), 65–77. doi:10.1037/sgd0000081.

The Trevor Project. (2022). 2022 National Survey on LGBTQ Youth Mental Health. www.thetrevorproject.org/survey-2022/assets/static/trevor01_2022survey_final.pdf.

Toomey, R. B. & Russell, S. T. (2016). The role of sexual orientation in school-based victimization: A meta-analysis. *Youth & Society*, 48(2), 176–201. doi:10.1177/0044118X13483778.

Weidle, B., Skarphedinsson, G., Højgaard, D. R., Thomsen, P. H., Torp, N. C., Melin, K., & Ivarsson, T. (2022). Sexual obsessions in children and adolescents: Prevalence, clinical correlates, response to cognitive-behavior therapy and long-term follow up. *Journal of Obsessive-Compulsive and Related Disorders*, 32, 100708. doi:10.1016/j.jocrd.2022.100708.

Wetterneck, C. T., Singh, S., & Hart, J. (2014). Shame proneness in symptom dimensions of obsessive-compulsive disorder. *Bulletin of the Menninger Clinic*, 78(2), 177–190. doi:10.1521/bumc.2014.78.2.177.

Williams, M. T. (2008). Homosexuality anxiety: A misunderstood form of OCD in L. V. Sebeki (Ed.), *Leading-edge health education issues* (pp. 195–205). New York: Nova Publishers.

Williams, M. T. & Ching, T. H. W. (2016). Transgender anxiety, cultural issues, and cannabis in obsessive-compulsive disorder. *AACE Clinical Case Reports*, 2 (3), e276–e277. doi:10.4158/EP161356.CO.

Williams, M. T. & Farris, S. G. (2011). Sexual orientation obsessions in obsessive–compulsive disorder: Prevalence and correlates. *Psychiatry Research*, 187(1–2), 156–159. doi:10.1016/j.psychres.2010.10.019.

Williams, M. T., Taylor, R. J., Mouzon, D. M., Oshin, L. A., Himle, J. A., & Chatters, L. M. (2017). Discrimination and symptoms of obsessive–compulsive disorder among African Americans. *American Journal of Orthopsychiatry*, 87(6), 636–645. doi:10.1037/ort0000285.

Williams, M. T. & Wetterneck, C. T. (2019). *Understanding sexual obsessions (pp.23–26) in Sexual obsessions in obsessive-compulsive disorder: A step-by-step, definitive guide to understanding, diagnosis, and treatment* (M.T. Williams & C. T. Wetterneck, Eds). New York: Oxford University Press.

Willis, H. A. & Neblett, E. W., Jr. (2018). OC symptoms in African American young adults: The associations between racial discrimination, racial identity, and obsessive-compulsive symptoms. *Journal of Obsessive-Compulsive and Related Disorders*, 19, 105–115. doi:10.1016/j.jocrd.2018.09.002.

Zimet, G. D., Powell, S. S., Farley, G. K., Werkman, S., & Berkoff, K. A. (1990). Psychometric characteristics of the Multidimensional Scale of Perceived Social Support. *Journal of Personality Assessment*, 55(3–4), 610–617. doi:10.1080/00223891.1990.9674095.

18 Conclusion

What we know, what we don't, and where to next

Andrew G. Guzick and Eric A. Storch

Over the past three decades, we have developed a strong understanding of childhood obsessive-compulsive disorder (OCD), with robust evidence regarding its prevalence, mechanisms, and nuances in clinical presentation. This foundational knowledge has paved the way for heightened awareness, treatment development, clinical specialization, and understanding of the underlying processes that are likely to drive OCD in childhood and adolescence across biological, psychological, and interpersonal domains. This literature has shown clear developmental distinctions for this disorder, such as differences in comorbidity patterns (i.e., with chronic tic disorders [CTDs]), genetics, family history, insight, and parental accommodation among children. Some of these insights have led to clear paradigm shifts in the field that have translated to improved treatments; for example, there is a consensus among OCD experts regarding the importance of targeting family accommodation in treatment that was not always universally recognized in the past.

In contrast, with the exception of CTDs, a developmentally sensitive understanding of the proposed "related" disorders is still in its very early stages. It is understandable why this may be the case; OCD and CTDs both have a frequent onset in the pre-pubescent period, and thus more child-focused professionals have directed their attention towards these populations relative to body focused repetitive behavior disorders, illness anxiety, body dysmorphic disorder (BDD), or hoarding problems. As described throughout this book, however, each of these "related" disorders have clear developmentally relevant components.

Take BDD as a particularly salient example. Body image issues are especially sensitive during adolescence as puberty begins, interests in dating accelerates, and more value is placed on the beliefs and opinions of their peers. Clearly, studying BDD during this phase of life is of utmost importance. Relative to OCD, however, a nuanced understanding of developmental factors has a much slimmer research base.

A less intuitive case to study during childhood is hoarding. As described in Chapter 8, however, the little we do know about hoarding during childhood points to several salient developmental components that

DOI: 10.4324/9781003517429-18

warrant consideration by clinicians and researchers. Excessive collecting and saving are extremely common early in childhood and co-occur with some of the most common neuropsychiatric conditions during this period (e. g., ADHD). Further, among adults with clinically significant hoarding, they most often recall these problems beginning during adolescence. There is a clear need for a better understanding of hoarding in childhood and adolescence to identify early risk factors for the development of hoarding disorder, as well as the underlying mechanisms of hoarding during this time to inform early intervention. Our hope is that many of the lessons learned in childhood OCD will provide a useful framework for studying these potentially related conditions. By providing a text with a summary of where the field is, it will be a launching pad for clinicians and researchers interested in deepening an understanding of these related disorders.

Across all these conditions, however, there is still a remarkable amount of work to be done. For all the recent advances in imaging and biomarkers, these findings have translated to minimal advancements in neurobiologically based treatments for youth with OCD. Similarly, despite advances in our understanding of several psychological factors that contribute to childhood OCD (e.g., sensitivity to disgust or other sensory experiences), exposure and response prevention therapy that was grounded in early theoretical work continues to be the dominant paradigm of OCD treatment in children and adults. Because exposure and response prevention is so effective, it has been difficult to show definitive incrementally useful strategies to enhance treatment outcomes beyond amplifying family involvement. Regardless, a meaningful portion of youth do not experience adequate benefits from evidence-based therapies, and thus there is clear room for improvement. Innovative theoretical models of OCD will hopefully pave the way for treatment innovations in the future. Among the very effective treatments that *do* exist for childhood OCRDs, they are rarely disseminated in community settings. Much more work is needed to uncover the major barriers and facilitators to widespread implementation.

Another clear future direction for this field is in improving inclusivity and cultural diversity in our studies. By and large, the research reviewed in this text is biased towards samples that disproportionately reflect families from White, educated backgrounds. Partnering with individuals from more diverse communities in formulating our research questions and reaching out to those traditionally excluded from this research and is paramount to developing a culturally sensitive understanding of OCD.

The goal of this book was to provide a comprehensive review on the classification, nature, development, and mechanisms of OCRDs in childhood. These disorders are highly impairing and typically onset in childhood or adolescence, though are often overlooked during this time. We hope this book provides a useful guide to OCRDs in childhood and draws attention to developmental considerations and transdiagnostic processes of these conditions during childhood and adolescence.

Index